Research Methods in Kinesiology

Research Methods in Kinesiology

Kent C. Kowalski
Tara-Leigh F. McHugh
Catherine M. Sabiston
Leah J. Ferguson

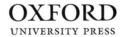
OXFORD
UNIVERSITY PRESS

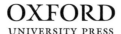

OXFORD
UNIVERSITY PRESS

Oxford University Press is a department of the University of Oxford.
It furthers the University's objective of excellence in research, scholarship,
and education by publishing worldwide. Oxford is a registered trade mark of
Oxford University Press in the UK and in certain other countries.

Published in Canada by
Oxford University Press
8 Sampson Mews, Suite 204,
Don Mills, Ontario M3C 0H5 Canada

www.oupcanada.com

Library and Archives Canada Cataloguing in Publication
Kowalski, Kent C. (Kent Cameron), 1970–, author
Research methods in kinesiology / Kowalski, McHugh, Sabiston, and Ferguson.

Includes bibliographical references and index.
ISBN 978–0–19–902068–3 (softcover)

1. Kinesiology—Research—Methodology—Textbooks. 2. Textbooks.
I. McHugh, Tara-Leigh F., 1978–, author II. Sabiston, Catherine, 1975–,
author III. Ferguson, Leah, author IV. Title.

QP303.K69 2018   613.7072'1   C2017-904256-4

Cover image: © Hero Images/Getty Images
Cover and text design: Laurie McGregor

Oxford University Press is committed to our environment.
This book is printed on Forest Stewardship Council ® certified paper
and comes from responsible sources.

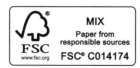

Printed and bound in the United States of America

1 2 3 4 — 21 20 19 18

Contents

8   Data Analysis in Qualitative Studies   152

9   Evaluating the Merits of Qualitative Research
Studies in Kinesiology   177

10   Mixed Methods Research   198

Preface and Acknowledgements

When you're young and think about writing a book, many potential topics come to mind. Maybe you dreamed of telling tales of Wonder Woman or Spider-Man saving the world from the latest cosmic threat. Your imagination might have wandered up to the most majestic mountain tops or to the depths of the deepest oceans as you created songs about mythical creatures that inhabit such inaccessible places. Perhaps you even tried your hand at writing a short romance novel about Ken and Barbie (weaving in, of course, their choices in the latest fashions). While these are just a few possible examples of stories you might have wanted to tell, our guess is that none of you grew up thinking, "One day I sure would like to write a research methods textbook!" Well . . . we didn't either. In fact, our guess is that even *reading* a research methods text wasn't all that high on your priority list.

Yet here we are. *We* having committed the past couple of years to writing a research methods text. And *you* reading this text (most likely because your course instructor required you to). No amount of cartoons, figures, or references to *Star Wars* can hide the fact that we are about to begin a journey of research methods together.

But why research methods? For us, it is the realization that pretty much anything we know about anything involves the research process in some way. Consider your favourite kinesiology course, whether it be biomechanics, exercise physiology, sport psychology, or any other. Regardless of the course, it was shaped by research. While we typically think of research as involving experiments in a lab or filling out a questionnaire, which it most certainly *can*, research actually encapsulates much, much more. For example, we might have a favourite Olympic athlete and become curious about her or his performances over the past few years. What might we do to satisfy our curiosity? We could look up her or his statistics online. We could read a personal memoir or daily blog. If we were really lucky, we might even speak with her or his coach directly and ask for details about previous training and competitions. In each of these cases, we would be engaged in the research process as we attempted to learn something new.

But what would happen if we went to a website that published the athlete's stats incorrectly, read a memoir that distorted history from almost every possible perspective other than that of the writer, or received misleading information from the coach because she or he was afraid you'd steal all his or her "secrets"? In these cases, your "research" could lead to very faulty conclusions about your favourite Olympic athlete.

At the end of the day, we hope that this book provides you an opportunity to be exposed to a wide range of research in kinesiology, as well as some skills and knowledge that assist you in telling the difference between "good" and "bad" research. As you'll find out, even determining what good and bad research looks like depends very much on context. In addition, as is the case with all great stories, we idealistically hope that this text offers a starting point for many great research adventures of your own.

Childhood dreams aside, this book also represents a passion for research and teaching that we share as co-authors. Each of us has taught numerous university research methods courses in kinesiology over the years; in many ways this text is a manifestation of our experiences

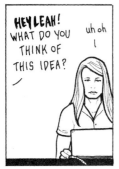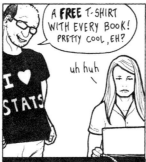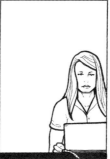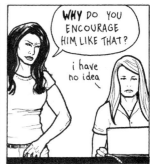

working with hundreds of students and our own research programs that span a wide range of research methodologies. But mostly, this is the text we always wished were available to us and our students when teaching our research methods courses.

There are many excellent books available on the topic of research methods; however, none we have found have been ideal for the research methods in kinesiology courses we teach. The available options tend to be predominantly focused on *either* quantitative research methods *or* qualitative research methods. In other cases, particularly those in which quantitative and qualitative methods are given equal weighting, the available options tend not to be specific to kinesiology. Finding a book with Canadian-specific examples as a centrepiece has also been a challenge for us.

In the end, we decided to write our own research methods text, one that represents the way we teach research methods in our courses. Ours is an approach that emphasizes and values quantitative, qualitative, and mixed methods approaches to research (if you're not familiar with these terms, you will be soon!), and one that emphasizes kinesiology-related examples specific to the Canadian context. We also weave an emphasis on Indigenous research and Indigenous research methodologies throughout the text, as we feel that we could not even contemplate writing a book focused on the Canadian context without a focus on Indigenous worldviews and ways of knowing.

Although we hope that our text can be read and enjoyed by all, it is written primarily to be used in introductory research methods in kinesiology courses taught in Canadian universities and colleges. As you read through the book, there are a number of features that might stand out, a few of which we highlight below.

First, our intent is to cover a wide range of topic areas relevant to kinesiology research. A more specific overview of the text content is provided at the end of Chapter 1, but we begin with an overview of quantitative, qualitative, and mixed methods research and an introduction to how researchers' philosophical worldviews shape the research process. The remainder of the text covers topics such as how to develop a study purpose, research ethics and ethical decision-making, and specific quantitative, qualitative, and mixed methods research designs. We also have specific chapters on participatory action research approaches and various choices researchers have in communicating their research findings to a wide range of audiences.

Second, we begin each chapter with clear *learning outcomes*, similar to what you might find at the start of a class on a particular subject. These learning outcomes are meant to provide a frame of reference for each chapter and to identify the key knowledges and skills we hope you take from each chapter. At the end of each chapter we include a list of *discussion questions* that link back to the learning outcomes and identify other areas of focus within each of the chapters.

Third, key terms are shown in **bold** font throughout the book, indicating particularly noteworthy concepts. Being able to define the bolded concepts is important; therefore, all bolded concepts are also listed again in a glossary at the end of the book along with accompanying definitions.

Fourth, in large part because we value engagement with content materials, we include many exercises and case studies throughout the book. Our intent through the exercises and case studies is to encourage you to reflect on the content presented in each chapter, to open up avenues for new discussion, and to provide you tangible experience with the research process. Many of these exercises and case studies have been used in our research methods classes over the years and we find them extremely valuable for students. However, we want to emphasize that they do not represent a comprehensive list of all materials that could be used to facilitate the application of research methods content. Rather, these exercises and case studies are designed as supplementary materials for instructors, because we recognize that there are many wonderful and knowledgeable teachers who have already developed highly effective approaches to helping students apply research methods content in their own courses.

Fifth, because an emphasis on the Canadian context is core to our text, we include a number of research and professional highlights. The research highlights provide concrete examples of excellent, and diverse, research *studies* being done across Canada. They also provide exemplars of specific content being discussed within each chapter. Alternatively, the professional highlights focus on specific *people* within Canada who exemplify some aspect of the research process within the field of kinesiology. The professional highlights are by no means an exhaustive list of all the top researchers in Canada (that would take a book equally as long just to list them!), but instead are meant to represent diversity in focus, geographical location, interest areas, and kinesiology-related careers. In many cases the people we highlight are indeed researchers; however, we also highlight some professionals working in the field to demonstrate how research is relevant to anyone working in any field within kinesiology in Canada.

We would be remiss not to thank the many students, teachers, colleagues, and researchers who have shaped our thinking about research methods over the years. Learning about the research process itself is an ongoing journey, and the content of this text would be very different had we not been influenced by the experience, guidance, critical analysis, and questions of others. Although there are far too many people to specifically identify, we'd like to thank Dr Peter Crocker, currently a professor at the University of British Columbia, in particular for inspiring us all towards a passionate approach to our own research programs. In addition, we are very grateful to everyone we've had the pleasure to work with at our publisher Oxford University Press for their professional guidance and support. It would be hard to envision what this text would have looked like without their wisdom and insight.

In the end, we hope that you enjoy the research process as much as we do.

1 Introduction to Research in Kinesiology

Learning Outcomes

By the end of this chapter, you should be able to:

- Discuss how the research process is important to understanding the current knowledge base in kinesiology.

- Describe a variety of research methods used in kinesiology.

- Identify implications that different philosophical worldviews have on the research process.

It is enormously easier to present in an appealing way the wisdom distilled from centuries of patient and collective interrogation in Nature than to detail the messy distillation apparatus. The method of science, as stodgy and grumpy as it may seem, is far more important than the findings of science.

—*Carl Sagan*

Introduction: Current Knowledge in Kinesiology

Carl Sagan was a Professor of Astronomy and Space Sciences and Director of the Laboratory for Planetary Studies at Cornell University who wrote eloquently about both scientific knowledge and the process of science. The quote that starts this chapter is from his 1997 book *The Demon-Haunted World: Science as a Candle in the Dark* in which he emphasized the importance of openness, curiosity, and excitement in the search for knowledge. While we as kinesiologists might not be trying to discover distant galaxies or answering questions related to the existence of life on other planets, Sagan's wisdom nonetheless has much relevance to us in kinesiology-related fields. Ultimately, while knowledge of "facts" is essential for professionals to perform competent and ethical work, understanding how knowledge within a field is generated is important because it allows us the skills to critique an existing body of knowledge. Perhaps even more exciting, an understanding of the research process provides kinesiologists the background needed to answer questions that *no one* knows the answer to yet.

There are a number of realities in kinesiology that are generally accepted to be "true." It is known that weight training can result in strength gains for athletes and that physical activity and a healthy diet can decrease obesity among youth, as just two examples. But have you ever considered how these facts, among others, have become known as truths to the field? Sometimes what we "know" is based on our own experiences in the world. For example, in your own experience you might have improved at shooting a basketball as a result of a lot of practice, thereby leading you to believe that practice can make someone better at basketball. But personal experience is limiting, because we don't always improve as a result of practice (sometimes more practice actually makes us worse at something!). Also, why is it that certain types of practice are more effective than other types of practice, as coaches and teachers know based on their work with athletes and students? Similarly, how do some people perform and learn movement skills better than others? Ballet is a skill that some people seem to be more adept at learning and performing at the highest level. Depending on each of our personal experiences, the answers to these types of questions can vary substantially.

However, not everything we know is based solely on personal experience. Perhaps we gained knowledge from a conversation, class, or practice with a teacher or coach. Perhaps we read about something online or in a magazine, journal article, or book. If we haven't experienced something directly, we tend to believe (and rely on) information gathered from outside sources, particularly if that information comes from an "expert" (e.g., professor, certified coach, or physician). But should we? Greg Easterbrook, the author of *The Kings of Sports: Football's Impact on America* (2013) and former author of the Tuesday Morning Quarterback column for ESPN.com, sometimes used the phrase "Trust us, we're experts" to lead into a discussion of how wrong experts are in their thinking. We can rely on accurate information from outside sources only to a point, beyond which we need to be able to critique that information ourselves.

The field of kinesiology continues to grow and expand enormously, resulting in a new and exciting body of knowledge, particularly as kinesiology programs in Canada become increasingly multidisciplinary and research focused. For example, it is now believed that physical activity during the growing years can have a beneficial effect on bone health and potentially decrease the risk of osteoporosis and related fractures later in life (Baxter-Jones, Kontulainen, Faulkner, & Bailey, 2008). Also, there is new evidence that strength training one limb can actually help preserve the strength of the opposite limb even when it is injured and immobilized (Magnus et al., 2013). These types of findings represent an exciting time for kinesiology, especially for practitioners working in fields of rehabilitation and health promotion.

Not only are new discoveries being made all the time, but we often learn that what was previously accepted as "fact" might actually be fallacy. For example, it wasn't all that long ago that many people believed (and were taught that) women couldn't pole vault effectively because of a relatively low centre of mass and weak upper-body strength compared to men. However, women's participation in pole vault has exploded in the past 20 years, most definitely proving the "experts" wrong . . . so much so that the women's world record in pole vault is now over five metres! Another example is that bed rest is no longer the recommended prescription for recovery for most injuries (this was believed many years ago, but sounds absurd to us today). This advancement in thinking about injury care has led to an increasing recognition of the role of physical activity in rehabilitation and the emergence of professions like physical therapy and athletic therapy.

The main point is that an understanding of the processes of science and research are essential to everyone in kinesiology, regardless of their particular interest areas and future professions. One of the most exciting aspects of kinesiology is the variety of fields within it. We see professionals with kinesiology-related backgrounds at almost every turn in our lives, with the most obvious examples including fitness trainers, athletic and recreation directors, physical education teachers, and exercise therapists. However, many who graduate with kinesiology degrees also go on to other professional programs, such as physical therapy, occupational therapy, dentistry, nursing, medicine, and community health and epidemiology, to name just a few. In fact, most kinesiology undergraduate programs are an almost ideal stepping stone for most health science programs. But the impact of kinesiology on a wide range of professions certainly doesn't stop there. Kinesiology graduates can also be found on the police force, as firefighters and border service officers, among leaders in business and government, working as clinical psychologists and school counsellors, and within many other professions. Knowledge of research methods enables professionals to critique an existing body of knowledge as well as build on that knowledge, both of which are essential for any profession to flourish. In essence, knowledge of research methods is a critical skill to develop for all professionals and students.

An important milestone in kinesiology research in Canada was the development of university kinesiology programs. The development of these programs provided the impetus for hiring researchers with a specific interest in kinesiology and sparked an increased focus on kinesiology research in Canada over the past 50 years. Digby Elliot (2007) provided a historical review of the first kinesiology programs developed in Canada. In the late 1960s, Simon Fraser University and the University of Waterloo independently developed their kinesiology programs, which since have sparked the emergence of many kinesiology programs in Canada (and even programs like the one at the University of British Columbia that had originally adopted

Case Study

You are a university student taking a biomechanics class that is required for your university degree. One day there is a visiting scholar, Dr Fastball, giving a guest lecture on the biomechanics of pitching a baseball. Dr Fastball claims that he has discovered that a certain combination of joint angles among the legs, hips, spine, shoulder, and wrist can enable a pitcher to throw a fastball exceeding 200 km/h (over 124 mph). Knowing that even elite Major League Baseball pitchers rarely can throw more than 160 km/h (100 mph) you are skeptical, although intrigued by Dr Fastball's claims.

Discussion Questions

1. What questions might you ask Dr Fastball to adequately critique the merits of his claim?
2. How would you go about testing for yourself whether or not what he claims is indeed correct?

other terms, such as human kinetics, have recently been renamed using the term *kinesiology*). The main impetus of the name change to kinesiology was a recognition that the field involves more than physical education teacher training. While teacher training remains an important aspect of kinesiology, the name kinesiology itself refers to the *study* of movement; hence research is now more easily recognized as core to the discipline.

Introduction to Research Methods in Kinesiology

The terms *science* and *research* are not new, and certainly not exclusive to the field of kinesiology. However, both terms are commonly used by researchers in kinesiology. In an effort to distinguish between them, Thomas, Nelson, and Silverman (2011) defined science as "a process of careful and systematic inquiry" (p. 10), whereas they described research as "a structured way of solving problems" (p. 17). Others (e.g., Baumgartner & Hensley, 2012) link the term *science* more to the formation of a theory that is developed based on the facts, whereas research refers to the discovery of those facts. Perhaps the easiest way to differentiate between them is to think of **science** as the discovery of knowledge and **research** as a specific method used to discover that knowledge. Regardless of the definitions, it is clear that science and research are intimately tied together.

Creswell (2014) identified three approaches to research: quantitative, qualitative, and mixed methods research designs. These three research approaches represent the majority of research studies conducted in the field of kinesiology to date; however, each research approach differs in underlying assumptions, the types of questions asked, the specific methods used, the type of data that results from the research, and subsequent analysis of the data. All three approaches will be covered in more detail in chapters that follow. As an introduction, each is briefly discussed below, accompanied by some examples of studies conducted by researchers at Canadian universities. This introduction is meant to highlight some of the key characteristics that differentiate among quantitative, qualitative, and mixed methods research approaches.

Quantitative research requires the generation of numerical (i.e., quantitative) data to answer research questions. Hence, quantitative research designs are typically described by researchers (e.g., Creswell, 2014; Thomas, Nelson, & Silverman, 2011) as best suited to questions related to the testing of theory (e.g., links between motivation and behaviour proposed by self-determination theory; Deci & Ryan, 2000), status on variables (e.g., obesity rates in Canada), differences among groups (e.g., physical activity levels in boys compared to girls), and relationships among variables (e.g., research at Acadia University on the relationship between family social influence and physical activity; Shields et al., 2008). As a result, quantitative research designs are fundamentally based on the premise that the data generated be as precise as possible. This precision, or validity (a term you will read much more about in later chapters), is necessary so that any conclusions that are made based on the research are accurate and can be applied to populations beyond the study sample. For instance, researchers at the University of British Columbia (i.e., Masse et al., 2016) recently found that the physical activity parenting practices most often employed by parents in Canada and the United States are not the practices emphasized in current research measures. As such, they argue that the predictive validity of such measures requires further examination. Researchers conducting quantitative studies attempt to be as objective as possible, typically use large sample sizes, focus heavily on the measurement of variables, and use statistics for their data analysis.

The Canadian Health Measures Survey (CHMS) is an example of a large-scale quantitative approach to research (Tremblay & Gorber, 2007). The CHMS, conducted between the years 2007 and 2009 was designed to study the health and wellness of Canadians. The researchers' goal was to produce baseline data for a variety of health indicators. Measurement of variables ranged from physical activity; to blood pressure; to muscular strength, endurance, and flexibility. A method used to enhance objectivity was the assessment of physical activity via the use of accelerometers, which participants wore for seven days. One published study based on the CHMS data presented the physical activity levels of 2832 Canadian adults between the ages of 20 to 79 years (Colley et al., 2011). Data were shown in the form of average daily minutes of activity at various levels of intensity and by the number of step counts per day. Results showed that only 15% of adults were meeting physical activity recommendations and that a large number of people spent the majority of their waking hours being sedentary.

Although quantitative research studies typically have large sample sizes, they do not always *require* large sample sizes. Experimental studies in particular can require a great deal of time and resources to test the effectiveness of treatments, programs, or interventions; as a result, experimental studies often rely on much smaller sample sizes. For example, Moreside and McGill (2012) recruited students at the University of Waterloo for their hip joint range of motion intervention study. Twenty-four participants were randomly assigned to four separate experimental groups, with interventions (e.g., stretching or core endurance exercises) occurring over a 6-week period. They found that hip rotation range of motion could be improved by a variety of intervention methods. Objectivity was attained through randomization of participants to groups, as well as by having the measurements of key variables conducted by a research assistant who did not share the results with the primary researcher who was present. These strategies helped to reduce the probability that their findings were simply a result of researcher bias and expectations. Even though the specific study design and sample size differed substantially between the Moreside and McGill study and the CHMS, both represent quantitative approaches to research because data collection methods resulted in numerical data that were then analyzed through the use of statistics to answer their research questions.

Qualitative research, in contrast to quantitative research, is based on the generation and interpretation of non-numerical (i.e., qualitative) data. Patton (2002) identified three main sources of qualitative data, including open-ended interviews, direct observation, and written documents. In addition to these traditional sources, there is also an increased use of arts-based research methods (Sullivan, 2005) as a form of data collection. Because the resulting data are non-numerical, qualitative research is particularly well-suited to understanding peoples' meanings of experience (e.g., the wheelchair dance experiences of children with spina bifida; Goodwin, Krohn, & Kuhnle, 2004). Qualitative research differs from a quantitative approach in that the design of the studies is often emergent and flexible, the data are typically collected in the participants' natural setting, themes are generated from the data collected, and the researcher is acknowledged as being an integral part of the research process (Creswell, 2014).

While the results of qualitative research can certainly be written up in journal articles, as are quantitative research results, they can also be represented in other ways, such as poems, theatre, and musical performance, to name just a few options (Sparkes & Smith, 2014). And because of the focus on understanding the complexity of peoples' experience, sample sizes in qualitative research tend to be much smaller than in quantitative research.

An example of a qualitative approach is a study conducted by researchers at the University of Alberta that explored the physical activity experiences of young adolescent girls (Clark, Spence, & Holt, 2011). To answer their research questions, they interviewed eight participants (aged 10 to 11 years) twice each in the girls' school setting. The two interviews occurred approximately one year apart. As part of developing trusting relationships with the girls prior to the interviews, the lead researcher also participated in a number of the girls' activities (e.g., art and physical education classes) during the weeks prior to data collection. Participants also completed either collage or drawing exercises prior to the first interview as a way to facilitate depth and richness within the subsequent interviews. Once collected, the interview data were then transcribed verbatim (i.e., typed out word for word) and analyzed using a thematic analysis that resulted in two main themes: (a) "Physical activity lets girls shine" and (b) "Taking care of myself, inside and out." In taking a qualitative approach to their research, Clark et al. were able to provide a rich, in-depth understanding of girls' physical activity experiences.

Another example of a study using a qualitative approach was conducted by Mosewich and colleagues (2009) on women track and field athletes' meanings of muscularity. They conducted focus groups followed by one-on-one interviews with four adult and four adolescent athletes from a variety of track and field events. A somewhat unique aspect of their work was that they had each of the participants complete a photography project between the focus group and one-on-one interviews as a way for the athletes to visually represent their muscularity experiences. The photographs were also used to facilitate discussion in the one-on-one interviews. A thematic analysis resulted in four main themes, including (a) "Many faces of muscularity," (b) "A blurred line between appearance and performance," (c) "A culture of comparison," and (d) "A journey towards self-acceptance." A qualitative study was particularly useful in showing the complexity of women athletes' experiences of muscularity. In both the Clark et al. (2011) study and the Mosewich et al. study, understanding of the participants' experiences was facilitated by presenting direct quotations from the interviews throughout the results, which is a strategy often used by qualitative researchers to facilitate a reader's entry into the participants' world of experience.

Mixed methods research is becoming increasingly common within kinesiology. As might be expected, a mixed methods research approach combines quantitative and qualitative research methods. This combination can take many forms, including research designs that prioritize either one or both of quantitative and qualitative methods, research designs in which quantitative and qualitative methods are conducted either simultaneously or one following the other, and programs of research in which both quantitative and qualitative studies are conducted over a longer period of time, all aimed at answering a broader research question (Creswell & Plano Clark, 2011). In essence, a mixed methods approach is used by researchers who see value in using *both* quantitative and qualitative data to answer their research question(s).

An example of a mixed methods approach is a study conducted by Ferguson and colleagues (2014), who used both quantitative and qualitative research methods to better understand the role of self-compassion in young women athletes' psychological well-being. In their study, a quantitative phase preceded a qualitative phase. The quantitative phase specifically focused on

Research Highlight

Research led by Nick Holt, a Professor of Physical Education and Recreation at the University of Alberta, is focused on the psychosocial dimensions of youth sport, physical activity, and physical education. He and his colleagues have numerous peer-reviewed publications and have utilized a wide range of research methodologies to help us better understand various study areas in kinesiology. Two of his studies with more unique methodologies are worth particular mention as a way to highlight some of the diversity found in kinesiology research. In a first example, Holt and colleagues (2008) conducted a study on children's perceptions on places to play and be physically active. To answer their research question, they used a "mental mapping technique" to assess perceptions of urban environment among 168 students from grades K to 6. The children created the mental maps by drawing images of the places they could play and be physically active in their neighbourhood. While the children were drawing, the researchers asked clarification questions about the children's images to further enhance their understanding. Some of the mental maps created by the children are presented in the published article, and they exemplify the benefits of artistic practice in answering research questions. In a second example, Holt et al. (2013) were interested in implementing and evaluating sport-based after-school programs for children in low-income areas in Edmonton. Their study took place over a three-year period and included a wide range of activities including initial work to identify the research questions and build relationships within the community, delivery of sport camps in partnership with the school board, the development of after-school programs with principals and teachers, and interviews with adult stakeholders including coaches, school board members, and others. A number of the children participating in the program were also interviewed. The combination of spending a great deal of time working with the community and use of multiple research strategies greatly enhanced the research team's ability to develop an effective and enjoyable physical activity program for low-income students. Taken together, Dr Holt's research is an example of how researchers often use a variety of research approaches to answer different types of research questions in their particular area of interest.

Further Readings

Holt, N. L., McHugh, T.-L. F., Tink, L. N., Kingsley, B. C., Coppola, A. M., Neely, K. C., & McDonald, R. (2013). Developing sport-based after-school programmes using a participatory action research approach. *Qualitative Research in Sport, Exercise and Health, 5,* 332–55. doi:10.1080/2159676X.2013.809377

Holt, N. L., Spence, J. C., Sehn, Z. L., & Cutumisu, N. (2008). Neighborhood and developmental differences in children's perceptions of opportunities for play and physical activity. *Health & Place, 14,* 2–14. doi:10.1016/j.healthplace.2007.03.002

presenting statistical relationships among measured variables, whereas the qualitative phase focused on athletes' experiences of self-compassion and psychological well-being. There were a few distinguishing features between the quantitative and qualitative phases, including the sample sizes (i.e., 83 in the quantitative phase, 11 in the qualitative phase), the methods of data collection (i.e., questionnaires in the quantitative phase, interviews in the qualitative phase), and analysis of data (statistics in the quantitative phase, a thematic analysis in the qualitative phase). Despite these differences between the phases, the quantitative and qualitative approaches each informed the general research question in a unique way. Across the two studies, a complex picture of possible ways that self-compassion might work to enhance psychological well-being for women athletes was presented.

An example of a mixed methods approach across a series of studies is the work on positive youth development in sport by Leisha Strachan (University of Manitoba), Jean Côté (Queen's University), and Janice Deakin (University of Western Ontario). In a qualitative study exploring positive youth development in elite sport contexts, Strachan, Côté, and Deakin (2011) used both interviews and observations as data collection sources with their sample of five elite youth sport coaches. Perhaps most interestingly, 123 athletes of these same coaches had participated in a previous quantitative study on personal and contextual outcomes associated with youth sports (Strachen, Côté, & Deakin, 2009). Their research showed that it is important to focus on positive identity, empowerment, and support in youth sport programs as ways to help prevent burnout and enhance enjoyment from the athletes' perspectives (based on the quantitative study). However, it also showed that coaches can play an important role in creating an appropriate environment in which to promote positivity for their athletes (based on the qualitative study). It is only when *both* studies are considered that a more complete picture emerges of ways to positively impact youth sport development. Across his program of research, Dr Côté in particular has used a variety of quantitative and qualitative methodologies, including different types of interview approaches, observation, video-task analysis, and questionnaires, to answer research questions focused on sport and physical activity performance and participation.

Components of a Research Design

The sources that are used to collect data in a research study, whether the measurement of physiological variables, one-on-one interviews, or arts-based methods, are informed by the specific research approach that is taken (i.e., quantitative, qualitative, or mixed methods). In short, the research approach and methods employed in a study are inherently linked. A researcher taking a qualitative approach is not going to rely on objective numerical data to gain a rich understanding of breast cancer survivors' body image experiences, just as a researcher conducting a quantitative study on the effects of a dynamic stretching program on endurance athletes' training recovery will likely have little need for poetic transcriptions (i.e., participants' words transformed into poems). As discussed in the previous section, the quantitative approach to research requires the application of appropriate quantitative methods, while the qualitative approach requires appropriate qualitative methods. Further, the mixed methods approach will utilize a variety of methods that are appropriate to either quantitative or qualitative research at different stages of the research.

But how do researchers choose both their approach and the corresponding methods? As will be shown throughout this book, there are several decisions to make and steps to take when planning and designing a research study. However, playing a fundamental role in the type of approach and choice of subsequent methods is a researcher's **philosophical worldview**, which represents a set of beliefs related to her or his general orientation of the world and the nature of research (Creswell, 2014). More specifically, a philosophical worldview dictates what a researcher believes (or does not believe) counts as knowledge. For example, a researcher might believe that the stories children tell about their experiences in physical education class are or are not important and valuable as knowledge. This belief permeates the entire research process from beginning to end.

Two concepts that align closely with a philosophical worldview are ontology and epistemology. Whaley and Krane (2011) provide a "primer on ontologies, epistemologies, and methodologies" (pp. 395–7) that we find quite useful. In essence, **ontology** refers to someone's belief in the nature of truth and reality. For example, if we accept that there is an objective physical reality separate from our own personal existence, that belief reflects a particular ontological stance. Alternatively, **epistemology** refers to someone's belief about how we acquire knowledge about that truth and reality (and even whether we can or should go about acquiring that knowledge). For example, valuing personal experience in the quest for knowledge reflects a particular epistemological stance. As Whaley and Krane describe, the ability for researchers to understand and appreciate various types of research depends largely on their epistemology, rather than simply not understanding a particular method (e.g., questionnaires, interviews, observations). If we look at the definition of philosophical worldview provided in the previous paragraph, it essentially represents an integration of both ontology (i.e., "general orientation to the world") and epistemology (i.e., "nature of research"). Hence our choice is to use the term *philosophical worldview* throughout this book to encompass a researcher's set of beliefs that guide her or his orientation to science and research (see Figure 1.1).

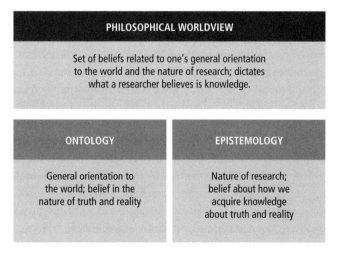

PHILOSOPHICAL WORLDVIEW

Set of beliefs related to one's general orientation
to the world and the nature of research; dictates
what a researcher believes is knowledge.

ONTOLOGY

General orientation to
the world; belief in the
nature of truth and reality

EPISTEMOLOGY

Nature of research;
belief about how we
acquire knowledge
about truth and reality

Figure 1.1 The relationship between philosophical worldview, ontology, and epistemology.

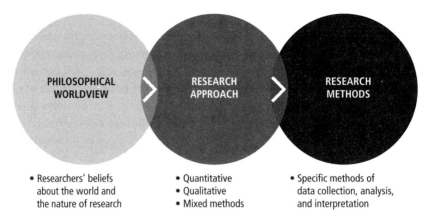

Figure 1.2 Three components of research designs.

While many philosophical worldviews exist, each uniquely providing a framework to guide the research process, Creswell (2014) identified four worldviews that are common in the literature: (a) postpositivism, (b) constructivism, (c) pragmatism, and (d) transformative. Another philosophical worldview that is becoming increasingly visible in Indigenous health research in Canada is two-eyed seeing. These five philosophical worldviews are common to the multidisciplinary field of kinesiology research in Canada and will be discussed in turn. Philosophical worldviews have inherent assumptions about knowledge that drive the research approach and distinct methods or procedures used in research, as shown in Figure 1.2.

Philosophical Worldviews as Guiding Frameworks of Research

Postpositivism is a common philosophical worldview in kinesiology research that is premised on the notion that there is a single reality or objective truth to be discovered through research. Inherent to postpositivism are the assumptions of determinism (causes determine effects) and reductionism (ideas can be reduced to small testable research questions), as well as a reliance on theory to uncover objective reality. An example of a postpositivist approach to research would be reflected in a study testing that enhanced strength and flexibility (the causes) result in increased parallel bar performance in gymnastics (the effect). Researchers with postpositivist worldviews are guided by the scientific method as a rigorous way to answer research questions. One popular approach to the scientific method described by Thomas et al. (2011) consists of four steps: (a) developing the problem, (b) formulating the hypothesis, (c) gathering the data, and (d) analyzing and interpreting results. Following these pre-defined steps aids in uncovering truth in the research process while remaining objective and unbiased. Researchers who adopt a quantitative approach to their research operate from a postpositivist worldview, since the characteristics of the quantitative approach (e.g., numerical data, measurement of variables, large samples, and statistical analyses) align with the philosophy of objectivity and finding one single truth in research.

Constructivism is another philosophical worldview that guides many kinesiology research programs. Constructivism is based on the notion that multiple realities exist and that meaning is varied and complex. For example, researchers with a constructivist philosophical worldview would likely adopt a stance that there is no distinct set of emotions that are similarly experienced by all people; instead they might view the experience of emotions as unique to each individual (e.g., what you experience as competitive anxiety might be very different from what someone else experiences as competitive anxiety). Therefore, in contrast to postpositivism, which is guided by the philosophy that there is one objective reality to be discovered, researchers with a constructivist philosophical worldview operate from the position that meanings of experience are subjective and socially constructed. That is, individuals engage with their world and make sense of it based on their own personal, social, cultural, and historical perspectives. Researchers with a constructivist worldview seek complexity of views rather than reducing or narrowing ideas down to a single testable idea. True to the belief that meanings are varied and multiple, researchers with a constructivist worldview recognize that their own realities and views shape the research process; they are not objective scientists but rather are closely connected in constructing and interpreting their findings. Kinesiology researchers with a constructivist worldview take a qualitative approach to exploring and understanding human movement, often incorporating open-ended discussions and interactions with other people to understand their personal, social, cultural, and historical worlds.

While postpositivist and constructivist philosophical worldviews include strong beliefs on the status of reality (i.e., single and objective or multiple and varied), a pragmatic worldview is somewhat different. **Pragmatism** is premised on the idea that researchers need to be concerned with solutions to problems; therefore, there is no commitment to any single notion of reality. Rather, truth and knowledge are viewed as what works at the time to address the research problem or question. Researchers with a pragmatic worldview are concerned about application, or doing what works. They recognize that questions related to the nature of reality are indeed important but are willing to set aside those types of questions temporarily (or permanently) in their research. Thus, rather than commit to one type of research approach and corresponding method over another, pragmatists incorporate all approaches that are appropriate and necessary to understand their research problem. Specifically, pragmatists adopt a pluralistic approach to their research, engaging in mixed methods research to incorporate both quantitative and qualitative approaches into their programs of research. A mixed methods approach works best for researchers with a pragmatic worldview because aspects from both quantitative and qualitative methods will provide the best understanding in their research, and ultimately the best solution to their research problem.

A **transformative** philosophical worldview is based on the notion that research needs to be closely connected with politics and have an action agenda to advocate for marginalized peoples, such as those who experience inequity based on gender, race, ethnicity, disability, sexual orientation, and socioeconomic status. Researchers with a transformative worldview focus on reform and change through their research, and they have the underlying objective to better the lives of the participants involved in their research. In order for action to take place, transformative research is inherently collaborative whereby researchers and study participants work together throughout the research process in order for change to occur and to be meaningful to the participants. The collaboration can be seen at all stages of the research process, including the development of research questions, data collection and analysis, and experiencing the reform and change as an outcome of the research. Researchers with a transformative worldview often adopt a qualitative approach to their research when working directly with study participants, though a quantitative approach can also add important elements, as is often seen through the use of numerical data to justify reform and change (e.g., statistics showing low participation or high risk). Researchers with a transformative worldview often focus on research topics of particular relevance to racial and ethnic minorities; persons with disabilities; members of the lesbian, gay, bisexual, transgender, and queer communities; and Indigenous peoples.

Two-eyed seeing is rooted in the belief that there are many ways of understanding the world, some represented by various Indigenous knowledge systems and others by European-derived sciences. Introduced to the research world by Mi'kmaw Elders Albert and Murdena Marshall, two-eyed seeing reflects the "bringing together" of knowledge by using the analogy of two eyes, with one eye seeing from the strengths of Indigenous ways of knowing and the other eye seeing from the strengths of Western ways of knowing (Bartlett, Marshall, & Marshall, 2012). Researchers with a two-eyed seeing worldview suspend judgment on the various ways of knowing, recognize that all knowledge systems are equitable, and embrace sharing knowledge from both Indigenous and Western knowledge systems. Two-eyed seeing draws upon Indigenous and Western knowledge in a way that addresses the needs of the individuals and/or community with whom researchers are working, without pitting one knowledge source against the other or favouring one perspective over the other. As such, this worldview is premised on respect, reflection, and co-learning. A two-eyed seeing philosophical worldview is particularly valuable in allowing for diversity of perspectives and valuing that all views contribute something unique and important.

It is important to gain an appreciation for philosophical worldviews, such as those presented in Table 1.1, as they are foundational to any research design. The philosophical orientation that researchers adopt about the world and the nature of knowledge will dictate the type of research that they do and the types of research that they value. For instance, researchers who believe that both Indigenous teachings about the land and Western physical activity adherence theory offer value (i.e., two-eyed seeing) when implementing a physical activity program for Indigenous youth will develop a very different study from researchers who want to determine which of three training programs provides the greatest strength gains for athletes (i.e., post-positivism). As another example, researchers who embrace the notion that our lives are socially constructed and that meanings are varied (i.e., constructivism) will adopt a qualitative approach and corresponding methods of data collection when exploring the lived experiences of adults with spina bifida. Alternatively, other researchers might be less interested in philosophical debates regarding the status of knowledge, truth, and reality and instead focus on problem solving (i.e., pragmatism), such as determining the best rehabilitation program for individuals living with multiple sclerosis. Finally, researchers who are fundamentally driven by an action agenda and are focused on reform (i.e., transformative) will respond to the removal of bike paths and associated increases in sedentary behaviours in a First Nations community by working collaboratively with community members to initiate change toward improved health. These are just a few examples highlighting the links between philosophical worldviews and the types of research approaches that might follow.

Table 1.1 A summary of the main philosophical worldviews.

WORLDVIEW	MAIN FEATURES	MAIN RESEARCH APPROACH
Postpositivism	• A single reality or objective truth discovered using scientific method • Determinism • Reductionism • Theory testing	• Quantitative
Constructivism	• Multiple realities exist • Meaning is varied and complex • Subjective and socially constructed • Seek complexity of views • Researchers' own realities and views shape the research process	• Qualitative
Pragmatism	• Focused on solutions to problems and consequences of actions • No commitment to any single notion of reality • Application-focused • Pluralistic	• Mixed methods
Transformative	• Closely connected with politics and advocacy • Empowerment-oriented • Focused on reform and change • Collaborative	• Quantitative • Qualitative
Two-eyed seeing	• Mutual strengths of knowledge from Indigenous and Western ways of knowing • Equity in knowledge systems • Premised on respect, reflection, and co-learning	• Quantitative • Qualitative

The bottom line is that what "counts" as knowledge to researchers will influence their entire program of research. Philosophical worldviews provide researchers with a guiding framework that informs their research approach (quantitative, qualitative, or mixed methods), specific strategy of inquiry within that approach, and particular methods used in their research.

Research Abstract Exercise

Although a researcher's philosophical worldview will influence her or his entire research process, many researchers do not explicitly specify a guiding philosophical framework when presenting their research. As such, a researcher's worldview can remain largely hidden from her or his research. Applying your knowledge of postpositivism, constructivism, pragmatism, transformative, and two-eyed seeing worldviews, identify a philosophical worldview that might underlie each of the research studies described in the following research abstracts:

Continued

1. Community design can have a positive or negative influence on the physical activity level of residents. The complementary expertise of professionals from both planning and public health is needed to build active communities. The current study aimed to develop a coordinated framework for planners and public health professionals to enhance the design of active communities. Planners and public health professionals working in Ontario were recruited to participate in a concept mapping process to identify ways they should work together to enhance the design of active communities. This process generated 72 actions that represent collaborative efforts planners and public health professionals should engage in when designing active communities. These actions were then organized by importance and feasibility. This resulted in a coordinated action framework that includes 19 proximal and 6 distal coordinated actions for planners and public health professionals. Implementation of the recommended actions has the potential to make a difference in community design as a way to enhance physical activity in community members. This coordinated action framework provides a way to address physical inactivity from an environmental and policy standpoint (adapted from Bergeron & Lévesque, 2014)

2. Renal transplant recipients have reduced peak aerobic capacity, muscle strength, arterial function, and an unfavourable cardiovascular disease risk profile. This study compared the effects of 12 weeks of supervised endurance and strength training (with 16 participants) versus usual care (with 15 participants) on peak aerobic capacity, cardiovascular and skeletal muscle function, cardiovascular disease risk profile, and quality of life in renal transplant recipients (age range = 42 to 68 years). Peak aerobic capacity and exercise hemodynamics, arterial compliance, blood pressure, muscle strength, lean body mass, cardiovascular disease risk score, and quality of life were assessed before and after 12 weeks. The change in peak aerobic capacity (endurance and strength training: 2.6 vs. usual care: −0.5 mL/[kg·min]), cardiac output (endurance and strength training: 1.7 vs. usual care: −0.01L/min), leg press (endurance and strength training: 48.7 vs. usual care: −10.5 kg) and leg extension strength (endurance and strength training: 9.5 vs. usual care: 0.65 kg) improved significantly after endurance and strength training compared with usual care. The overall change in quality of life improved significantly after 12 weeks of endurance and strength training compared with usual care. No significant difference was found between groups for lean body mass, arterial compliance, blood pressure, or cardiovascular disease risk score. Supervised endurance and strength training is an effective intervention to improve peak exercise aerobic capacity and cardiac output, muscle strength and quality of life in clinically stable renal transplant recipients (adapted from Riess et al., 2014).

3. Implementation of heart failure guidelines in long-term care settings is challenging. Understanding the conditions of nursing practice can improve management, reduce suffering, and prevent hospital admission of long-term care residents living with heart failure. The aim of the study was to understand the experiences of nurses managing care for residents with heart failure. Five focus groups, totalling 33 nurses working in long-term care settings in Canada, were audiorecorded, then transcribed verbatim, and entered into the qualitative data analysis program NVivo9. A complex adaptive systems framework informed this analysis. Thematic content analysis was conducted by the research

team. Triangulation, rigorous discussion, and a search for negative cases were conducted. Nurses characterized their experiences managing heart failure in relation to many influences on their capacity for decision-making in long-term care settings: (a) a reactive versus proactive approach to chronic illness; (b) ability to interpret heart failure signs, symptoms, and acuity; (c) compromised information flow; (d) access to resources; and (e) moral distress. Heart failure guideline implementation reflects multiple dynamic influences. Leadership that addresses these factors is required to optimize the conditions of heart failure care and related nursing practice (adapted from Strachan et al., 2014).

Now consider how each of the research studies described above might look if guided by a different philosophical worldview. Would the research focus remain the same? How might the methods change? Is there any implication for the conclusions drawn at the end of the abstract?

Text Content Overview

This text covers quantitative, qualitative, and mixed methods research approaches used in kinesiology, with a specific focus on the Canadian context. All research begins with a question that remains unanswered (or one that has not been answered adequately). Once the decision has been made to begin the research process, a host of ethical issues invariably arise that require adequate knowledge, skill, and judgment for researchers to successfully navigate through. Hence, prior to a more in-depth discussion on the three specific approaches introduced in this first chapter, we provide chapters on how to identify a research question and study purpose (*Chapter 2*) and ethical considerations in research (*Chapter 3*), which are important to all approaches to research, regardless of whether they be quantitative, qualitative, or mixed methods.

Chapters 4 to 6 focus specifically on quantitative research approaches, covering a wide variety of quantitative research designs, ways to analyze quantitative data (i.e., statistics), and criteria used to judge the merits of quantitative research. There are many different forms of quantitative research, and through our discussion you will learn things like what it means to "randomly assign" participants to groups in an experimental research study (and why doing so

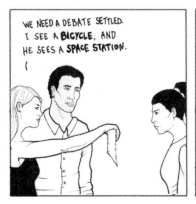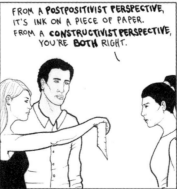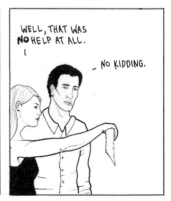

is particularly critical to intervention studies). You will also be introduced to terms like reliability and validity, which lie at the heart of all quantitative research approaches in kinesiology.

We then switch our focus to qualitative research approaches in *Chapters 7 to 9*. Similar to quantitative research approaches, a wide range of qualitative research designs will be introduced. We will cover strategies of inquiry such as phenomenology and ethnography (which, although commonly used in research articles, might be terms you are unfamiliar with). You will learn things like why qualitative research often includes a section describing the researchers' backgrounds and perspectives and why "reflexivity" is key to that understanding. You will also be introduced to terms like trustworthiness and credibility, which are criteria often used to evaluate the quality of qualitative research in kinesiology.

Chapter 10 then builds on the discussion of mixed methods approaches from earlier in this chapter. There are many ways to combine quantitative and qualitative approaches to answer kinesiology-related research questions, and together they can add both breadth and depth to our understanding of a particular topic area. You will learn about some of the potential strengths, challenges, and opportunities that mixed methods research approaches offer to those conducting research in kinesiology.

In *Chapter 11* you will be introduced to participatory action research (PAR), which is particularly well-suited to research questions that require collaborative and action-based methods to achieve success (i.e., research that stems from a transformative philosophical worldview). You will learn why the guiding assumptions underlying PAR might be particularly well-suited for work with Indigenous communities and to researchers who value an Indigenous worldview.

We conclude the book with a discussion of options researchers have to translate their research findings for various audiences (*Chapter 12*). Dissemination of research results to the community is becoming increasingly important, as is the recognition that writing up research solely in journal articles is somewhat limited because of the audience they are designed to reach. Hence, strategies for communicating the results of research to others, including audiences both with and without research backgrounds, will be presented. Featured will be a range of innovative forms of knowledge translation, such as online videos, fictional narratives, poetic transcription, and ethnodrama.

While perhaps somewhat ambitious, ultimately we hope that this book encourages you to evaluate information in kinesiology with openness, curiosity, and skepticism. Although they

Writing Exercise

What types of research approaches are most common in the journal articles that you have read? What types of skills and knowledge would be useful to be able to critique the findings you have read about in those articles? Write down some of the specific challenges professionals (e.g., physical therapists, coaches, teachers) working in kinesiology-related fields might have in understanding journal articles. Of course, if you haven't ever read a journal article, now would be a good time to explore a few.

Professional Highlight

Heather Moyse, Occupational Therapist and Olympic Champion

Profile: Two-time Olympic gold medalist Heather Moyse completed a B.Sc. Honours degree in kinesiology and a Master's degree in occupational therapy. In 2010 she received a Young Alumni Award from the Faculty of Applied Health Sciences at the University of Waterloo for her accomplishments as an athlete, her commitment to continuing education, volunteerism, and public service, as well as her leadership in the field. Heather is a multi-sport athlete, having competed in three Olympics in the sport of bobsleigh (2006 Turin Winter Olympics, 2010 Vancouver Winter Olympics, and 2014 Sochi Winter Olympics), being a member of the Canadian National Senior Women's Rugby team, and representing Canada in the 2012 Pan-American Cycling Championships. She is well-known as an inspirational speaker and for her humanitarian work. Heather is also a shining example of a professional committed to kinesiology across its many dimensions.

Further Resource

Heather Moyse's website: http://heathermoyse.com

might seem to be at present, science and research need not be intimidating. As Carl Sagan (1997) wrote:

> I know personally, both from having science explained to me and from my attempts to explain it to others, how gratifying it is when we get it, when obscure terms suddenly take on meaning, when we grasp what all the fuss is about, when deep wonders are revealed.

To this end, throughout this book we offer some of the basic building blocks to help you evaluate current knowledge in the field and provide some insight into how you might begin answering your own questions. The world of kinesiology is beautiful, exciting, and mysterious . . . and ready to be explored.

Summary

Chapter 1 focused on providing students with an introduction to research in kinesiology in a variety of ways. The first section encouraged students to question known "facts" in the field of kinesiology, showing how current knowledge in kinesiology is intimately tied to an understanding of the research process. The second section introduced a wide variety of research methods using Canadian examples from sport, exercise, health, and physical education to demonstrate how research is relevant and important to a variety of careers in kinesiology-related fields. Five philosophical worldviews were highlighted (i.e., postpositivism, constructivism, pragmatism, transformative, and two-eyed seeing), and the implications these worldviews have on the research process were discussed. The third section provided an overview of topics covered in the remainder of the text, with the goal of fostering students' openness, curiosity, and excitement for the research process (and desire to keep reading).

Discussion Questions

1. Why is the research process important to understanding the current knowledge base in kinesiology?
2. What are key characteristics of (a) the three research approaches and (b) the five philosophical worldviews used in kinesiology?
3. How does a researcher's philosophical worldview shape her or his chosen research approach and choice of research methods?
4. Why is it important to critically evaluate research studies and the findings of research?
5. What topic areas interest you in kinesiology? What research approach(es) and philosophical worldview(s) might be a good fit for your interest areas?

Recommended Readings

Bartlett, C., Marshall, M., & Marshall, A. (2012). Two-eyed seeing and other lessons learned within a co-learning journey of bringing together Indigenous and mainstream knowledges and ways of knowing. *Journal of Environmental Studies and Sciences, 2,* 331–40. doi:10.1007/s13412-012-0086-8

Elliott, D. (2007). Forty years of kinesiology: A Canadian perspective. *Quest, 59,* 154–62. doi: 10.1080/00336297.2007.10483544

Sagan, C. (1997). *The Demon-haunted world: Science as a candle in the dark*. London, UK: Headline.

Credit

2 Identifying a Research Question and Study Purpose(s)

Learning Outcomes

By the end of this chapter, you should be able to:

- Describe the process of identifying your research topic.
- Identify strategies to narrow your interests to a specific research question and purpose for your study.
- Discuss *why* literature is used and *how* it is used in research.

It is really important to do the right research as well as to do the research right. You need to do "wow" research, research that is compelling, not just interesting.

—George Springer, Chairman of the Aeronautics and Astronautics Department at Stanford University

The Research Topic

The research topic and related purpose and questions make up the foundation of a study. In essence, they are the reason you are engaging in research in the first place. This process of identifying a research problem can be both the most frustrating and the most rewarding part of the research process. It can be frustrating because coming up with "the" most important problem in a certain area can be a daunting task, especially when it feels like everything has been done already. Alternatively, it can also be extremely rewarding when a problem is identified because it is like a mission achieved, with the excitement of the remainder of the research process ahead.

Research topics are narrowly focused and represent clearly defined focal areas related to an important complex problem(s). The identification of a research topic usually comes from the researcher's interests, experiences, coursework, and academic background. For example, students in kinesiology usually have diverse backgrounds in sport and exercise or employment experiences, and across a variety of courses with sociology, psychology, physiology, anatomy, biomechanics, physics, epidemiology, geography, and public health and policy underpinnings. Being familiar with existing research is also critical to identifying a topic, a purpose, and research questions. Familiarity with existing research is garnered primarily throughout a review of literature, including a critical review of what has been done, what has not been done, and the strengths and weaknesses of existing studies. Just a few examples of the topics that might be pursued by kinesiology researchers include:

- Sport drinks and recovery
- Risk of concussion in contact and non-contact sport
- Caffeine and exercise performance enhancement
- Type of exercise and mental health
- Active videogame use and improvements in ventilatory threshold
- Sport training and immune function regulation
- Work-related muscle strain and standing desks
- Policies to increase number of minutes of physical activity in schools
- Standardized physical education fitness testing and body image
- Muscle fibre type, mitochondrial function, and aging

Given the breadth of the knowledge base in kinesiology, topics in the field also vary tremendously and are often initiated based on what the researcher enjoys the most from the courses and experiences she or he has had. Other ways of identifying topics can include having conversations with professors and graduate students, reviewing research that is done at the university, and paying attention to controversial issues in areas of interest. It is only through searching and reading existing research and knowledge that interesting topics will be identified. Using this type of approach, scientists recently discovered a lymphatic system for the central nervous system that essentially links the brain to the immune system. The vessels were not known and had escaped detection in spite of the lymphatic system being

Writing Exercise

Think about your own background experiences in work, school, recreation, and sport. Write down your answers to the following questions.

1. What are some kinesiology-related topics that you are most interested in learning more about? What courses have you enjoyed the most? What areas of these courses have most interested you?
2. Think about where these interests come from. Are they based on conversations with your parents/guardians as you were growing up? Are they questions you have had since playing sports when you were young? Are they related to jobs you have had? Are they related to observations you have while going about your day-to-day activities?

Make a list of the topics that you would be interested in studying and keep re-visiting this list as you read through this chapter and even the rest of the book.

thoroughly mapped out throughout the body. This discovery will change the way the systems are described in textbooks and taught in coursework, and this knowledge will have significant implications for neurological diseases such as Alzheimer's and multiple sclerosis (Louveau et al., 2015). It's hard to believe that parts of the human body are still being discovered, but this is just one example demonstrating the "black hole" of topics that could be researched.

Once you have identified a topic area, you need to identify a related problem that can be researched. Things to consider when drafting your topic into a problem include specifics of the topic, populations, time periods, locations, and theory and practice applications. For example, if you are interested in the topic of exercise performance you could explore aerobic and strength training exercises (*specifics of the topic*) among older adults (*population*) in Halifax (*location*) to explore if cardiac output is a key regulator of exercise performance based on testing Hill's muscle model (*theory*). The key to homing in on these specific elements may rest in your critical review of existing literature, the strengths and weaknesses identified within published papers, and gaps in the literature. In the next section, strategies for identifying the research problem are presented.

The Research Problem

Once you have identified a general topic for your research, it is important to come up with a problem and related research questions. The **research problem** represents the foundational need for the study and describes the context for the study and the issues that exist in literature, theory, and/or practice (Creswell, 2014). Effective problem statements answer the question *"Why does this research need to be conducted?"* Probably the most important step in coming up with the problem is to gain knowledge about what is already known on the topic. Research review papers, meta-analyses, and textbook chapters offer good starting points because they are summaries of what has been done to date. It is also important to delve into the literature and get acquainted with all kinds of research studies that have been done on the general topic of interest. When you are reading through the review papers and original studies, take note of not only what has been done previously . . . but also more importantly of *what has not been done*.

There are many reasons why a topic has not been studied, including that it has limited scope or interest, it is too challenging to study appropriately, it might take too much time (which is difficult for undergraduate or graduate students given they do want to finish their degrees!), it is not feasible, or it could be unethical. When reading the review papers and textbook chapters, you can also identify the references within and read those papers, or locate current research papers on the topic. Overall, it is important to use a variety of sources to home in on an area of interest to you and also of value to the larger kinesiology research and practice community.

In addition to finding a problem of interest to you and of value to others, there are other guidelines to keep in mind at this stage in the research process. Specifically, the research problem should be (a) challenging, but neither too difficult nor too easy; (b) worthwhile and important; and (c) feasible with respect to your time, expertise, and available resources (e.g., equipment, finances, study participants).

There are different types of problems that can be identified and that ultimately direct the research process and outcomes. Generally, research problems can have descriptive, predictive, and explanation bases.

Problems that are **descriptive** in nature include the need for describing a phenomenon, event, condition, or circumstance whereby no attempt is made to link information or explain outcomes. An example of descriptive research could be the need to describe levels of physical activity among adults in Canada. The Canadian Fitness and Lifestyle Research Institute (CFLRI) is one organization that compiles descriptive data for research and practice and publishes reports such as the *Physical Activity Monitor*. Based on descriptive data from 2013 (Bulletin 1: Physical activity levels of Canadians), more men (55%) than women (51%) self-report that they are active, and physical activity levels decline with advancing age (60% of young adults aged 20 to 34 years report being active compared to 48% of older adults aged 65 or older).

Predictive research problems are based on the premise that there is a need to identify relationships among **variables**, which are attributes or characteristics that may vary over time or across cases. In addition to simple relationships, one might also be able to propose a direction of relationship such that certain variables predict an *outcome* (i.e., the main focus of the study). For example, there are many risk factors for sports injury including training, functional range of motion, anxiety levels, environmental factors (e.g., playing surface, weather), and type of sport. Researchers could combine measures related to these and other variables to predict a person's risk for or susceptibility to sustaining a sport injury (the outcome). Another example of predictive research problems would be risk of cardiovascular disease. There is strong evidence that age, sex, cholesterol level, smoking status, and blood pressure are predictors of cardiovascular disease. Individuals can answer questions related to these personal and health conditions and can obtain a risk score using online resources (e.g., https://www.cvdriskchecksecure.com/FraminghamRiskScore.aspx).

Research problems arguably at the highest level of sophistication and scientific advancement include those with explanatory bases. **Explanation problems** exist when researchers can make claims about cause and effect, or attempt to answer problems of *why* events and behaviours happen. A classic example of causal claims is the experimentation that was (and continues to be) done around cigarette smoking and lung cancer. Also, think about all the advances in sporting equipment that have taken place over time, such as the design of swimwear for racing or the technology changes that have been done in the sport of bobsledding (e.g., the material in the sled; the form and function of the helmet and racing suits). All of these equipment advances are a result of experiments conducted to address explanatory research problems.

Use of theory

In addition to reading the literature (discussed in more detail later in this chapter), it is also important to gain knowledge and identify problems through relevant theories. A **theory** is an explanation of observed patterns or supposition about a relationship among phenomena. Theories are generally derived from observations, experimentation, and reflective thinking and are composed of verifiable, testable statements or propositions (Mood & Morrow, 2015).

Theories often include relational statements that connect two or more variables such that knowing something about one variable can help to understand the other.

As an example, a common theory in sport and exercise psychology research is the Theory of Planned Behaviour (TPB; Ajzen, 1991). As described by Ajzen, exercise (or any health behaviour) can be directly explained by one's intentions to engage in the behaviour and one's perceptions of control over the behaviour. In turn, exercise intentions are explained by one's attitude towards the behaviour and perceptions of the social norms relative to the behaviour. Based on this theory (see Figure 2.1), researchers can make problem statements that pertain to the relationships outlined. For example, a key problem that arises with the use of the TPB has to do with the intention-to-behaviour gap, such that some people do not exercise in spite of their best intention to do so and their high perceptions of behavioural control (i.e., they think they can control their exercise behaviours). So questions that arise could be *"Under what conditions do intentions lead to behaviour change?"* or *"Is the intention-to-behaviour gap different for males and females or for people with chronic disease?"*

As can be seen from this example, theories can be used to provide a blueprint or framework to guide research problems and questions. Theories can also be more abstract directives that offer a foundation for connecting other frameworks. For example, Fitts' law is a characterization of human movement used by researchers in motor control and learning to examine speed and accuracy of movement (Fitts, 1954). According to Fitts' law, a speed–accuracy trade-off occurs in which the time required to accurately and rapidly move to a target area increases

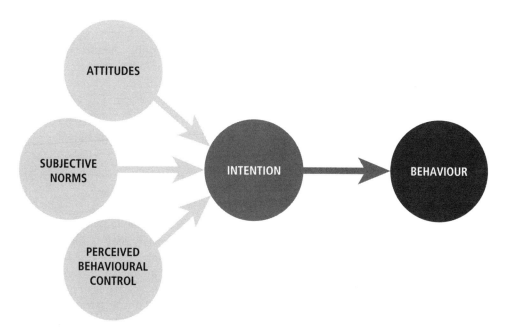

Figure 2.1 Example of theory in research: The Theory of Planned Behaviour

Adapted from: Ajzen, I. (1991). The theory of planned behavior. *Organizational Behavior and Human Decision Processes, 50,* 179–211, and Arbour, L., & Cook, D. (2006). DNA on loan: Issues to consider when carrying out genetic research with aboriginal families and communities. *Public Health Genomics, 9,* 153–60.

as a function of the ratio between the distance to the target and the width of the target (i.e., a person must increase movement time to maintain accuracy as the difficulty of the movement increases). This proposition has been studied among a range of participants using a number of different tasks such as walking through narrowing doorways, aiming at targets, and pointing (Passmore, Burke, & Lyons, 2007). There is also some evidence of conditions in which the theory may be violated (e.g., movement time is shorter when aiming at the farthest target in a group), leading to more work in the area and the possibility of adaptations to the theory. For example, researchers in kinesiology programs across Canada have studied precues, advanced knowledge and planning, and learning effects as reasons to explain shorter movement times on the aiming and accuracy on the last target in an array (e.g., Blinch, Cameron, Hodges, & Chua, 2012; Glazebrook, Kiernan, Welsh, & Tremblay, 2015). The work on the violation of Fitts' law helps researchers identify new research problems and provides a foundation for testing other theories or perhaps combining theoretical frameworks.

The use of theory in the development of the problem will differ depending on the researchers' philosophical worldviews and research approach, which were introduced in Chapter 1. In studies using quantitative approaches, theory is generally used to guide the entire research process from the problem, purpose, and hypothesis generation through to analysis and discussion. Dr Kathleen Martin Ginis espouses the use of theory in her research with a predominant focus on individuals with spinal cord injuries. In reading her work, it is clear that she uses theory to inform the literature searches, purpose statements, and measures that are used in her research. In research with qualitative approaches, theories may be used to inform the research problem and purpose, but they can also be used as an outcome following the research process such that the gathering of data informs a theory (Charmaz, 2006). This theory generation process can then be the impetus for future research testing and confirming the theory.

Professional Highlight

Dr Kathleen Martin Ginis, Professor, Kinesiology, University of British Columbia—Okanagan

Profile: Dr Martin Ginis conducts research targeting psychosocial influences on, and consequences of, physical activity participation. She focuses on understanding and modifying theory-based determinants of physical activity and the psychosocial benefits of physical activity. Recently, she has focused her research on physical activity participation among people with spinal cord injury (SCI). For example, Dr Martin Ginis and her research team have developed and tested a measure for physical activity among men and women with SCI. She has also led the creation of a large community-university partnership program for individuals with SCI that promotes physical activity through onsite fitness facilities, telephone-based guidance for physical activity, and an evaluation of barriers to physical activity in the community. Her research program led to the development of "SCI Action Canada," which brings together researchers, specialists, service groups, and community members focused on advancing physical activity knowledge and participation among

Canadians living with SCI. Her research also formed the development of the "Physical Activity Guidelines for Adults with SCI" (http://sciactioncanada.ca). In addition, Dr Martin Ginis and her research team published a "SCI Get Fit Toolkit," which is an evidence-based resource tailored for adults with SCI (http://sciactioncanada.ca/guidelines/docs/sci-get-fit-toolkit-brochure-r.pdf). The toolkit includes activities for manual- and power-chair users, strategies to overcome physical activity barriers for adults with SCI, as well as action plans and safety tips. Taken together, Dr Martin Ginis' research exemplifies the use of theory, the importance of measurement, and the value of creating collaborations among researchers, community professionals, and participants with the aim of improving physical activity opportunities for people with SCI. Many of her colleagues and former graduate students also hold positions at universities across Canada, including Amy Latimer-Cheung (Queens University), Kelly Arbour-Nicitopoulos (University of Toronto), and Heather Gainforth (University of British Columbia).

Further Readings

Martin Ginis, K. A., Arbour-Nicitopoulos, K. A., Latimer-Cheung, A. E., Buchholz, A. C., Bray, S. R., Craven, B. C., . . . Horrocks, J. (2012). Predictors of leisure time physical activity among people with spinal cord injury. *Annals of Behavioral Medicine, 44,* 104–18. doi:10.1007/s12160-012-9370-9

Martin Ginis, K. A., Latimer-Cheung, A. E., Corkum, S., Ginis, S., Anathasopoulos, P., Arbour-Nicitopoulos, K. P., & Gainforth. H. (2012). A case study of a community-university multidisciplinary partnership approach to increasing physical activity participation among people with spinal cord injury. *Translational Behavioral Medicine, 2,* 516–22. doi:10.1007/s13142-012-0157-0

Martin Ginis, K. A., Phang, S. H., Latimer, A. E., & Arbour-Nicitopoulos, K. P. (2012). Reliability and validity tests of the Leisure Time Physical Activity Questionnaire for People with Spinal Cord Injury. *Archives of Physical Medicine and Rehabilitation,* 93: 677–82. doi:10.1016/j.apmr.2011.11.005

Types of reasoning

A research problem is also developed and approached using reasoning. The two types of reasoning in the scientific approach include deductive and inductive reasoning. **Inductive reasoning** involves using observations of specific events and circumstances to make predictions about general principles that are tied together and united into theory. Take for example the hotly debated topic of stretching before running. Based on numerous experiments and observations, people were instructed to stretch before they engaged in exercise. More recently, this need for stretching has been dispelled, with researchers observing that stretching does not reduce injury and may be unnecessary (Simic, Sarabon, & Markovic, 2013). These discrepancies in research findings and inductive reasoning help advance science, and only time will tell what (if any) additional revisions to theory on stretching, injury, and performance will be required.

Deductive reasoning is the opposite approach to the development of scientific knowledge compared to inductive reasoning. Using a deductive approach, researchers start with concrete

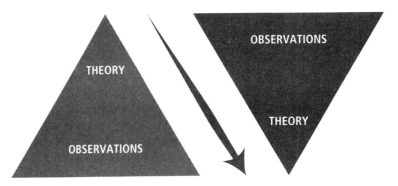

Figure 2.2 Deductive (depicted on the left) and inductive (depicted on the right) reasoning.

generalized information often contained within a theory and use this information to explain specific events or circumstances. Going back to the theory of planned behaviour (Ajzen, 1991), researchers could use the theory to develop **research questions** and **hypotheses** pertaining to the relationships outlined in the theory (see Figure 2.1). For example, many researchers have tested the proposition that positive attitudes toward exercise (e.g., belief that exercise is good for you) and higher subjective norms (e.g., belief that people around you value exercise) relate to higher intentions for exercise. In this way, the theory informs initial research questions and hypotheses, the hypotheses are then tested, and the results can be compared across studies to confirm (or refute) the theory.

The general analogy of inductive and deductive reasoning is illustrated in Figure 2.2.

The Literature Search and Review

Throughout this chapter so far, we have made reference to the importance of the literature review to identify the research topic and research problem(s), and we will be discussing the importance of the literature review for identifying and defining the purpose statement, variables and concepts of interest, hypotheses, and research questions. But what is a literature review and how do you go about doing one?

The literature review is like a synopsis of what researchers know based on studies that have already been done on similar, relevant topics. In this way, it situates the current study within an ongoing textual discussion and dialogue related to the topic. Of course, summarizing everything that has been done on a topic could take months or years to accomplish (for example, there are nearly one million references for self-esteem!), and the review is not meant to be exhaustive as long as it is up to date and timely. The key is to try to include the critical papers that justify your chosen topic, narrate the problem you are trying to address, and identify complementary as well as juxtaposing perspectives. Baumgartner and Hensley (2012) offer a number of helpful strategies in the process of reading and writing research. They highlight the importance of the iterative nature of working between an idea and the literature in a back and forth manner that culminates in a clear focus on a unique topic that is both valuable and interesting.

Sources for the literature review

One of the first steps to conducting a literature review is to identify key words. Think about the words or clues you would use to describe your topic of interest to friends during a game of charades. Once you have generated a list of at least three key terms, use this list to search for literature sources. Search tools can include the university library catalogue, online search engines such as Google Scholar, and computerized databases that capture research in kinesiology (e.g., ERIC, PsychInfo, Web of Science, SPORTDiscus, PubMed), and published graduate theses and dissertations (e.g., ProQuest). You can also identify specific journals in the field of kinesiology that are central to your research topic (e.g., *Medicine and Science in Sport and Exercise* is one of the leading journals for kinesiology topics generally, and there are other more specific journals such as *Journal of Sport & Exercise Psychology, Sociology of Sport, Journal of Motor Development, Measurement in Physical Education and Exercise Science*). Finally, you can use the reference sections from any published document to identify more sources.

The main sources in a literature review include research articles, book chapters, meta-analyses, conceptual articles, and published reports that provide foundations for the topic, problem, and purpose. Review papers are particularly helpful because they summarize a group of empirical published studies that focus on a similar topic, target sample, or situation. Once sources are identified, it is a matter of reading and re-reading publications to get a critical evaluation of the area of research. Specifically, homing in on a research problem and questions (as well as the target sample, methods, and possible analyses) is an iterative process that is informed by a constant reflection and reading of the literature. This process helps researchers refine ideas and may even send them down new paths of research interests.

Reading research

Reading and processing the fundamentals of a research publication can take time to master. Thomas, Nelson, and Silverman (2011) identify some suggestions for reading the literature:

- Get familiar with a small number of publications that are important in your field of interest. These key publications can be identified by a professor or researcher in the area, a librarian, or even by the number of citations that they have garnered (even though the latter is not always an indication of good quality research!).
- Do not get bogged down by research that is peripheral to your interests. Stick to what you like and what you feel you can read based on your knowledge and background.
- Read the article to capture the big picture and ideas rather than trying to identify the eternal truths. Be critical and cautious.
- The abstract is an excellent starting point to any study. It provides a summary of the research background, purpose, method, results, and conclusion. If you read the abstract and it sparks some interest or curiosity, continue to read the article.

- Do not get overwhelmed with trying to understand the details of the statistical analysis. It is important to look at the data and to think about what it all means in practical terms, rather than focusing solely on the statistical significance.
- Pay attention to the discussion and the ways that researchers explain, defend, and refute their findings. This section of the article usually includes an explicit discussion of the strengths and limitations of the work, offers ideas for future research, and (ideally) provides implications of the findings to the general field of study.

Organizing the literature

There are many ways of organizing the literature and you should find what works best for you. If you are a visual person, you might try to create a **literature map**, which is a visual representation or figure that draws together the existing studies and identifies how your topic is situated within the broader body of research. There are open source software tools to help organize your literature map such as the Visual Understanding Environment (http://vue.tufts .edu) or Popplet for use on your tablet (http://popplet.com). The idea is to represent the literature in a way that offers a visual representation of what is known about your topic and how the literature sources fit together to home in on the problem and purpose statement. You can also develop an **annotated bibliography**, which is a summary and critique of the articles and book chapters and documents you have identified. You first write out the citation (i.e., the authors, date, journal article title, journal title, volume, issue, and page numbers) and then a descriptive and evaluative paragraph (i.e., the annotation). In this paragraph, the goal is to inform yourself and others of the value and relevance of the reference to your topic, and the quality of the sources cited. There are many online guides to developing an annotated bibliography, such as the one presented at the University of Toronto (http://www.writing.utoronto.ca/advice/ specific-types-of-writing/annotated-bibliography).

Another approach to summarizing the articles and research sources you have read is to think about ways the studies are similar (and different) in terms of theoretical approaches, problems and purpose statements, research questions, methodologies, findings, and implications. Creating tallies based on your interests could be an effective way of visualizing your review. For example, if you were interested in the effect of a specific type of protein supplementation

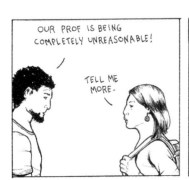
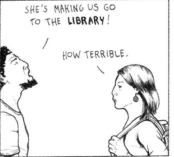
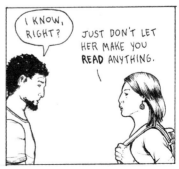

Table 2.1 Sample chart for summarizing research studies.

AUTHORS	PURPOSE	DESCRIPTION OF PARTICIPANTS	MEASURES	PROCEDURE	MAIN FINDINGS
Study 1					
Study 2					
Study. . .					

on exercise performance, you might conduct a literature review and find 10 studies that use similar protein sources (such as whey) and that all explore performance as running times. You could summarize the studies as follows: *Out of the 10 research studies exploring the effectiveness of protein supplementation on running performance, three studies reported statistically significant differences in run times favouring the protein supplementation with differences in time of 1.2 minutes, 2.1 minutes, and 2.2 minutes.* This type of summary is likely facilitated by creating a chart that identifies the key features of the literature sources that you have identified and read. A sample chart is provided in Table 2.1. This type of chart should have as many rows as there are identified research studies, but the column headings can be altered based on your interest. For example, you might add a column for a summary of the key strengths and limitations of the studies.

Summarizing Research Exercise

Thinking about your topic of interest, develop a map of some literature on the topic. Specifically, identify 10 to 15 articles that support your topic and illustrate them in a map. Draw lines to connect sources that discuss similar ideas.

Using the same articles, create a summary chart using the headings in Table 2.1 as a guide. Once you have completed the literature map and the summary chart, review both approaches to determine which method you feel is more helpful to you in summarizing and organizing the articles you have identified on your topic of interest.

Writing the literature review

Once you have read the key articles, and have identified 20 to 40 articles of relevance to your topic, it is time to summarize the articles in a formal literature review. You can use your literature map to guide the sections of your review or draft a table of contents with the key areas that you want to write about. An outline is extremely helpful at this point of the research process. This outline should be developed with an understanding that there are three main parts to a literature review, including an introduction (a statement of the problem that creates interest for the reader), the body (identifying what is and what is not known about the problem), and the conclusion (a summary of the existing studies that culminates with the purpose statement, research questions, and/or hypotheses). Creswell (2014) identifies the general approach to writing the introduction as a deficiency model because a main goal of this section of the research paper is to identify the gaps in the literature, or deficiencies, that set the foundation for the current research study.

The introduction is an opportunity to "sell your idea" to the reader and to provide the context of the study. The introduction section, which is usually one paragraph in length, can include providing the reader with summary statistics that highlight the importance of the topic. For example, an opening statement such as "Fifty percent (50%) of Canadians will suffer from a mental health problem before the age of 40 years" would be a strong argument justifying the need for a study exploring the preventative effects of physical activity on anxiety. As another example, statistics from the Canadian Cancer Society could be an alarming way of demonstrating the need for more research on the prevention of cancer, given that one in two individuals in Canada is affected by cancer as a patient or caregiver. If our protein supplementation study summary were based on empirical evidence rather than a fictitious example, we could start our introduction of the literature review with something to the effect of "Several studies have demonstrated that run times can be enhanced by an average of nearly two minutes with the ingestion of certain protein supplements." Aside from attracting attention to the importance of the problem of interest, the introduction paragraph should also be used to identify variables or phenomena that will be further described throughout the body of the literature review. We will describe what we mean by *key variables* (important focus in a quantitative study) and *central phenomenon* (the main interest in a qualitative study) in detail later in this chapter.

The body of the literature review should be organized in a meaningful, straightforward, and clear and concise way. The organization of the literature review can take many forms, but needs to be logical and represent a flow of ideas. The important elements of the pending study (usually identified as the key variables or central phenomenon, as well as target sample characteristics, contexts and situations, historical periods, etc.) can be described using subheadings or clearly articulated sentence structures that end each paragraph with a summary statement. For example, if researchers are interested in studying the effects of protein supplementation on endurance performance, the body of the literature review is likely to have a paragraph (or two) on different types and sources of protein supplementation, a paragraph (or two) on different ways of assessing endurance performance, and then maybe a paragraph on sex or gender differences and similarities in protein metabolism and endurance performance (if researchers are interested in whether the effects are different for males and females). Within each of these subtopic paragraphs, it is important to identify what is known about the topic, why it is important, what has not been done (and why), and to end with a summary of the topic that usually hints at how gaps in the literature will be addressed. This latter point is critical for a logical flow of ideas. The key to writing these paragraphs is to offer details on some studies that may be most relevant to the topic while summarizing a group of studies that are similar in the use of theory, participant characteristics, methodologies, and/or findings.

The final section of the literature review is the summary of what is known and what is still unknown or needs more study, including the presentation of the research purpose, questions, and hypotheses. These central elements of the research study will be discussed more in the next sections.

A final feature of the practice of writing a literature review is to understand how to properly cite study findings. Keep in mind that plagiarism is not tolerated in research (and academics) and needs to be avoided at all stages of the research writing process. It is good practice to first summarize what other authors state in your own words, and then use your own summaries when you are writing your literature review. When you summarize any information or ideas that are not your own, citation is essential. Citation means referencing or giving credit to the researcher(s) who originally identified the ideas or conducted the research you are summarizing. There are a number of different citation styles that are used in kinesiology research, and a full summary or review of each citation style is beyond the scope of this text. However, a few examples include the American Psychological Association (APA), Modern Language Association (MLA), Vancouver, and Chicago citation styles. It is important to use the citation guidelines that are common in your field of study (or required in your class), and your professor or supervisor can help identify the appropriate approach. Most journals also have a standard citation style that may dictate which style you use for your final product.

In summary, the literature review is essential for the foundation of the research study. Day and Gastel (2006) provide a good reference for strategies in writing research papers and can be a very useful source to find tips that will assist you writing (and reading) science coherently.

Purpose

The literature review concludes with a statement of the study purpose. According to Creswell (2014), the purpose statement is the most important statement in an entire research study. The purpose of a study needs to be clear and concise, and ultimately states the intent of the study. The purpose statement should also identify all the variables or phenomena/concepts in the study.

The study variables and phenomena

The identification of variables is particularly important when conducting a quantitative research study, and there are several types of variables that should be considered. The **independent variable** is the variable that is manipulated (i.e., treatment variable). When the problem is founded on prediction, the independent variable (IV) is also identified as the predictor or correlate. The **dependent variable** is the variable that is being affected and represents the outcome being assessed as a result of the independent variable(s). The dependent variable (DV) is also often the main focus of the study (i.e., the variable researchers are interested in changing). Let's go back to the example on predicting sport injury. We identified several factors that might relate to susceptibility of enduring an injury including training, functional range of motion, anxiety levels, environmental factors, and type of sport. A potential purpose statement based on that topic area might be: "To determine if playing on artificial turf increases susceptibility of sport injury among varsity soccer players." In this purpose statement, we are "manipulating" the playing surface (e.g., we could look at university athletes who play on artificial turf and compare them to athletes who play on natural surfaces), which would be the independent variable. Our dependent variable in this example would be sport injury, which could be measured by number of injuries sustained among varsity soccer players in a season as the outcome.

Now let's make the above study example a little more detailed by including differences in injury risk for junior versus senior soccer players. If so, age would be considered a **moderator variable** (also called a categorical variable or effect moderator), which is a variable of interest that cannot be manipulated (i.e., we can't ask our participants to change their age or playing status for the purpose of our study). Other common moderator variables in kinesiology might be sex and race/ethnicity. A moderator variable is studied specifically to examine whether the presence of this variable changes the relationship of the independent and dependent variable. We could also identify **control variables** in our study. These are variables that could influence the outcome or results of our study. They are measured variables, but are not a main focus of the study. Control variables in our example might be level of competition and type of athletic footwear. Additionally, we could make our purpose statement more complex by examining a **mediator variable** (i.e., a variable that is proposed to at least partially explain the relationship between an independent and a dependent variable). For example, we could test playing surface as a mediator in the relationship between weather conditions and sport injury, such that the moisture level of the surface (e.g., slippery and wet playing fields) might at least partially explain any association between weather conditions and injury. Finally, there might be other variables that explain the relationship in our study that we have not measured. These unmeasured variables, which are not controlled for in the study, are called **extraneous variables**. Extraneous variables are often identified in the discussion section of the study write-up when researchers attempt to make sense of their findings. For example, it could be that functional movement skills, flexibility, and joint angles (e.g., ankles, knee) as well as psychological variables (e.g., proneness to anxiety) could influence risk of injury; however, it is possible that measuring these variables was not considered when the study was initially developed. Extraneous variables are often then measured in future studies. In fact, the identification of these types of variables is a great way to start with a new topic and new research questions for another study.

A review that might be of interest based on the example provided above is a systematic review of studies linking playing surface to sport injury that was published by Balazs and colleagues in the *American Journal of Sports Medicine* in 2014. Their conclusion, based on a summary of 10 studies (that were deemed by the authors to be of high quality) and a total of 963 anterior cruciate ligament (ACL) injuries in soccer and football, was that the risk of ACL injury was higher on artificial playing surfaces for football but that there was no apparent higher risk for soccer. The authors of the review recommended that more studies are needed to better understand the discrepancy in risk of ACL injury for football versus soccer players. As such, a new purpose statement on this topic awaits!

In a qualitative study, in contrast to quantitative research, the focus is more on a **central phenomenon** as the main concept in the research. A central phenomenon is a key construct or a focal area that the researcher tries to better understand, explore, and describe. The aim is to advance one's understanding of this central phenomenon rather than trying to understand associations among variables or comparing groups, which is common in quantitative studies.

Literature searches will help to identify what variables or central phenomenon should be studied. In particular, it is useful to pay attention to the discussion and future directions sections of published works. In these two sections particularly, researchers who have already invested time and resources identify what they could have done differently to improve their work. You can then draw from their insight to help develop your own study.

Theories are an additional resource for identifying variables or a starting point to identify a central phenomenon. For example, in the Theory of Planned Behaviour (TPB) model depicted in Figure 2.1, the independent variables could be any or all of attitudes, subjective norms, and perceived behavioural control variables; the dependent variable could be exercise behaviour; and the mediator in that model could be identified as intention to engage in exercise. As a general rule in figures representing theoretical models, variables with arrows heading away from them to other variables are often independent variables, variables that have arrows heading both to and away from them are often defined as mediators, and variables at the end of the diagram with arrows heading only to them are the dependent variables. The TPB might also be used to inform a central phenomenon, such as "intentions to exercise" in a qualitative study, or could be used in the discussion section as a way of making sense of findings related to a central phenomenon not otherwise identified in the theory.

The particular features of purpose statements are specific to the research approach (i.e., quantitative, qualitative, and mixed methods). These features are presented below along with strategies for writing different purpose statements within each of the three research approaches.

Quantitative research purpose statement

It should be clear from the above discussion that identifying an effective purpose statement for a research study is essential. As guidance, the writing of a purpose statement for a quantitative study should generally follow the strategies identified in Figure 2.3.

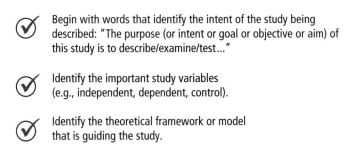

Begin with words that identify the intent of the study being described: "The purpose (or intent or goal or objective or aim) of this study is to describe/examine/test…"

Identify the important study variables (e.g., independent, dependent, control).

Identify the theoretical framework or model that is guiding the study.

Identify the participants targeted for the study.

Mention the strategy of inquiry (e.g., survey research, experimental).

Figure 2.3 General strategies for writing a quantitative research purpose statement.

A template purpose statement for quantitative studies could look something like this:

> In line with the *psychosocial model of stress* [theory/model], the *purpose* of this *experimental survey* [strategy of inquiry] study is to *test the relationship* that *stress* [independent variable] is related to *immune function* [dependent variable] and that the relationship is mediated by *physical activity* [mediator variable], controlling for *age, sex, and socioeconomic position* [control variables] among *older adults* [participants].

Writing Exercise

Applying your knowledge of the purpose statement so far, identify the independent, dependent, mediator, and/or moderator variables in the following statements, and identify at least two potential control variables and one possible extraneous variable for each:

1. The study objective was to determine, within adults age 18 to 64 years, whether moderate-to-vigorous physical activity (MVPA) accumulated in bouts is more strongly associated with metabolic syndrome than an equivalent volume of MVPA accumulated sporadically (Clarke & Janssen, 2014).
2. In this study, the relationship between exercising at low, moderate, and high intensity, cerebral oxygenation, and cognitive performance (measured as reaction time and accuracy) was examined in young adults (Mekari et al., 2015).
3. This longitudinal study examined the association between participation in school sport during adolescence and mental health in early adulthood (Jewett et al., 2014).
4. This study examined how access to fast food restaurants, less healthy/healthier food outlets, and supermarkets relate to measured levels of overweight and obesity among grade five and six students (Larsen, Cook, Stone, & Faulkner, 2015).
5. During childhood, physical activity is likely the most important modifiable factor for the development of lean mass. However, the effects of normal growth and maturation must be controlled. The purpose of this study was to investigate the independent effects of physical activity on total body and regional lean mass accrual, while accounting for the confounding effects of growth and maturation (Baxter-Jones, Eisenmann, Mirwald, Faulkner, & Bailey, 2008).

Qualitative research purpose statement

Purpose statements in qualitative research focus on the central phenomenon to be explored rather than specific variables. As such, a qualitative purpose statement narrows the focus to one central concept.

The writing of a purpose statement for a qualitative study should generally follow the guidelines presented in Figure 2.4.

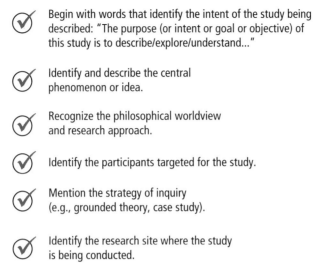

Begin with words that identify the intent of the study being described: "The purpose (or intent or goal or objective) of this study is to describe/explore/understand..."

Identify and describe the central phenomenon or idea.

Recognize the philosophical worldview and research approach.

Identify the participants targeted for the study.

Mention the strategy of inquiry (e.g., grounded theory, case study).

Identify the research site where the study is being conducted.

Figure 2.4 General strategies for writing a qualitative research purpose statement.

A template purpose statement for qualitative studies could look something like this:

The purpose of this *phenomenological* [strategy of inquiry] *constructivist qualitative* [philosophical worldview and research approach] study is to understand the *emotional experiences* [central phenomenon or idea] among *adolescent girls* [participants] involved in *sport* [research site].

Writing Exercise

Identify the central phenomenon in the following study aims, and identify which guidelines for qualitative purpose statements have been used and what information is missing:

1. Although a growing presence within sport, elite athlete mothers have minimal presence within sport psychology research, particularly within the context of sociocultural expectations concerning motherhood and sport. The purpose of this study was to extend this understanding by examining how news media constructed elite athlete identities of prominent athlete mothers during the 2012 Olympic year (McGannon, Gonsalves, Schinke, & Busanich, 2016).

2. Medical advances have reduced mortality in youth with congenital heart disease (CHD). Although physical activity is associated with enhanced quality of life, most patients are inactive. By addressing medical and psychological barriers, previous literature has reproduced discourses of individualism that position cardiac youth

Continued

> as personally responsible for physical inactivity. Few sociological investigations have sought to address the influence of social barriers to physical activity, and the insights of caregivers are absent from the literature (Moola, Fusco, & Kirsh, 2011).
> 3. Survivorship is one of the least studied and thus least understood aspects of a breast cancer experience. Defined as a lifelong, dynamic process, survivorship begins when people have completed medical treatment for breast cancer yet live with the memories of their treatment and the possibility of a cancer reoccurrence. The numbers of women surviving breast cancer are growing, which means research on survivorship is imperative. In this article, I examine dragon boat racing for breast cancer survivors. Dragon boat racing has been adapted to a woman-centred, community-based leisure pursuit focused on life after medical treatment for breast cancer (Parry, 2008).

Mixed methods research purpose statement

The mixed methods purpose statement contains information from both the quantitative and the qualitative objectives. The statement should follow all of the guidelines outlined above for the different research approaches and also include a rationale for using a mixed methods approach. The details of mixed methods research will be covered in later chapters. However, one feature that is important to the directives of the purpose statement is whether the study follows a concurrent or sequential design. As the names imply, a **concurrent mixed methods research design** is conducted with the qualitative and quantitative phases going on at the same time, whereas a **sequential mixed methods research design** involves either the quantitative or the qualitative phase conducted first and informing the other phase.

The writing of a purpose statement for a mixed methods study should generally follow the guidelines of both quantitative and qualitative purpose statements. These considerations are identified in Figure 2.5.

A template purpose statement for mixed methods studies could look something like this:

> The purpose of this two-phase *sequential* [or concurrent] mixed methods study was to first explore and identify themes about *reasons for drop-out* [central phenomenon] *among youth involved in competitive sport* using *field observations and semi-structured individual interviews* [strategies of inquiry] with *youth and their parents* [participants]. Based on the themes, the second phase of the study was to *develop and test* a *survey* [strategy of inquiry] that could be used to identify *youth* [participants] most at *risk for drop-out* [dependent variable].

Regardless of the research approach, the purpose statement identifies the reason for conducting the study that has been justified through extensive literature searches, practical experience, and theory. The more information that is included in the purpose statement, the clearer the study intent.

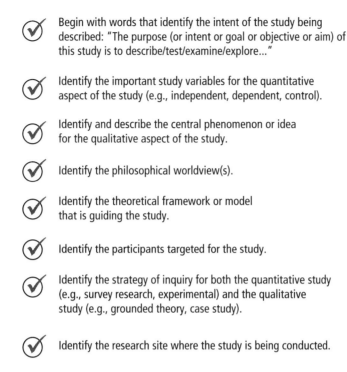

Begin with words that identify the intent of the study being described: "The purpose (or intent or goal or objective or aim) of this study is to describe/test/examine/explore…"

Identify the important study variables for the quantitative aspect of the study (e.g., independent, dependent, control).

Identify and describe the central phenomenon or idea for the qualitative aspect of the study.

Identify the philosophical worldview(s).

Identify the theoretical framework or model that is guiding the study.

Identify the participants targeted for the study.

Identify the strategy of inquiry for both the quantitative study (e.g., survey research, experimental) and the qualitative study (e.g., grounded theory, case study).

Identify the research site where the study is being conducted.

Figure 2.5 General strategies for writing a mixed methods research purpose statement.

Writing Exercise

It is important to get lots of practice in writing a purpose statement. Thinking of the topic and problem you identified earlier during the reading of this chapter, write a purpose statement for each of a quantitative, qualitative, and mixed methods study. Don't forget to label your participants (e.g., who will be included in your study?), identify your independent and dependent variables (e.g., the minimum variables needed for a quantitative research study) as well as other variables if appropriate, the concept or phenomena of interest, and your research approach.

The Research Questions and Hypotheses

Following your statement of the research purpose, it is important to present research hypotheses or questions that emanate from the literature review and theory and further guide the research process. As a general rule, quantitative and mixed methods research approaches use hypotheses, whereas qualitative research approaches use questions. There are no hypotheses in qualitative studies given the nature and purpose of the research approach.

A **hypothesis** is a prediction that is derived from theory, literature, or speculation about the outcome of a study. The **research hypothesis** (also called the alternative hypothesis) can be a statement about what treatment group might have higher scores (e.g., it is hypothesized that men who are in the yoga intervention will have better mental health scores compared to men in the control condition; it is expected that individuals who are in the drug condition will perform better compared to individuals in the placebo, or no drug, condition) or statements about the strength or direction of a relationship (e.g., it is expected that there will be a significant negative correlation between alcohol consumption and sport performance; it is expected that the relationship between number of training hours and sleep will be positive among varsity athletes). Research studies would be conducted to test the hypothesis. The results of the study would then either refute or support the research hypothesis.

The **null hypothesis** states that the independent and dependent variables are not related (e.g., there will be no significant correlation between alcohol consumption and sport performance) or that there are no significant differences between groups (e.g., men who are in the yoga intervention and men in the control condition will have similar mental health scores; individuals who are in the drug condition will perform equally to those in the placebo condition). The null hypothesis is the basis for all statistical analyses that will be done to examine the purpose statement and research questions. There will be much more on null hypothesis testing in later chapters.

Research Highlight

Sabiston et al. (2009) conducted a qualitative study to explore the experiences of physical activity motivation and change in a group of overweight women involved in a dragon boating intervention. The central research question could be described as "What does dragon boating mean to women who are inactive and overweight?" whereas sub-questions were directed at factors related to experiences of dragon boating, such as "What are the reasons that women get involved in dragon boating?" "What are the women's barriers to physical activity?" and "How do the women describe their social support for physical activity?" These sub-questions were part of the researchers' interview guide, and led to varied responses from the women in the study. The researchers reported that groups of women shared similar experiences in dragon boating. Specifically, based on the interview data collected throughout the intervention, women were identified as those who: (a) consistently struggled with negative self-perceptions and body image; (b) experienced positive self-perceptions; and (c) developed more positive self-perceptions and body images throughout the program. Across these profiles, there were distinct changes in the physical self, social support, and main motivational outcome following participation in the dragon boat program.

Further Reading

Sabiston C. M., McDonough M. H., Sedgwick W. A., & Crocker P. R. E. (2009). Muscle gains and emotional strains: Conflicting experiences of change among overweight women participating in an exercise intervention program. *Qualitative Health Research, 19,* 466–80. doi:10.1177/1049732309332782

For qualitative studies, a **research question** is a broad inquiry statement about the central phenomenon. The research question is really the question that can be asked at the broadest level of a study and represents a question that gets at the complex set of factors that are relevant to the central phenomenon. Generally, researchers should typically ask one or two central research questions, each of which can then be followed up with a few sub-questions. The sub-questions should be more focused than the general question and together should provide an overview of the questions needing answered heading into the study.

In a mixed methods study, the elements of research hypotheses and research questions are combined. Researchers could write separate quantitative hypotheses and qualitative research questions, and attempts should be made to link the study approaches with a mixed methods statement. Alternatively, researchers could choose to write questions that reflect the content and procedures of sequential or concurrent mixed methods rather than combining quantitative research hypothesis and qualitative research questions. This latter approach would enhance the importance of connecting the different phases of the study (Creswell, 2014).

Writing Exercise

Using the topic and purpose statements that you have drafted throughout this chapter, write:

1. A quantitative research hypothesis and null hypothesis
2. A qualitative central research question and three to five sub-questions
3. A mixed methods research question

Case Study

Veronique is a 14-year-old girl starting high school next year. Veronique is a healthy young girl with a very supportive network of family and friends; however, she is experiencing some concerns around her appearance. Veronique began to experience this discomfort when she noticed rapid changes in her body including the development of breasts, hips, some weight gain, and her period. She is extremely anxious about starting high school, as she is feeling very uncomfortable in her new body and is worried that she will be negatively evaluated by others and maybe even teased about her development. Veronique is worried that she is much larger than her peers and the women she sees in the media. One of Veronique's best friends, Daria, recently expressed to Veronique that she is experiencing similar concerns. In an attempt to reduce her concerns, Daria downloaded the most popular social media applications (apps) on her phone, including a photo-based app that allowed her to Photoshop her images, making her look thinner, eliminating her acne, and enlarging her breasts. Daria believes that these photographs are making her feel better

Continued

about herself; thus, she takes several selfies a day and posts them on numerous social media platforms. Daria encourages Veronique to download the app and to take selfies herself, but Veronique is skeptical about this suggestion.

Discussion Questions

1. Based on your new knowledge of research designs, how would you study the selfie phenomenon?
2. How would you formulate your research question(s) to examine the selfie phenomenon?
3. Identify your hypotheses.
4. What research methods would you use to measure the number of selfies taken per day?
5. What methods would you use to examine the *type* (e.g., was Photoshop used or not?) of selfies taken per day?
6. What sample would you target to better understand the selfie phenomenon?
7. Are there other variables (e.g., control, moderator) that should be considered?
8. If the number of selfies taken is the independent variable, what are some dependent variables that the researcher should consider?

Summary

Chapter 2 focused on identifying the research topic and key words used to target the topic of interest. The chapter guided an understanding of how to identify a topic that contributes to the literature and is interesting, and how to conduct a literature review on the topic. Furthermore, a description of the main variables of interest was offered to highlight the distinction between independent and dependent variables as well as moderator, mediator, control, and extraneous variables. Following a description of how to identify the problem and topic, the importance and meaning of a purpose statement was discussed. The methods of writing a clear and concise statement of purpose for quantitative, qualitative, and mixed methods studies were reviewed in the chapter. Research questions and/or hypotheses were discussed as flowing from the purpose statement and distinctions between descriptive, predictive, and explanatory research questions were covered. Finally, this chapter summarized the use of literature searches and methods used to make sense of the potential masses of literature on topics of interest.

Discussion Questions

1. When you begin the research process, people around you will no doubt ask you what you are studying. It is important that your description of your research topic is a direct, short, simple, and quick summary. This is called an "elevator pitch" because you think about how to describe your topic to someone with no knowledge of your area of interest in a short period of time. How would you describe your topic area to a stranger riding in the elevator with you? Give yourself about 30 seconds.

2. Can you identify the key similarities and any differences related to writing a quantitative and qualitative research purpose, questions, and hypothesis(es)?
3. How would you describe some uses for theory in a research study?
4. Why and how is the literature search used in a research study?

Recommended Readings

Baumgartner, T. A., & Hensley, L. D. (2012). *Conducting and reading research in kinesiology* (5th ed.). New York, NY: McGraw-Hill.

Creswell, J. W. (2014). *Research design: Qualitative, quantitative, and mixed methods approaches* (4th ed.). Thousand Oaks, CA: Sage.

Day, R. D., & Gastel, B. (2006). *How to write and publish a scientific paper.* Westport, CT: Greenwood.

Credit

Chapter epigraph reprinted with permission from Dr George Springer.

3 Ethics

Learning Outcomes

By the end of this chapter, you should be able to:

- Discuss reasons why ethical standards are important to the research process in kinesiology.

- Describe core ethical principles and ethical guidelines and how they shape research planning, data generation, data analysis, and knowledge translation.

- Identify unique ethical considerations for engaging in research with Indigenous peoples.

- Describe a process of ethical decision-making as a professional in kinesiology-related disciplines.

- Apply an ethical decision-making process to an ethical dilemma in kinesiology.

Ethical Standards in Research

Engaging in ethical research is perhaps the most important responsibility of researchers. Ethics policies for research involving humans are focused on respecting the rights of study participants and protecting them from harm. Therefore, the terms *ethics* and *respect* are often used interchangeably. Not all people involved in research would know if they have been treated unethically, but most people would know if they have been disrespected. Although research can result in a number of benefits, it often involves risks to participants. As a result, ethics should not be viewed as a single event, but rather as an ongoing process involving various considerations for research planning, data generation, data analysis, and knowledge translation.

Ethics policies in Canada

Research ethics policies have been developed, in part, in response to historical practices of unethical treatment of people in research. Possibly the most internationally recognized examples are the "medical experiments" that were conducted by Nazi researchers during World War II (Annas & Grodin, 1995). Thousands of people were tortured and murdered when subjected to experiments, such as the high-altitude experiments, which apparently were meant to examine the limits of human endurance at extremely high altitudes. People were placed in low-pressure chambers that were intended to represent high altitudes, which subsequently led to severe injuries and death. The unethical experiments conducted by Nazi researchers led to the development of the Nuremberg Code, which is often referred to as the ten commandments of ethical human medical research.

The Tuskegee and Willowbrook experiments also garnered international attention for the unethical treatment of people (Rothman, 1982). The Tuskegee syphilis experiments, which took place in Alabama from 1932 to 1972, examined the effects of untreated syphilis among approximately 400 black men. Although penicillin was identified as a treatment for syphilis during the 1950s, and despite the establishment of the Nuremberg Code in 1947, the Tuskegee experiment continued until an article written in the *Washington Star* alerted Americans and ignited uproar among citizens. Infectious disease was also the focus of the Willowbrook study conducted on Staten Island, New York, where new residents of the Willowbrook institute for people with intellectual impairments were unknowingly and systematically infected with hepatitis viruses. Researchers argued the ethical nature of their protocol by stating that hepatitis was endemic to Willowbrook and that all patients would eventually contract the disease. They argued that purposefully infecting patients with hepatitis would provide opportunities for researchers to monitor the course of the disease, which would lead to less severe complications associated with the disease.

In Canada, there are also examples of the unethical treatment of people in research. For instance, in 1998, researchers from Baylor College of Medicine in Texas conducted a study in Newfoundland and Labrador that included family members who had a greater-than-average risk for a genetic heart defect. Longtin (2004) described how the researchers became known as the "Texas Vampires" because they "bled" participants to collect their DNA samples, and then vanished without ever sharing the results of their study. As well, in the 1940s and 1950s "nutrition research" by Canadian researchers resulted in Indigenous children being denied basic health care and dietary requirements (Mosby, 2013). Particularly concerning is that more than 1000 children in residential schools were given less than half of their daily nutritional requirements and used as the "baseline" against which to test various vitamin supplements.

In an effort to prevent further research atrocities like these and others, as well as to ensure that *all* study participants are respected and protected from harm in future research, various policies have been developed to guide and support the ethical practices of Canadian researchers. Most notable is the second edition of the *Tri-Council Policy Statement: Ethical Conduct for Researchers Involving Humans* (TCPS 2), released in 2010 and updated in 2014. The TCPS 2 is a joint policy of the three federal funding agencies in Canada (i.e., Canadian Institutes of Health Research [CIHR], the Natural Sciences and Engineering Research Council of Canada [NSERC], and the Social Sciences and Humanities Research Council of Canada [SSHRC]). All researchers funded by these agencies, of which there are many from kinesiology in Canada, are required to adhere to the TCPS 2. The policy is informed by three core **principles** that convey the value of human dignity (see Figure 3.1):

1. Respect for Persons: *Respect for Persons recognizes the intrinsic value of human beings and the respect and consideration that they are due.*
2. Concern for Welfare: *The welfare of a person is the quality of that person's experience of life in all its aspects.*
3. Justice: *Justice refers to the obligation to treat people fairly and equitably.*

(Canadian Institutes of Health Research, Natural Sciences and Engineering Research Council of Canada, and Social Sciences and Humanities Research Council of Canada, 2014)

These three core principles are interdependent, and all research studies will differ in terms of how the principles are applied. For instance, *Respect for Persons* incorporates the obligation to respect the autonomy of individuals who are directly involved in research as participants (e.g., face-to-face interviews), as well as those whose data (e.g., biological materials) are being used in research. Given that individuals can participate in research in a variety of ways, the application of the *Respect for Persons* principle will depend on the context of the research. The research context is also important to consider when applying the *Concern for Welfare* principle. It refers to the manner in which researchers work to protect the welfare of participants by ensuring that the benefits of participation outweigh the risks. Again, depending on the specifics of the study (e.g., there might be physical pain because of certain experimental procedures or emotional discomfort as a result of talking about sensitive information in interviews), researchers must account

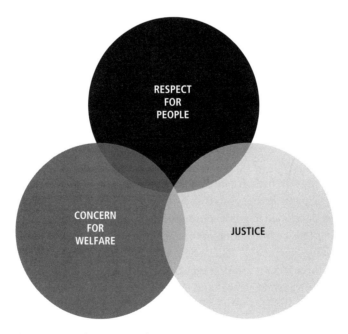

Figure 3.1 The three core ethics principles.

for a number of considerations to ensure that *Concern for Welfare* is appropriately applied. Lastly, in terms of *Justice*, it is important to note that there are certain groups (e.g., children, prisoners, elderly) that have, at times, been treated inequitably and unfairly in research. As such, if researchers are engaging such groups in their research, it might be necessary to provide special attention and additional considerations when working to honour the principle of *Justice* in their research.

By applying the three core principles, researchers can strive to achieve two important ethical standards. Specifically, (a) researchers need to provide the necessary protection of participants and (b) research needs to result in shared benefits, whereby the research meets the needs and priorities of both researchers *and* participants. The three core principles serve as a foundation for the various ethical **guidelines** outlined in the TCPS 2, some of which are described below. The wide breadth of guidelines outlined in the TCPS 2 might be challenging to remember, but they can easily be accessed to inform research practices (for further information see http://www.pre.ethics.gc.ca/pdf/eng/tcps2-2014/TCPS_2_FINAL_Web.pdf). It is realistic to expect that all those who engage in research with humans should be familiar with the three core principles and to recognize that they serve as a foundation to guide all research processes.

Most Canadian universities have adopted the guidelines of the TCPS 2 and are guided by the same three core principles. In addition to the TCPS 2, all Canadian universities that govern research have their own research ethics boards (REBs) and human research ethics policies. All researchers, including undergraduate students and graduate students conducting research, are required to adhere to the ethics policies that have been developed by their respective universities. As well, when researchers are engaging in biological or medical research, they will also likely need to apply for biohazards approval from their university. By engaging in a biohazards review process, and obtaining biohazards approval, researchers can demonstrate that they are committed to ensuring that their research adheres to established safety guidelines and regulations. A **biohazard** is any organism, or its derivative, that could negatively influence another organism. Researchers in kinesiology commonly work with biohazards, including blood, sweat, and saliva; researchers must consider how such biohazards are appropriately handled, stored, and disposed. Research lead by Neary, Malbon, and McKenzie (2002) at the University of New Brunswick included various types of biohazards. They examined the relationship among cortisol measured in saliva, serum, overnight urine, and 24-hour urine samples to determine which is most appropriate for monitoring recovery from the physiological stress caused by exercise training. Findings from their research suggest that salivary sampling should be used as the method of choice because of the ease of repeated sampling and its non-invasive nature. The findings may have important implications for studying physiological stress caused by exercise training, but perhaps more relevant to this chapter and its focus on ethics, the researchers described how such biohazards were collected and stored (e.g., blood samples frozen at −80°C).

Depending on where the research is taking place, researchers may also be required to adhere to organization- or community-specific ethics policies. For instance, hospital-based research requires medical institution ethical clearance. Also, those who want to conduct research in the Northwest Territories require a Scientific Research Licence that can be obtained through the Aurora Research Institute. As part of this licence, researchers need to demonstrate that they will adhere to specific ethical principles for engaging in research in the north (e.g., researchers should become familiar with traditions and cultures of local communities). Ethics guidelines for northern research can be found in various documents including Ethical Principles for the Conduct of Research in the North that was developed by the Association of Canadian Universities for Northern Studies (for further information see http://acuns.ca).

It is critical to remember that there is no single ethics policy that can provide answers to all ethical issues that may arise in the research process. As well, ethics policies or guidelines are indeed just that, *guidelines*. It is researchers' responsibility to apply guidelines to their research. The following examples from the TCPS 2 are not an exhaustive list but a sample of guidelines that can be drawn upon during research planning, data generation, data analysis, and knowledge translation. More specifically, guidelines discussed below include conflicts of interest, process of consent, and privacy and confidentiality.

Conflicts of interest

Identifying a study question and purpose is one of the first phases of the research process, and researchers need to consider if there are any conflicts of interest that could arise from their proposed question and purpose. A conflict of interest might occur when the study places researchers, or the university they are associated with, in a conflict with their duties related to research, personal, or institutional interests. For instance, a conflict of interest could arise from researchers' economic investments (e.g., a researcher is a shareholder in a specific fitness centre that wants to fund the study) or interpersonal relationships (e.g., a researcher's sister is the coach of a team from which the data collection needs to occur). When faced with potential conflicts of interest, researchers can draw upon Article 7.4 of the TCPS 2, which states:

> Researchers shall disclose in research proposals they submit to the REB any real, potential, or perceived individual conflicts of interest, as well as any institutional conflicts of interest of which they are aware that may have an impact on their research. Upon discussion with the researcher, the REB shall determine the appropriate steps to manage the conflicts of interest.

It is best to try to avoid research that could present a conflict of interest. However, despite good intentions, conflicts might still arise. Consider the Nancy Olivieri case (Thompson, Baird, & Downie, 2001):

> In 1996 Nancy Olivieri, a researcher with the University of Toronto and Hospital for Sick Children, was engaging in clinical trials to test a drug that could treat people with blood disorders. Through her research she found evidence of unexpected medical risks associated with the drug, including the progression of liver fibrosis. She informed her governing REB as well as the pharmaceutical company that made the drugs and that supported the trials. The REB instructed her to inform participants about her concerns, but the pharmaceutical company indicated that

Dr Olivieri had signed a confidentiality agreement and informing the participants about concerns would violate the agreement. In spite of the agreement, Dr Olivieri informed the participants about her concerns, and the drug company terminated the trials.

This case led to ongoing legal battles between the researcher, the university, and the pharmaceutical company.

Although many ethical issues are relevant to the Dr Olivieri case, Somerville (2002) highlights a number of interests that could create potential conflicts of interest. First, there were the interests of the participants in that they had the right to know the risks associated with their participation so they could provide ongoing informed consent (the importance of the *process of consent* is discussed in more detail below). Second, Dr Olivieri had the responsibility to inform participants of risks because of her commitment to the core principle *concern for welfare*. Third, the pharmaceutical company had interests in protecting its drug. Fourth, the REB had the right to know of the study's risks and to respond to such risks. Fifth, the general public had, and continues to have, interests in the ethical integrity of research. But the most encompassing potential conflict of interest was perhaps with the university who had interests in (a) protecting the academic freedom (the freedom to pursue research and communicate the findings without restriction) of Dr Olivieri, (b) ensuring her research was conducted ethically, and (c) sustaining opportunities for funding because the pharmaceutical company was potentially going to give the university over $90 million for a new research facility (Sommerville, 2002). This complicated case demonstrates the ethical challenges that can occur with respect to conflicts of interest. There are no ethics policies that can provide specific answers with respect to how to proceed when such conflicts arise, but the TCPS 2 provides guidelines (e.g., Article 7.4 noted above) for how researchers should proceed when there is a possibility for such conflict.

Process of consent

Researchers must ensure participants' free, informed, and ongoing consent throughout the research process. With respect to the need for free or voluntary consent, Article 3.1 of the TCPS 2 states:

(a) Consent shall be voluntary, (b) Consent can be withdrawn at any time, (c) If a participant withdraws consent, the participant can also request the withdrawal of their data or human biological materials.

At first glance, it may seem relatively easy to apply this ethical guideline. However, there are various influences that could compromise the extent to which participation is free or voluntary, including offering participants incentives (e.g., money or gift cards) for their participation. The TCPS 2 neither discourages nor promotes the use of incentives, rather it stipulates that incentives should not be so large that participants subsequently disregard the risks associated with the study.

Case Study

Dr Strong is testing a new muscle-enhancing drug that could be used to treat people with muscular dystrophy (MD). For the clinical trial experimental group, she is seeking participants who have MD and, for the control group, those who do not have MD. The two-month drug trial could lead to a medical "break through" for those living with MD, but the drugs may also have negative health side effects (e.g., nausea, fatigue).

Discussion Questions

1. What would be the consequence of offering an incentive of $10 to potential participants? What if the incentive were $1000? What if it were $100,000? Would the amount offered as an incentive change the type of participants likely to volunteer for the study?
2. What if the risks of the study were even greater? Would the amount of incentive offered be of even more consequence?
3. Considering the TCPS 2 guidelines regarding the process of consent and incentives, what do you think would be an appropriate incentive amount to offer participants in this study? Justify your answer.

Note: Ethics policies can provide researchers with a resource to guide the answers to their questions, but ultimately it is up to the judgment of the researchers, pending approval from ethics boards, to decide on what is or is not appropriate in terms of incentives.

Additional ethical considerations related to consent might arise when the intended participants of the study lack the capacity to understand their rights and potential consequences of their participation. In particular, when the intended research participants are children or those living with permanent intellectual impairment, consent from authorized third parties (e.g., parents or guardians) must be sought and maintained. Participant assent, or their willingness to participate, might also be required. As stated in Article 3.10 of the TCPS 2:

> Where an authorized third party has consented on behalf of an individual who lacks legal capacity, but that person has some ability to understand the significance of the research, the researcher shall ascertain the wishes of that individual with respect to participation. Prospective participants' dissent will preclude their participation.

When designing a study, researchers need to be aware of the extra ethical considerations that are required when involving those who may lack the capacity to provide free, informed, and ongoing (i.e., throughout the research process) consent.

Although free and informed consent is generally required in research, there are some research questions that necessitate alterations to consent requirements. Partial disclosure or deception might be necessary in kinesiology research that seeks to understand how people respond or behave in certain situations. Alterations to the requirement for consent might be possible if various conditions, as outlined in Article 3.7A of the TCPS 2, can be demonstrated.

For example, researchers must be able to demonstrate that the study does not involve more than minimal risk to participants and that the welfare of participants is not adversely affected because of the alteration of consent. As well, researchers must demonstrate that partial disclosure or deception is *necessary* to answer the research questions and to conduct the study. If partial disclosure or deception is necessary, it is typical for a debriefing or full disclosure to be provided to participants at the conclusion of the study. Janes and colleagues (2016) from Memorial University of Newfoundland examined the effect of stretching knowledge or deception on successive force output following static stretching. Their research involved two groups of male participants, a biased group and a deception group. The biased group included participants that were familiar with the static stretching literature and the potential impairments on subsequent force production, and the deception group included individuals who were not aware of the static stretching literature and were falsely informed (i.e., deceived) that static stretching would increase subsequent force production. The bias or deception effects that were noted in their study were generally small, suggesting that there is no knowledge or deception advantage to static stretching. This research example demonstrates how deception is sometimes necessary in kinesiology-related research. Although participants in the deception group were falsely informed about static stretching, upon completion of the study the participants were debriefed and informed of the general findings of the existing static stretching literature. This additional step is important, because debriefing and informing participants after a study are an important part of the ethical process when using deception.

Privacy and confidentiality

Privacy and *confidentiality* are two terms that are often used in our day-to-day discourse, and they are particularly meaningful terms when referring to research ethics. A person's **privacy** refers to her or his right to be free from intrusion by others, and throughout all phases of the research process researchers must consider how they will work to protect the privacy of participants. The ethical duty of **confidentiality** refers to researchers' obligation to safeguard entrusted information. Taken together within a research context, respect for *privacy* requires that researchers treat participants' personal information in a *confidential* manner. The ethical duty of confidentiality has been outlined in Article 5.1 of the TCPS 2:

> Researchers shall safeguard information entrusted to them and not misuse or wrongfully disclose it. Institutions shall support their researchers in maintaining promises of confidentiality.

During the design of the study, researchers should outline the strategies that will be used to safeguard personal information. For example, participants might be given identifiers, such as a participant code (e.g., number) or pseudonym (e.g., false name) at the onset of the study to protect their privacy. To further safeguard information, when data are being generated and collected, paper copies of such information should be stored in a locked location. Paper documents should be shredded when they are no longer needed. Electronic files should be password protected on devices that are also stored in a locked location.

There are limits on the extent to which privacy can be guaranteed, and it is the researchers' responsibility to clearly articulate the strategies that will be taken to support their duty of confidentiality. For example, when data are generated in a focus group (e.g., multiple participants share their insights in a group setting), researchers cannot control the actions of other participants or the possibility that a participant might be recognized by or known to another participant. Similarly, an ethical challenge regarding confidentiality could arise if some participants in a qualitative study want to use pseudonyms and others want to forgo the use of pseudonyms because they would like to be recognized for the knowledge (e.g., direct quotes) that they have contributed to a study. As part of the research planning, researchers need to prepare for the various ethical challenges regarding privacy and confidentiality that could arise within their study.

Research with Indigenous Peoples

When describing research ethics within a Canadian context, it is critical to explore the unique ethical considerations for engaging in research with Indigenous peoples. Many Indigenous peoples in Canada, and Indigenous peoples globally, are distrustful of research since it has been at the root of colonialist practices that have resulted in exploitation. In addition to the "nutrition research" described earlier in this chapter, an early 1980s arthritis research study involved the collection of blood samples from over 800 people from the Nuu-chah-nulth First Nations in British Columbia. Participants consented to participate in scientific research focused on arthritis, only to find out that their blood samples were subsequently used for other research purposes, including the isolation of mitochondrial DNA for determining ancestry (Arbour & Cook, 2006). Given that research is inextricably linked to colonialism, it is not surprising that research "is probably one of the dirtiest words in the indigenous world's vocabulary" (Smith, 2012, p. 1).

When engaging in research with Indigenous peoples, there is no single "best" ethics policy to guide researchers. However, as noted below, there are certain policies that are commonly used by those engaging in research with Indigenous peoples. In addition, Indigenous communities might have their own specific ethics policies to guide research conducted with members of their community, and it is researchers' responsibility to adhere to such policies. In terms of federal policies, chapter nine in the TCPS 2 is one of the most recently developed ethics policies for engaging in research with Indigenous peoples. As previously stated, most Canadian universities have adopted the guidelines of the TCPS 2; therefore, it is not surprising that this policy is a leading guiding document for research involving Indigenous peoples.

Chapter nine of the TCPS 2 describes how the core principles of *Respect for Persons*, *Concern for Welfare*, and *Justice* are applied to research with Indigenous peoples. Justice refers to treating people equitably and fairly. When applying this principle to research with Indigenous peoples, justice can be compromised when there is a real (or perceived) power imbalance between the researcher and participants. It is essential that researchers acknowledge the historical practices that might impact justice in their current studies. In addition to the core principles, there are also specific ethical considerations described in the chapter. For example, the requirement of community engagement with Indigenous peoples is necessary under certain conditions, including when research is conducted on First Nations, Métis, or Inuit lands or when Indigenous identity is required to participate in a study.

Respect for community customs and codes of practice is also necessary when engaging in research with Indigenous peoples. There may be instances whereby the customs of a community do not allow for the study of cultural ceremonies, and it is the researcher's responsibility to become informed about, and adhere to, such codes of practice. The principles outlined in chapter nine of the TPCS 2 serve to support the development of ethical research processes for engaging in research with Indigenous peoples in Canada, and they may also be useful when engaging in research with Indigenous peoples in other countries.

In addition to adhering to a specific ethics policy (e.g., TCPS 2) when engaging in research with Indigenous peoples, researchers should also consider incorporating the OCAP (ownership, control, access, and possession) principles into their work. Released by the National Aboriginal Health Organization in 2005, the OCAP principles were developed with a focus on First Nations peoples but are relevant to research involving all Indigenous peoples in Canada, as well as many Indigenous peoples globally. The *ownership* principle acknowledges the relationship between a First Nations community and its cultural information or data. This principle states that any information collected from First Nations peoples is owned by the community. The *control* principle outlines how First Nations peoples and their respective communities have the right to control all aspects of research (e.g., generation of research questions, data management) that impact them. First Nations peoples also have the right to

Research Highlight

Community engagement and respect for community customs were two ethical considerations exemplified in a photovoice study by researchers and Indigenous community partners at the University of Alberta (i.e., McHugh, Coppola, & Sinclair, 2013). Their study explored the meanings of sport to urban Indigenous youth, and the researchers engaged Indigenous community partners throughout the entire research process. For example, community consultations were held in order to generate a relevant and respectful research question for urban Indigenous youth, and an Indigenous community partner played a crucial role in supporting data generation (e.g., facilitating sharing circles), data analysis, and interpretation of findings. In addition, in an effort to ensure the respect for community customs, the Indigenous partner who facilitated the sharing circles was offered a package of tobacco as a way to acknowledge and support cultural tradition. Furthermore, to thank participants, and to respect community customs, a feast of meats, cheeses, fruits, and vegetables were offered to all research participants during the sharing circles. This example of a research project with an Indigenous community demonstrates how ethical considerations outlined in the TCPS 2 (i.e., community engagement, respect for community customs) were incorporated into a research study.

Further Reading

McHugh, T.-L. F., Coppola, A. M., & Sinclair, S. (2013). An exploration of the meanings of sport to urban Aboriginal youth: A photovoice approach. *Qualitative Research in Sport, Exercise and Health, 5*, 291–311. doi:10.1080/2159676X.2013.819375

Professional Highlight

Dr Lucie Lévesque, Professor, School of Kinesiology and Health Studies, Queens University

··

Profile: Dr Lévesque's research is focused on enhancing the accessibility of physical activity opportunities for youth, and more specifically youth within Indigenous communities, to eliminate health disparities related to physical inactivity. Her work emphasizes the use of participatory and community-based research approaches, particularly when working with Indigenous peoples in Canada. Dr Lévesque is one of the researchers involved in the long-standing Kahnawake Schools Diabetes Prevention Program (KSDPP), which serves as a framework for researchers and community partners interested in using community-based and participatory research approaches to address health. The KSDPP is focused on decreasing the incidence of type II diabetes in the community of Kahnawake by implementing physical activity and healthy eating initiatives. Although her program of research is primarily Canadian-based, she also collaborates with Mexican researchers and students to support their work focused on obesity prevention and physical activity promotion.

Further Readings

Lévesque, L., Guilbault, G., Delormier, T., & Potvin, L. (2005). Unpacking the black box: A deconstruction of the programming approach and physical activity interventions implemented in the Kahnawake Schools Diabetes Prevention Project. *Health Promotion Practice, 6,* 64–71. doi:10.1177/1524839903260156

Paradis, G., Lévesque, L., Macaulay, A. C., Cargo, M., McComber, A., Kirby, R., . . . Potvin, L. (2005). Impact of a diabetes prevention program on body size, physical activity, and diet among Kanien'kehá:ka (Mohawk) children 6 to 11 years old: 8-year results from the Kahnawake Schools Diabetes Prevention Project. *Pediatrics, 115,* 333–39. doi:10.1542/peds.2004-0745

---

access any information about themselves regardless of where the information is held, and this right is reflected in the principle of *access*. The principle of *possession* refers to the rights of First Nations peoples to physically possess all and any research data that are collected. The OCAP principles are foundational to many research programs involving Indigenous peoples in Canada, and therefore the principles are reflected in most ethics policies (e.g., TCPS 2). By applying the OCAP principles, it may be possible to support ethical research processes with Indigenous peoples.

Animal Research Ethics

The focus of this chapter has been on engaging in ethical research with humans. However, in an ethics chapter focused on kinesiology research, we would be remiss not to mention animal research ethics. Animal models are used extensively in kinesiology research to provide unique insight into biological structure and function, and to understand how the body functions in states of both health and disease. For example, studies using canines and rats have investigated the mechanisms underlying effects of exercise training and aging on the cardiovascular system. The impacts of exercise on gut microbiota have also been examined through research that has included the use of mice. For instance, research led by Jennifer Lambert from the University of Calgary examined if exercise influences the gut microbial profile in normal and diabetic mice (Lambert et al., 2015). The authors highlighted that the most interesting finding was the observed interaction between exercise and diabetic state on specific bacteria (i.e., *Bifidobacterium* spp.), where exercise was associated with lower abundance in diabetic mice and greater abundance in nondiabetic mice. This example is particularly relevant to a chapter on ethics because it demonstrates how animal models can be used in kinesiology research. Importantly, Lambert et al. (2015) stated that ethical approval was granted by the University of Calgary Animal Care Committee, and they described how their research conforms to the Canadian Council for Animal Care's guidelines. Similar to national level policies (e.g., TCPS 2) that support the ethical practices of research involving humans, the Canadian Council on Animal Care (CCAC) has developed nationally and internationally recognized policy statements for the experimental care and use of animals in research. These various policy statements identify the necessary requirements and ground rules for research conducted within Canadian universities. Embedded within the various policy statements identified by the CCAC is the Three Rs tenet:

1. *"Replace:* Avoid or replace the use of animals wherever possible."
2. *"Reduce:* Employ strategies that will result in fewer animals being used and which are consistent with sound experimental design."
3. *"Refine:* Modify husbandry or experimental procedures to minimize pain and stress."

Canadian Council on Animal Care (2015, p. 4)

The Three Rs tenet is recognized internationally and guides Canadian researchers who use animals for research purposes. It is the responsibility of researchers to ensure that animals are only used when best efforts to identify an alternative have been explored. When animals are indeed included in research, it is imperative to employ humane methods and to use the smallest number of animals necessary to obtain valid information.

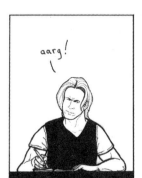 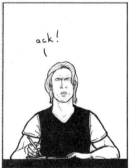 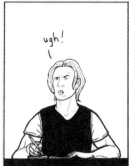 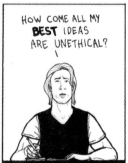

Ethical Decision-Making

Ethics policies and considerations are important for all individuals working with humans (and/or animals), regardless of involvement in research activities. For example, a kinesiologist working with a client to improve fitness needs to be aware of ethical situations that can arise as much as a researcher collecting data on a group of athletes. In order to abide by the ethics standards of practice, professionals need to have an effective *ethical decision-making process*.

While ethical decisions can cause a great deal of stress for professionals, as well as those impacted by the decisions they make, sometimes the most appropriate ethical choice is fairly clear. For example, if you were a researcher interviewing children about their motor coordination skills and learned that one of them was in need of protection from harm, breaching confidentiality is the clear ethical (and lawful) choice. However, having an effective ethical decision-making process is important in *all* situations, because it can help minimize the damage (and maximize benefit) to the community, the profession, and a professional's career that can result from actions taken. As another example, let's say that you were conducting a qualitative study and collecting interview data on body image in adolescent females and there was a consistent message in the interviews that at a particular school the physical education teacher was offering negative body comments and inappropriate commentary/dialogue specific to girls' bodies. An advisable action plan would likely include speaking to a counsellor at the school about the situation. Doing so would likely cause stress for you as a researcher, because you would be keenly aware that it could put another professional's career at risk. Alternatively, not disclosing in this same situation would violate your ethical obligation as a researcher to act in the best interest of the young women in the study. In other words, ethical situations are often very difficult to navigate through.

Some of the most challenging situations professionals face are when there is no clearly correct ethical choice, as is the case in an **ethical dilemma**. An ethical dilemma is a situation that requires ethical action, but the professional is required to perform *two or more mutually exclusive actions* (Welfel, 2012). This means that a professional is required to do two (or more) things . . . but if she or he does one thing, she or he cannot do the other.

Consider the following:

> You are a kinesiologist who has worked with an international level athlete for the past five years. She is at Canadian Olympic trials and suffers an injury, and, as a result, she is now at risk of missing the afternoon final. Because of the established relationship she has with you (and her confidence in your skills), she calls you unexpectedly for help. You would like to meet with her immediately in order to give her the best chance possible to make the Olympic team. However, you have another appointment with a research participant who is coming to meet you for the first time in 15 minutes for an important study you are conducting, and you have no way to contact him if you miss his appointment.

The above scenario would likely present an ethical dilemma for you as a kinesiologist. You would likely want to help the athlete to qualify for the Olympics, which in addition to giving her a best chance at success would also prevent potential harm to your relationship with her (e.g., if you didn't help her, she might think you didn't care). However, as a researcher you have a professional and ethical responsibility to uphold promises made and professional obligations to study participants. This can be especially important when meeting someone for the first time, because it might be her or his first experience with research and your profession. A missed appointment might thereby put your own integrity and the credibility of the research profession at risk.

In situations like the one presented above it is particularly important to have a good ethical decision-making process to refer to. And despite the best attempt to make an ethically defensible decision in an ethical dilemma, there is sometimes no clearly "right" ethical choice to make. As a result, professionals can experience what has been termed **ethical residue** following the decision; essentially meaning that they will wonder if the correct choice was made. However, fear of making wrong decisions does not absolve professionals from making choices in ethical dilemmas, because the choice not to act is itself an ethical decision.

Given the complexity of ethical decision-making, it is probably no surprise that there is no one "right" way to make an ethically defensible decision and that there are many different ethical decision-making models. The steps presented in Figure 3.2 represent *one option* for an ethical decision-making process that professionals could follow, which includes a number of steps common to many ethical decision-making models (e.g., the ethical decision-making process outlined in the *Canadian Code of Ethics for Psychologists*, which was developed by the Canadian Psychological Association in 2000).

We can use the following example to highlight various steps in the model, and to describe how the model could be applied by a professional:

> You are a well-known and respected certified personal trainer in Regina, Saskatchewan. Ahmed, a hockey player with a professional team in Toronto, Ontario, hears that you work with a number of athletes and that you developed a new type of exercise training program shown to be effective in your research. He ends up working with you to prepare him for his professional season. He goes on to win player of the year and buys you a $1000 gift certificate as a "thank you gift."

1 Develop ethical sensitivity	2 Consult code of ethics	3 Search ethics literature
4 Develop self-awareness	5 Apply ethical principles	6 Develop alternative courses of action
7 Consult with colleagues	8 Take action	9 Reflect upon the results of your actions

Figure 3.2 An ethical decision-making process for professionals.

Prior to presenting each step in the decision-making model, you are encouraged to complete the following Writing Exercise to gain insight into some of your initial responses related to the case study.

Writing Exercise

Write down your answers to the following questions, which would be important to reflect upon if you were the personal trainer who was offered a thank you gift such as the one described in the scenario above:

1. What ethical issues are relevant in this case study (if any)?
2. What actions would you take if you were faced with this scenario as a professional?

Note: Throughout the remainder of this section on ethical decision-making, tips and strategies as to how you would go about answering these questions are provided. However, reflecting on your answers in advance of this discussion will allow you a chance to critique the strengths and weaknesses to your own approach.

Step 1: Develop ethical sensitivity

The first step to effective ethical decision-making in any situation is being sensitive to ethical issues (Malloy, Ross, & Zakus, 2003; Welfel, 2012). Critical to this step is the need to recognize that the choices we make as professionals affect other people. For example, not understanding the ethically relevant issues when conducting research with Indigenous peoples has the potential to do much harm, as history has demonstrated.

As the personal trainer working with the hockey player in the scenario presented above, you would want to carefully consider who would be affected by a decision to accept or not accept the $1000 gift certificate. Because the gift has a monetary value, the most obvious people affected would be you and your client; however, your decision could also impact the expectations of other clients, the financial well-being of your and/or your client's family (especially if similar gifts became common), the reputation of the personal training business you work for, other personal trainers who do research on the effectiveness of exercise training programs, and the integrity of the profession itself. In most cases, ethical issues are so challenging because they have the potential to impact so many others. Recognizing this early in situations is one of the most important facets to being an ethical professional. Also, being proactive can be particularly useful in helping to avoid more challenging ethical situations in the future. For example, explaining confidentiality protections and limitations at your first meeting with a participant or client is one type of discussion often recommended by a profession's code of ethics.

Step 2: Consult code of ethics

A professional code of ethics is designed specifically to offer professionals a guide in their ethical decision-making. As stated by Beauchamp and Childress (2009) in the context of biomedical ethics, "Health care professions specify and enforce obligations for their members, thereby seeking to ensure that persons who enter into relationships with these professionals will find them competent and trustworthy" (p. 7). In other words, a code of ethics helps ensure the credibility of a profession and offers protection for the clients they serve. However, a significant challenge in developing a code of ethics is that it does not (and can not) cover all situations that professionals encounter, and therefore needs to be interpreted, modified, and applied by professionals (Welfel, 2012). Having said this, consulting a profession's code of ethics is an excellent place to start for guidance when considering ethical decisions.

As an example where codes of ethics can be extremely useful, consider a situation in which you are a professional (e.g., personal trainer/physical therapist/coach/mental training consulting/occupational therapist) who has developed a close relationship with one of your clients. Although certainly not your intent in the beginning, you find yourself strongly attracted to your client and would like to begin a romantic, sexual relationship. Recognizing, at minimum, that this is a situation fraught with ethical implications (i.e., Step 1: being ethically sensitive), you decide to consult codes of ethics for guidance. It might be surprising to learn that not all codes of ethics offer precisely the same guidance. Even within one profession, there can be some variation in codes of ethics. For example, while the Canadian Psychological Association (CPA, 2000) and Canadian Counselling and Psychotherapy Association (CCPA, 2007) agree that sexual intimacy with current clients is unethical, the CCPA is more explicit in stating that a minimum period of three years must pass following termination of the counselling relationship before a professional could even begin to consider entering into such a relationship. The CPA codes of ethics instead states that minimizing the potential for harm requires a "period of time following therapy during which the power relationship reasonably could be expected to influence the client's personal decision making" (Article II.27, p. 18). Contrast this with the Canadian Medical Association (CMA, 2004) code of ethics, which makes no explicit mention of sexual relationships, and instead relies on more general articles like, "Consider first the well-being of the patient" (Article 1, p. 1) and "Do not exploit patients for personal advantage" (Article 12, p. 2).

Returning to our hockey scenario, because it describes a personal trainer working in Saskatchewan, the *Code of Ethics* of the Saskatchewan Kinesiology and Exercise Sciences Association (SKESA, n.d.) is likely the governing code of ethics. Two relevant articles in the SKESA code of ethics are:

- Article One: Professional Integrity and Professional Development. *Members will ensure their professional integrity and judgment is not compromised by motives of profit, and will only enter into contracts and agreements when professional integrity can be maintained.*
- Article Five: Conflict of Interest. *Members shall not exploit any relationship established as a therapist to further their own physical, emotional, financial, political, or business interests at the expense of the best interest of the client. This includes ... securing or accepting significant financial or material benefit for activities which are already awarded by salary. ...*

While these articles do not explicitly offer a solution to the situation described in the hockey scenario, these articles strongly suggest that any decision related to accepting gifts from clients must not jeopardize professional integrity, as well as emphasize the need to prioritize the client's best interests.

Because articles in a profession's code of ethics are often (intentionally) general and might not cover a specific circumstance, a code of ethics in another field might offer additional guidance for professionals. For example, the following section from the Canadian Association for Music Therapy *Code of Ethics* (1999) offers a recommendation in terms of both what decision might be most appropriate in the hockey scenario and how to implement any action taken:

- Section II.40: Ethical Business Practices. *Accept from clients only gifts of minimal monetary value. When offered a gift by a client a music therapist would consider the possible consequences of accepting and refusing the gift ... When refusing a gift, a music therapist would make reasonable attempts to explain the reasons for his/her decision to the client.*

Not only does this section offer insight into whether or not accepting a $1000 gift certificate is likely appropriate, but it also provides guidance on additional factors that need to be considered in the decision that are not evident in the SKESA code of ethics (e.g., how to act on that decision in a respectful way that protects the relationships between professionals and their clients). As such, a promising approach to developing an ethical decision-making process is to gather resources from a variety of professional fields of practice.

Step 3: Search ethics literature

Another source to help with ethical decision-making is ethics texts and journal articles. The ethics literature is vast and covers a wide variety of topics ranging from confidentiality, to boundaries of competence, to harmful dual relationships with clients. In fact, research methods texts typically cover ethics specifically as a first step in offering guidance related to ethical issues specific to research. However, the ethics literature can be especially useful when a profession's code of ethics does not adequately address the specifics of a situation requiring ethical decision-making.

Demonstrating how the ethics literature can be useful within the hockey scenario presented earlier, Welfel (2006) specifically discusses accepting gifts from clients and suggests, " ... the ethics of accepting a gift from a client depends substantially on the circumstances under which it was offered (It also depends on the attitude of and impact on its recipient)" (p. 163). The implication is that accepting and receiving gifts depends a lot on context, suggesting that there is still no simple answer as to whether receiving a $1000 gift certificate would be appropriate or not. The ethics literature can also provide unique perspectives on an issue and fill in gaps not covered in a code of ethics. For example, Zur (2011) states that, "the fact that very expensive gifts are not a financial burden for wealthy clients is not a good enough reason to accept such gifts," which is clearly relevant to our case study given that the client is a professional athlete and likely (although not necessarily) has a relatively high income.

One of our most highly recommended ethics sources is Truscott and Crook's (2013) *Ethics for the Practice of Psychology in Canada*. While their book is framed in the context of clinical and counselling psychology, we feel it has much application for a wide range of professions in kinesiology (because, after all, most professions in kinesiology are helping professions in some way or another). Consider a situation in which you were asked to work with a client from a different culture from yours. Because of an increasing awareness of the importance of both cultural awareness and cultural competence among professionals and within professions, you realize that guidance might be critical to your work. Truscott and Crook offer an entire chapter devoted to providing services across cultures, which includes a number of gems for professionals, such as, "Indeed, commonly practiced professional services may be ineffective and even antagonist to the goals desired by persons who do not share the majority view of what constitutes desirable behaviour and lifestyle" (p. 149). However, this is only one among many valuable sources. And most importantly, the ethics literature can offer new insights, critical advice, and cautionary tales that can help professionals navigate through ethical situations.

Step 4: Develop self-awareness

Knowing the bias you bring to a situation that could impact your decision-making process is another important step in effective ethical decision-making. This step requires substantial self-awareness as a professional, because you would want to identify whether there are any other self-interests that you need to recognize. Relevant to the hockey scenario, if you were financially struggling with your personal training business, how might that impact your decision to accept or reject a $1000 gift certificate from a client? Similarly, what if you were someone who would enjoy the status that might come with having others know that you work with a professional athlete? Being aware of these types of self-interests would need to be considered when trying to make the most defensible ethical decision possible. As another example, understanding the stresses that one experiences when there is pressure to perform under tight deadlines can help someone avoid temptation to engage in forms of academic dishonesty such as plagiarism.

Step 5: Apply ethical principles

Ethical principles help to shape most codes of ethics in kinesiology-related professions. As such, it is important to apply fundamental ethical principles to a situation requiring ethical decision-making (Beauchamp & Childress, 2009; Welfel, 2012). Ethical principles also underlie many ethical standards in research, such as the ones discussed earlier, so it is particularly important to understand ethical principles. Some of the most common ethical principles identified as particularly important to effective ethical decision-making are:

- *Autonomy*: Freedom to make one's own choices and take actions based on one's own personal values and beliefs
- *Nonmaleficence*: Obligation not to inflict harm upon others intentionally
- *Beneficence*: Obligation to act for the benefit of others

- *Justice*: Fair, equitable, and appropriate treatment of others
- *Fidelity*: Fulfilling one's responsibilities of trust
- *Veracity*: Truthfulness

In fact, it is a conflict among ethical principles that makes a situation an ethical dilemma. For example, as a physician, in order to respect an athlete's own choice to play while injured (i.e., an honouring of autonomy), you might be exposing her or him to potential long-term harm that is preventable (i.e., a violation of nonmaleficence). Recent concussion guidelines in sport are an example where athletes' autonomy is sacrificed to protect them from further harm. Within an ethical dilemma, identifying the ethical principles in conflict, as well as the likely actions stemming from honouring each of the principles, can be critical to considering all possible options as a professional. Consider the following as a way to test your knowledge of how to apply ethical principles:

Writing Exercise

You are an occupational therapist who has been working with a client for approximately two months. The client is very committed to your program and has been very open to the various (and often challenging) therapies that you have recommended. However, at your very first session she made it clear that she didn't want anyone to know that she was seeing you as a client, because she was afraid that her boss would fire her if she knew about her impairment (your client told you that she's seen it happen at her current workplace before). One night you are attending a party at a friend's house and, not long after your arrival, your client walks in. You realize that she is the partner of one of your friends. Write down your responses to the following questions:

1. What ethical principles are relevant to the situation?
2. What two ethical principles are in conflict, making it an ethical dilemma for you as the occupational therapist?

Note: Understanding ethical principles and how they conflict is key to understanding ethical dilemmas.

Step 6: Develop alternative courses of action

When deciding on alternative courses of action, professionals will want to clearly detail (as best as possible) the probable costs and benefits of each possible action. At this point, *all* options should be brainstormed, as doing so can lead to unique solutions not previously considered. This step also provides a chance to reflect on who might be affected in the situation (in Step 1) and to identify how each action could influence them. The goal of professionals at this step is to create as extensive a list as possible. In the hockey scenario, the two most obvious potential courses of action are to either accept or not accept a $1000 gift certificate. However, there is a wide range of other potential actions that could be considered, such as using the money to start an athletic scholarship or suggesting a gift of small to no monetary value (among *many* other possibilities).

Step 7: Consult with colleagues

Consultation with trusted colleagues is a useful step in ethical decision-making because it can offer perspectives and options that a professional has not already considered. Trusted colleagues can often provide a more objective lens and help protect a professional against decisions that are closely entwined with personal bias or conflicts of interest. Having others to help researchers navigate through tricky ethical issues is one of the largest potential benefits of research teams. However, even though professionals are also bound to ethical standards of the profession, it is important to still consider other ethical issues in the consultation process. For example, consider how to consult with a colleague about your ethical dilemma in a way that does not disclose the identity of your client. Another good source of external consultation is the ethics boards of professions themselves (e.g., REBs), who can offer much guidance based on their knowledge of ethical issues and experience dealing with cases. Perhaps just as importantly, if you find yourself hesitant to consult with other professionals because of concerns over what they might think about your decision, that in-and-of-itself is a sign that alternative courses of action might need to be considered (Step 6). For example, if you were tentative about admitting to a colleague that you were accepting a $1000 gift certificate from a client, consultation with colleagues would probably be even more important.

Step 8: Take action

Once all of the previous steps have been completed, it is time to implement the chosen action plan. This should include informing the people who are going to be affected by your actions, as well as a commitment to assume responsibility for action(s). Ethical decision-making can be extremely difficult and complex, so it is critical that professionals learn from their experiences and take actions that are most defensible to other professionals. Documenting the ethical decision-making process can help in the defence of actions taken, especially to show an awareness of and commitment to ethical issues. Perhaps one of the best questions to ask yourself is *"Would I act this way in a 'well-lit' room?"* In other words, would you act the same way if *everyone* could hear and see what decisions you made? If not, it might be important to think twice (or three times) . . .

Step 9: Reflect upon the results of your actions

Reflecting upon the results of decisions in ethical situations is recommended in many ethical decision-making models (Cottone & Claus, 2000). As a standard of practice, your actions should be consistent with what someone demonstrating outstanding ethical virtues would characteristically do (Beauchamp & Childress, 2009). Ethical virtues include qualities such as compassion, discernment, trustworthiness, integrity, and conscientiousness and represent the qualities that professionals should be trying to develop in their pursuit of the profession's goals. These ethical virtues should govern *all* ethical decision-making, regardless of whether situations are explicitly covered in a code of ethics. However, ethical virtues are an especially useful standard against which to judge actions in cases that require a greater degree of interpretation of a profession's ethical standards.

Summary

Chapter 3 focused on introducing the necessary and central role of ethical standards within research. Drawing upon university and Tri-Council research ethics policies, Chapter 3 provided an overview of the ethical standards that should be considered for the various processes of research, including the planning, data generation, data analysis, and knowledge translation. Recognizing the unique history and status of Indigenous peoples in Canada, this chapter highlighted ethical considerations for engaging in research with Indigenous peoples. The chapter concluded with the presentation of an ethical decision-making model to guide professionals working in kinesiology-related fields.

Discussion Questions

1. Why are ethics standards important to the research process?
2. What are some guiding principles for engaging in respectful research with Indigenous peoples in Canada?
3. As a researcher, you are interested in studying sport and physical activity experiences of First Nations youth. Based on this research area, what are the OCAP principles that you would need to uphold? How would you apply each of the four principles?
4. What are some examples of common ethical dilemmas kinesiology-related professionals face? Identify the ethical principles in conflict in those ethical dilemmas.
5. You recently completed your undergraduate degree in kinesiology and are looking for a job as a personal trainer at a fitness centre. You go to your first job interview and are asked what you would do if you found out that one of the personal trainers you are working with is charging his clients more than the publicized cost for service, and that he is keeping the extra money for himself (without telling the fitness centre coordinator). You decide the best way to answer the question is to describe the steps you would take to make an ethically defensible decision in the situation. What are four ethical decision-making steps that you think would be particularly important to discuss as part of your answer to the interviewer's question?

Recommended Readings

Beauchamp, T. L., & Childress, J. F. (2009). *Principles of biomedical ethics* (6th ed.). New York: Oxford University Press.

Smith, L. T. (2012). *Decolonizing methodologies: Research and indigenous peoples*. New York, NY: Zed books.

Truscott, D., & Crook, K. H. (2013). *Ethics for the practice of psychology in Canada* (revised and expanded edition). Edmonton, AB: The University of Alberta Press.

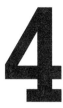

4 Quantitative Study Design

Quantitative Study Design

You have now defined your research topic, assessed the research problem, identified important questions, and stated your hypotheses. Perhaps without even knowing it, you have already informed the *design* of your study. As mentioned in Chapter 2, the purpose statement is the foundation for the design of your study. The design then informs the methods of measurement and assessment as well as the statistical analyses that will be needed to answer the research questions and test the hypotheses. Within a postpositivist philosophical worldview, researchers use quantitative strategies to answer questions that are founded on determining associations, comparing groups, developing and testing measures, and/or theory verification. In this way, quantitative designs can be used to address descriptive, predictive, and explanatory research problems. It is the type of design, and the inherent features of each design, that will distinguish between these research problems.

Before delving into the various study designs that researchers might choose from, there are a few terms that will be used consistently throughout the next three chapters. The most important aspect of conducting a quantitative study is to ensure you are studying something meaningful and valuable, and that you are actually measuring your variables accurately and consistently. Hence, **validity** is a general term used to reflect the degree to which we can have confidence in our conclusions based on the research we conduct. There are a number of types of validity that we will focus on in our discussion of quantitative research, including logical validity, construct validity, internal validity, and external validity. **Logical validity** refers to the quality of researchers' arguments, their application of theory to support the needs for the study, and the appropriate interpretation of results based on the data. For example, if you conducted a research study, we might ask, *"Have you provided convincing justification for all the actions and outputs of your study?"* **Construct validity** refers to whether the measures used by researchers assess/test what they intended to measure. For example, measuring a child's height on a growth chart mounted to the wall would give you a measure of height in centimetres; as such, the growth chart presumably does indeed measure the child's height. **Reliability** is an important part of construct validity and indicates that the measure is consistent or repeatable; if any type of assessment is not consistent, then it cannot be trusted. For example, measuring the same child's height on the growth chart every hour throughout a day should give you a consistent value in centimetres, otherwise it would not be a valid measure of height (i.e., if we got a different result every time we tested a child's height, there's no way it would be an accurate measure other than on only a very few occasions). Logical and construct validity will be discussed in more depth in Chapter 6 when we provide applied examples of how to evaluate quantitative research.

The remaining focus of Chapter 4 is primarily on internal validity and external validity. When we talk about the research design of a quantitative study, we are essentially referring to its overall structure. However, before discussing internal validity and external validity specifically, we will briefly cover the overall structure of the research study (i.e., the design). There are typically five main research elements that researchers use to distinguish the design. All of these elements will be discussed throughout this chapter. The main research elements can be identified with five simple questions:

1. Are the people in the study assigned to groups?
2. How many measurements are being used?
3. What types of measures or observations are being used?
4. Is there an interest in generalizing the findings to other populations or settings?
5. Can you conclude that the findings are based on the manipulation of the independent variable?

The answer to the first question, *"Are the people in your study assigned to groups?"* dictates the main design of your study. If the answer is NO, you have what is called a **non-experimental** study design (i.e., the study of individuals where there is no intervention or manipulation; for example, giving a survey to a group of older adults in a recreation facility focused on balance) or **pre-experimental** study design (i.e., a researcher studies one group of individuals and provides an intervention during the study, but there is no other group to compare to the intervention group; for example, giving a group of master-level volleyball players a mindfulness program during the competitive season). If the answer is YES, the follow-up question is, *"Are the people randomly assigned to these groups?"* A further YES response means that you have a **true experiment** (i.e., a study in which there are two or more groups, and individuals are randomly *assigned* to the control and experimental groups; for example, a researcher might randomly *select* physical education teachers from across Canada, but then would need to also randomly *assign* each teacher to participate in either an online leadership

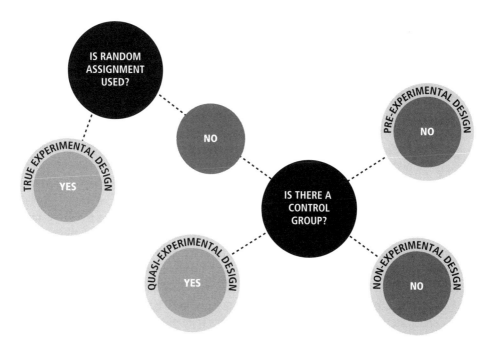

Figure 4.1 A schematic question and answer dialogue to assess research design.

program or no program and examine the effectiveness in teaching). A NO response requires one more question: *"Is there another group or multiple measures in your study?"* A NO here also suggests you have a non-experimental or pre-experimental study design, whereas a YES infers you have a **quasi-experimental** study design (i.e., there are two or more groups but no random assignment to control and experimental groups; for example, studying intact groups like athletes and non-athletes). A simple flow diagram related to these questions and answers is depicted in Figure 4.1. Further details on these types of research designs are presented throughout this chapter.

Experimental research design

The true experimental design may be the most powerful means of generating new knowledge and is the only quantitative design that can be confidently used to identify a cause-and-effect relationship. Typically, a true experiment is conducted in a laboratory within a controlled environment. This level of control helps to ensure the study's **internal validity**, which in essence is the overall quality of research. Internal validity specifically refers to the researcher's ability to claim that any change in an outcome is the result of a treatment or intervention (i.e., manipulation of the independent variable) and not a result of other factors related to the sample, the measures, the techniques, and other possible potential threats that will be discussed later in this chapter.

Within an experimental design, **external validity** (i.e., the potential application of the results of the study, or generalizability) is not as easy to claim given the trade-off needed to ensure internal validity. In other words, having a tightly controlled environment reduces the chances that the same findings would be observed in "real-life" settings where all the factors cannot be controlled. For example, we often hear that the benefits of moderate-to-vigorous exercise are so profound that if we could bottle them into a pill we would solve many health problems. So, let's say we are interested in testing a new drug that offers the same physiological and psychological benefits as running for 20 minutes a day at moderate-to-vigorous intensity. In an experimental study that ensures internal validity, we would need to have participants come to the laboratory and live in a controlled environment for an extended period of time. To strengthen our design further, after randomly assigning our participants to the experimental (e.g., exercise drug) or control (e.g., placebo drug capsule with flour in it) group, we might feed them all the same food, allow them to sleep the same number of hours per night, limit their exercise behaviour, control the ambient temperature in the room, give them the same amount of water, and keep everyone isolated from each other to avoid social contact. Notwithstanding the likelihood that no one would ever volunteer for this study, the findings would probably not be generalizable outside of our laboratory (and hence have low external validity) since we have controlled for many factors that are not easily controlled in the "real world." However, because of high internal validity, we could be confident that it was the drug and not something else that led to our conclusions on the health benefits. It is this type of trade-off between internal and external validity that researchers often face when conducting true experiments.

As might be apparent from the example above, a true experimental design has (a) at least one group that is called the **experimental group** (also called the treatment or intervention group), whereby the members of this group are exposed to some level of manipulation, as well as (b) at least one other group labelled the **control group** or placebo group, in which members are not exposed to the manipulation. The group membership is defined using a method of random assignment. Specifically, each person in the sample has an equal chance of ending up in the experimental and control groups, which helps to ensure that the groups are equivalent prior to the study manipulation. Methods for randomly allocating people to the groups include using chance methods such as flipping a coin or a random number generator. It is also important to note that people can also act as their own controls, in which case each participant is randomly assigned to the treatment/intervention or control (placebo) condition in any order. Dr Kerry Courneya at the University of Alberta has conducted numerous true experimental research studies testing exercise effects on health outcomes among cancer survivors.

The goal of a true experimental study design is to allow researchers to collect data and test their hypothesis with minimum influence or contamination from extraneous variables. As mentioned previously, this type of design can be used to claim a cause-and-effect relationship whereby it is logically determined that one factor has a predictable influence on another factor. To make this claim, **extraneous variables** need to be controlled (i.e., limit the influence). We discussed these variables as **control variables** in Chapter 2, and some common extraneous variables in kinesiology research include characteristics such as sex, age, race, and ethnicity; fitness level; physical activity history; health status; and health behaviours (e.g., tobacco, alcohol, or drug consumption). In our above example of the drug study, we would want to know all of this information about our participants so that we know to whom we can generalize

Professional Highlight

Dr Kerry Courneya, Professor and Canada Research Chair in Physical Activity and Cancer, Faculty of Physical Education and Recreation, University of Alberta

....

Profile: Dr Courneya's research is focused on physical activity and cancer including examining physical activity as a means for primary prevention, as a strategy used to help patients and cancer survivors cope with treatments and recover effectively after treatments, in aiding long-term survivorship outcomes related to quality of life, and examining the role of physical activity in preventing or delaying disease recurrence and optimizing survival. Dr Courneya has conducted hundreds of *experimental, quasi-experimental, and both longitudinal and cross-sectional non-experimental studies* with people diagnosed with cancer; the findings from this work have informed clinical guidelines for physical activity.

Further Readings

Courneya, K. S., Karvinen, K. H., McNeely, M. L., Campbell, K. L., Brar, S., Woolcott, C. G., . . . Friedenreich, C. M. (2012). Predictors of adherence to supervised and unsupervised exercise in the Alberta Physical Activity and Breast Cancer Prevention Trial. *Journal of Physical Activity and Health, 9*, 857–66. doi:10.1186/s12966-014-0085-0

Courneya, K. S., Sellar, C. M., Trinh, L., Forbes, C. C., Stevinson, C., McNeely, M. L., . . . Reiman, T. (2012). A randomized trial of aerobic exercise and sleep quality in lymphoma patients receiving chemotherapy or no treatments. *Cancer Epidemiology, Biomarkers & Prevention, 21*, 887–94. doi:10.1158/1055-9965.EPI-12-0075

Courneya, K. S., Stevinson, C., McNeely, M. L., Sellar, C. M., Friedenreich, C. M., Peddle-McIntyre, C. J., . . . Reiman, T. (2012). Effects of supervised exercise on motivational outcomes and longer term behavior. *Medicine & Science in Sports & Exercise, 44*, 542–9. doi:10.1249/MSS.0b013e3182301e06

our results. We certainly wouldn't want to market our drug to everyone and then find that it doesn't work, or even worse creates some adverse effects in older adults or people with a history of smoking, for example.

Within an experimental study (remember, this means random assignment of participants and inclusion of a control group), there are several specific research designs that can be used. These research designs are identified based on the specific type of research problem and question, as well as the number of measurement or assessment periods. *Any study that is designed with random assignment of participants, a control group, and manipulation of the independent variable is considered a true experiment.* Another common name for these studies is **randomized control trial** or RCT. The two main RCT design methods used in kinesiology research include (a) pre- and post-test designs and (b) post-test only designs.

A **pre- and post-test design** is used to examine change in the dependent variable that can be attributed to the independent variable. In this way, we want to see which group changes more as a result of the manipulation or treatment. The purpose statement for this type of design would be stated something like: The purpose of this experimental study is to examine changes in mood following a yoga, tai chi, or meditation activity. Participants might then complete a self-report survey on mood, be randomly assigned to an intervention group (e.g., yoga group, tai chi group, or meditation group), and subsequently complete the same self-report survey again after the intervention. We could then statistically compare the changes in mood for participants assigned to each group to determine the effects of the various interventions.

An important thing to keep in mind is that having a *pre-test* is not an essential condition of a true experiment. In a **post-test only design**, the independent variable is introduced to the randomly assigned experimental group participants, and then the effects of the "treatment" versus "no treatment" (or manipulation of the independent variable) are tested by looking at whether the groups are different. Our example of the exercise drug study described in this chapter would fit this description because participants are randomly assigned to the drug (experimental) or no-drug (control) group, they are exposed to the treatment for a month, and then tested (for the first time in the case of a post-test only design) to see if the two groups are different on the dependent variable(s) of interest. If the two groups were the same at the start of the study (something random assignment should take care of), then any differences in the groups following the intervention are probably due to our manipulation of the independent variable (which in our example is the exercise drug).

Research Highlight

A pre- and post-test experimental design was used in a study conducted at McGill University, and published in the *Journal of Sport & Exercise Psychology*, looking at whether different types of motivation for exercise were related to a number of performance outcomes (Scarapicchia, Garcia, Andersen, & Sabiston, 2013). In this study, inactive and healthy-weight women were randomly assigned to exercise at a self-selected pace on a treadmill beside another woman who was providing either intrinsic (e.g., "I really enjoy exercising") or extrinsic (e.g., "I am only here for the money") verbal statements. As such, the type of motivational verbal feedback (intrinsic or extrinsic) was the independent variable. The dependent variables that were assessed at pre-test and post-test included heart rate, rating of perceived exertion, time spent in moderate-to-vigorous exercise, and exercise continuance. Findings from the Scarapicchia et al. (2013) study suggested that women who exercised beside another woman providing intrinsic verbal cues, compared to extrinsic cues, had higher heart rate and ratings of perceived exertion (worked harder), spent more time at higher-intensity exercise, and continued to exercise when given the choice to stop. The researchers concluded, "Based on these findings, exercise motivation can be 'contagious' through verbal primes, suggesting that exercising with or around intrinsically motivated individuals may have beneficial outcomes" (p. 563).

Further Reading

Scarapicchia, T., Garcia, E., Andersen, R., & Sabiston, C. M. (2013). The motivational effects of social contagion on exercise participation in young female adults. *Journal of Sport & Exercise Psychology, 35,* 563–75.

Writing Exercise

Many experimental studies around the world are registered with ClinicalTrials.gov, a program that was established to provide information on existing and completed trials for patients, family members, and members of the public. While researchers can use the system to locate other competing or complementary studies going on and the details of these studies, patients can find information on a trial for a new drug or intervention that could help them live longer or improve their quality of life. Also, there are specific journals dedicated to experimental research, such as the journal called *Contemporary Clinical Trials*. Go online and look for an exercise intervention in the database (https://clinicaltrials.gov/ct2/home) or an experimental research journal (for example, visit: http://www.journals.elsevier.com/contemporary-clinical-trials/). Describe the trial using the questions and prompts below:

1. Where is the study being conducted?
2. What is the purpose of the study?
3. Identify the research hypothesis.
4. Identify the independent and dependent variables.
5. What is the experimental design?
6. Describe the participant characteristics.
7. How were the participants randomly assigned to the experimental and control groups?
8. How many groups are there?

Once you have described the study, think about a study you could conduct that would mimic the same design but answer a different research question. Provide answers to the same questions and prompts for your own study.

There are many other derivatives of the true experimental design. For example, many studies involve **between-groups** designs in which separate groups of participants are compared for each of the different conditions in the experimental study. In a simple between-groups design all participants are measured once, which was described earlier as a post-test only study. More complicated designs involve multiple testing sessions (i.e., **repeated measures**) for each participant; these types of designs are sometimes called a **within-subjects** design. In a between-groups design, it is important to randomize participants to conditions. In a within-subjects design, it is important to randomize the order of the conditions. Clearly, there are a number of ways to design a study that follows the guidelines of a true experiment. The key points to remember are that a true experiment includes (a) random assignment of participants, (b) a control group (either the participants themselves who are part of both conditions in a random order or another unique group of participants), and (c) the manipulation of an independent variable (i.e., a treatment).

Quasi-experimental research design

As the name implies, quasi-experimental studies are those that are "sort of" experimental in design. However, the big distinguishing feature from a true experiment is that there is no randomization to groups in a quasi-experimental research design. These studies usually involve

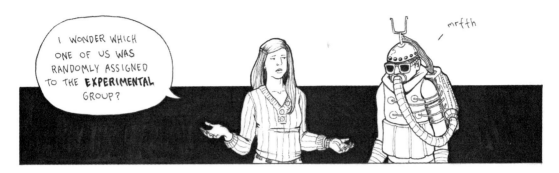

intact groups such as children in classrooms, people with memberships at different fitness centers, or men and women. As such, quasi-experimental studies are low on internal validity because the groups are not likely to be equivalent at the outset of the study. Hence, it is difficult to make claims in a quasi-experiment that any changes seen between the pre- and post-test are due only to the manipulation of the independent variable. However, quasi-experimental studies are often higher on external validity than true experiments because people are studied in a natural environment, making generalizability more feasible.

The basic formula for a quasi-experimental study is that (a) people are studied in real-world settings, (b) an independent variable is introduced or manipulated, and (c) there is a dependent variable (the effect) that is measured.

Pre- and post-test design methods are often used within the quasi-experimental framework when researchers do not have the ability to randomize participants to groups, or they want to use intact groups for convenience. An example of this type of research can be seen in a study published in the *Applied Physiology, Nutrition, and Metabolism* journal, which is the official journal for the Canadian Society for Exercise Physiology and the Canadian Nutrition Society. Supervised by A. William Sheel at the University of British Columbia, Guenette and colleagues (2006) conducted a study testing the effects of respiratory muscle training on maximal inspiratory pressure and time to exhaustion on a cycling task in men and women. The researchers had the participants complete a time-to-exhaustion cycling test at the beginning and end of the study, and they reported that the training had an effect on time to exhaustion. Also, there were no differences in the training effects for men and women. In this example, men and women are intact groups; in addition, there was no random assignment of participants to an experimental group and a control group. One way that this study could be conducted as an experimental design would be to randomly assign both men and women to one of two groups, such that the experimental group would receive the respiratory muscle training and the control group would not. Then the study procedures could follow the same protocol (pre-test measure of time to exhaustion, respiratory muscle training or no training manipulations, post-test measure of time to exhaustion).

Another type of study that is common in kinesiology research is called a **repeated measures** design. In this type of quasi-experimental study approach, there is only an experimental group with multiple levels of the independent variable (and usually only one dependent variable). Participants are essentially their own control group, and, in an ideal design, each participant is exposed to each condition (i.e., think "within-subjects design").

This framework is economical in both time and effort since the recruited volunteer participants are involved in the study several times. It is also more sensitive to revealing the effects of the experimental manipulation because there are fewer sources of variability that would be present compared to having different people in different groups (i.e., such as a between-groups design). Also, fewer participants are needed in a within-subjects design compared to a between-groups design.

A repeated measures design was used by Vanderloo and Tucker (2015) to examine the physical activity and sedentary behaviour of young children. The participants wore accelerometers (i.e., a device that measures movement in minutes and different intensities throughout the day) for five consecutive days during the time they were at the childcare centre. The researchers compared the activity levels of boys and girls. Among other important findings, Vanderloo and Tucker reported that physical activity levels peaked during the middle of the week and that the levels of sedentary behaviour and physical activity were not different between the boys and girls. Based on these results, the researchers offered practical recommendations that childcare centres could benefit from introducing more active play programs at the start and end of the week.

Of course, there are important factors that need to be considered when embarking on a repeated-measures study. The design works best when there is little connection or interaction between the levels of the independent variable. For example, if you are interested in testing different exercise intensities on heart rate, you have to be careful to ensure that participants doing high-intensity exercise have enough time to rest before doing low-intensity exercise (or else the potential effects of high heart rate could carry over to the effects of the low-intensity exercise). To minimize the possible effects that one manipulation has on the other, researchers should randomize the order of the manipulations. This means that each participant is exposed to each manipulation in a different order. Also, there should be sufficient, but not extensive, time between measurement sessions. This time between testing sessions is called a **wash-out period** and should be sufficient to wipe out the effects of the previous condition so that participants are essentially starting from their normal baseline at each session.

An example of randomized test administrations is illustrated in Table 4.1. In this example, the purpose of the study is to test the effects of diet composition on sleep quality among university students. The fictitious repeated-measures study involves 50 students who come into the lab and receive a food box that they are to consume for one week. While at the lab, they fill out a questionnaire on their sleep quality (pre-test measure). Then they leave the lab with their box of food that consists of one of three options: high-carbohydrate foods, low-carbohydrate foods, or food that they had previously reported as their "normal" diet. Eight days later, they return to the lab and complete the sleep quality questionnaire again (post-test measure). Then they wait a week (i.e., the wash-out period) before returning to the lab to get their next food box to help reduce the interaction of the manipulation effects. The procedure is repeated for a total of three times since there are three conditions. In total, each participant completes the pre-test three times, a week of diet manipulation three times, and a post-test three times. The key aspect of this example is that the ordering of the intervention for each participant is random.

Table 4.1 A depiction of randomization for three participants involved in a repeated-measures study comparing three diets on sleep quality.

PARTICIPANT	TESTING WEEK 1	TESTING WEEK 2	TESTING WEEK 3
1	No diet manipulation (CONTROL)	High-carbohydrate diet	Low-carbohydrate diet
2	Low-carbohydrate diet	No diet manipulation (CONTROL)	High-carbohydrate diet
3	High-carbohydrate diet	Low-carbohydrate diet	No diet manipulation (CONTROL)

Incidentally, a repeated measures study design method was used by Tikuisis, Jacobs, Moroz, Vallerand, and Martineau (2000) at Defence and Research Development Canada to examine the effects of carbohydrate substrate use in conditions of cold water immersion among women. Their study was specifically designed to inform prediction models of survival in cold exposure; more specifically, if a boat capsized in the Atlantic Ocean and the coast guard had some knowledge of the crew members' body composition and what they ate, could they predict how long they have to rescue the crew members before major adverse outcomes?

A final type of quasi-experimental study design is called a **single-subjects** design, or "*N* of 1," in which a single person or a small number of people are studied over a long period of time. In this type of study, the naturally occurring behaviour of an individual is examined over time. A "baseline behaviour" is assessed, a treatment is provided, and then once the treatment is withdrawn the behaviour is assessed again over a period of time. Let's say we are interested in knowing if behavioural counselling can help a sedentary person become more physically active. We would have the individual wear an accelerometer to assess physical activity over many days or weeks (until a habitual pattern could be determined), then we would implement behavioural counselling over several days or weeks (while continuing to assess physical activity), and then stop the behavioural counselling and continue to assess physical activity for many more days or weeks. The goal would be to examine whether the physical activity behaviour assessed before the intervention was better or worse than the physical activity assessed during and after the intervention.

Pre-experimental research design

A **pre-experimental design** is described as a study in which researchers examine *one* group of individuals and provide an intervention during the study. In a pre-experimental study, there is either the absence of a control group for comparison or a non-equivalent comparison group is identified during the study or after the intervention. Creswell (2014) identifies four different pre-experimental designs, which are depicted in Table 4.2.

Pre-experimental designs pose challenges to internal and external validity since many of the threats (described in the subsequent section) are not controlled in this type of study design. It may be less costly financially and in terms of time, as well as potentially pose less burden on participants, but this type of design should be used only with great caution in kinesiology research because of the challenges it poses for researchers hoping to identify causal relationships among variables.

Table 4.2 Some possible pre-experimental research designs with examples from kinesiology research and practice.

PRE-EXPERIMENTAL STUDY DESIGN	DESCRIPTION	EXAMPLE
One-time case study	Participants are exposed to an intervention (e.g., treatment) and then are assessed on the outcome of interest.	A researcher is interested in whether writing about an exhilarating experience improves mood. Participants are brought into the lab, asked to write down all the details about an exhilarating experience (e.g., skydiving, bungee jumping, heli skiing)–the writing is an intervention–and then complete a mood questionnaire.
Pre-test–post-test design with one group	Participants complete an assessment, are exposed to an intervention, and then complete an assessment.	The purpose of the study is to examine changes in reaction time following a maximal three-minute exercise test. Participants complete a reaction time test on a computer, cycle at maximal output for three minutes, and then complete the reaction time test.
Post-test only with nonequivalent groups	This design is used after an intervention is implemented with one group. Participants for a comparison are selected and both the experimental group and the comparison group(s) complete a post-test assessment.	Researchers are studying the effects of attending a health and wellness retreat on healthy eating among a group of individuals presenting with obesity. Participants who attend the summit are compared to a group who did not attend the summit on fruit and vegetable consumption, total fat, and fibre intake.
Alternative treatment post-test-only with nonequivalent groups design	Similar to the "post-test only with nonequivalent groups" design, in this approach participants are exposed to an intervention, a comparison group is identified and selected who are exposed to a different intervention, and both the experimental group and the comparison group(s) complete a post-test assessment.	Using the purpose from the study above, participants who attend the health and wellness retreat are compared to participants who attended a motivational speaker engagement on healthy diet.

Non-experimental research design

If there is no randomization to groups, no groups to randomize to, and no manipulation of the independent variable, researchers have a **non-experimental** study design. A non-experimental study relies on researchers' interpretation and observation to come to conclusions. As a result, non-experimental studies cannot be used to demonstrate cause-and-effect relationships; instead they can be used to report correlations or associations among variables of interest. Oftentimes, these studies are descriptive in nature, and they can be classified as either **cross-sectional** (participants assessed at one point in time) or **longitudinal** (following participants over time). Non-experimental designs are the only possible choice for researchers if there is interest in independent variables that cannot feasibly be manipulated. For example, if you were interested in aggression levels among Olympic athletes and non-athletes, you could not have a true experimental study because the independent variable for aggression is athletic status; but you can't very easily manipulate whether someone is an Olympic athlete or not.

Non-experimental study designs are used frequently among researchers in kinesiology. As one example, Katya Herman at the University of Regina published a study with colleagues in Quebec exploring factors related to sedentary behaviour among children aged 8 to 10 years (Herman, Sabiston, Mathieu, Tremblay, & Paradis, 2015). The data were drawn from the QUALITY study (see http://www.etudequalitystudy.ca), which is an on-going longitudinal study following children who are at risk for obesity because they live with at least one parent who is obese. The authors defined their dependent variable, sedentary behaviour, as exceeding two hours a day of screen time; a decision based on the Canadian sedentary behaviour guidelines for youth. Among other factors, children were more likely to be sedentary if they were older, male, ate dinner in front of the television, participated in limited physical education at school, and were more overweight. However, no matter how intuitively appealing, cause and effect cannot be inferred from their results (e.g., being overweight did not cause more sedentary behaviour) because of their use of a non-experimental study design.

As can be seen in the example of the QUALITY study, non-experimental research can use "natural" differences in a population (e.g., some people exercise and some do not, some people smoke and some do not) to understand *potential* effects of differences on dependent variables of interest. Classic examples of this type of research come from epidemiology, a field in which there is a focus on describing the state of health problems (e.g., what percentage of the Canadian population meets the strength training guidelines?), identifying factors that are related to diseases (e.g., participation in moderate-to-vigorous intensity physical activity and cancer risk), guiding public health resources and programming (e.g., walking school bus for children to safely and actively commute to school), and examining prevention strategies (e.g., what level of physical activity is needed to prevent heart disease?). Findings from epidemiological research have played a critical role in advancing science and practice, and offer further justification for the importance and relevance of non-experimental research studies.

Threats to Experimental Validity

Based on the discussion so far, you should be able to answer the question *"Are the people in the study assigned to groups?"* and identify whether a study is experimental, quasi-experimental, or non-experimental. We have also discussed the answer to the question *"How often/how many measurements are being done?"* that informs the study design. If you have an experimental study, you might use post-test only (one measurement) or pre- and post-test (two measurements). If your study is quasi-experimental, you can use pre- and post-test (two measurements) or repeated measures (more than two measurements) designs. If you have a non-experimental study, you could collect data as a cross-sectional (one measurement) or longitudinal (more than one measurement) study.

There are two other important study design questions that have been introduced throughout this chapter. One question focuses on the **internal validity** of the study: *"Can you conclude that the findings are based on the manipulation of the independent variable?"* Experimental studies have the highest level of internal validity, while non-experimental studies have the lowest level of internal validity. In the latter the data are collected in an uncontrolled, often non-systematic way. The second remaining study design question relates to **external validity**: *"Is there an interest in generalizing the findings to other populations, settings, or time?"* As described in this chapter, experimental studies often cannot claim high levels of external validity (i.e., the findings are not generalizable) due to the controlled nature of the study; yet quasi- and non-experimental studies have the potential for higher levels of external validity because they can be conducted in natural settings or with intact groups.

Throughout the remainder of this chapter, we will discuss ways that researchers can attempt to improve the internal validity and external validity in their studies. Unfortunately, there are no numerical values assigned to external and internal validity conditions so it is up to individual researchers to judge the study protocol and ensure that all conditions that undermine validity are considered. In the next section, these conditions, or threats, to internal validity and external validity are described.

There are many factors that can impede the validity of a study because there are various conditions that can impact dependent variables separate from any effects of the independent variable and/or limit the generalizability of findings from a research study.

Threats to internal validity

Factors that may alter the dependent variable separate from the effects of the independent variable are considered threats to internal validity. Researchers can identify these threats to internal validity and design their studies so that the threats are minimized. These threats are related to the study's experimental procedures, the treatment or manipulation of the independent variable, and/or the participant characteristics. The main threats to internal validity are based on the seminal list introduced by Campbell and Stanley (1963) and Creswell's (2009) suggestions for alleviating some of the threats.

1.   Threats related to the experimental procedure:

   *   *Testing:* Participants may become familiar with the test, and this experience might influence future performances. In kinesiology research, these practice or learning effects can often be seen if participants complete a novel task the first time and then become familiarized with the test so that their performance a second time will be enhanced. Also, doing a task once could offer incentive to improve, and this improvement would be independent of the manipulation. Ways of reducing the effects of testing might be to have a long period between testing and to use different measures for the second test (but this latter solution might also decrease internal validity since consistency in instrumentation is also important).

- *Instrument accuracy:* The measures used in kinesiology research need to be as reliable and valid as possible, which includes measuring tools and processes being in good working order. In some cases the dependent variable might change as a result of inaccurate calibration of a machine, inappropriate use of an instrument, differences in techniques in the first and follow-up measure(s), or even between-researcher differences in the data collection protocol. Key strategies to reduce instrumentation bias include having the same person complete the measures over time for the same participants, using the same machine and same calibration process, and following a guidebook for procedures outlining the data collection process to ensure all steps are identical across testing periods. Consistent calibration of the study equipment is also important.

2. Threats related to the treatment or manipulation:

- *Diffusion of treatments:* If participants in the experimental and control groups communicate with each other, the communication can impact the scores on the dependent measure. For example, if Sally and Sam are co-workers and they have been randomly assigned to different treatment groups (e.g., Sally gets a printed book about exercise, Sam gets daily text messages about exercise), they might speak over coffee one day and realize that the other is getting treated differently (or feels differently or perceives a certain effect). This type of communication between participants could influence the way either one or both of them respond on follow-up tests. If Sally feels that she is getting less than Sam (i.e., treated unequally), she might even express resentment or feel there is a rivalry between them and the rest of the participants in the two groups. These types of diffusion of treatment have been common in studies related to exercise interventions, wherein the control group participants were not able to exercise at all and the experimental group participants would get personalized training, equipment, attention from personal trainers, and additional resources. To help avoid diffusion of treatments, it is now common practice to provide the control group with *something* rather than nothing, such as the physical activity guidelines for Canadians. However, researchers should also attempt to keep the groups as separate as possible during the experiment and/or avoid sampling from intact groups (e.g., workplace) as much as possible to limit how much participants know one another. Also, **blinding** the participants to the condition can dramatically reduce the diffusion of treatment (i.e., hiding or concealing the condition/treatment/manipulation). In the exercise drug study presented earlier, we could have blinded the participants by having everyone take the same colour and size of pill capsule, with the only difference being that one is filled with our new drug and the other is full of flour. Using this type of strategy means that no one in the study would be aware of what group they were in and what they were taking. Ideally, researchers should also be blinded to the study manipulation (called a **double-blind study**, because both the researcher and participant are unaware of who has received the manipulation). In exercise experimental studies, it is challenging to blind the researcher since it is pretty obvious when a participant is exercising or not, or using the bicycle versus the treadmill! The bottom line is that the less people involved in the study know about each other and what group they are in, the better.

- *Halo effect:* When researchers have some expectation about the performance of participants and are in a position to assess performance, their knowledge of the experimental conditions could influence their judgment on outcomes or could influence the way they respond to the participants. For example, if a researcher knows that a participant is an athlete, she or he might push the athlete harder during a fitness test than participants who are non-athletes. A "halo" is anything that clouds researchers' impartiality or leads to coercing the participants. Double-blinding is one strategy that can help reduce the halo effect threat.

3. Threats related to the participants:

- *Maturation:* Participants in the study might mature naturally or change in many ways over time (e.g., gain or lose weight, get taller, develop better coordination, become more or less anxious and stressed). This growth, learning, or maturation can be of significant concern in studies of chronically ill patients or children, given their unpredictable and often rapid changes. For example, in the ongoing QUALITY study described earlier, the children were 8 to 10 years of age when the study started and are subsequently being followed through adolescence. There will be a number of changes that occur both within each participant and across participants that need to be accounted for in follow-up testing. However, there is some level of control within the QUALITY sample since all children were recruited at the same age. Standardizing age is often an important strategy when trying to limit the effects of maturation in particular.

- *History:* Events other than the experimental treatment can often affect the results of studies. Let's return to the example of Sally and Sam who are both in your study looking at whether getting daily text messages about exercise can increase overall time spent in moderate-to-vigorous physical activity compared to getting print material. You conduct your research and find that participants in both conditions increase physical activity. However, what you didn't know was that their workplace initiated an incentive program that gave all employees one hour of paid time per day to exercise, along with a free gym membership. The threat is that this type of event (i.e., an employer physical activity incentive program) can also act to facilitate improved physical activity levels but is unrelated to the independent variable manipulation (i.e., your text messages). One way of limiting history effects is to have randomization of your participants to groups, such that both groups have equal chances of being exposed to other events. However, no matter how conscientious they are in considering all possible influences, it is unlikely that researchers will be aware of all extraneous "historical" events.

- *Regression*: When participants who have extreme scores (i.e., extremely high or extremely low) are recruited for an experiment, sometimes their scores just naturally change in the direction of the mean (the average of scores). For example, the "soph-omore jinx" in sport (i.e., top rookies often struggle in their second year) is an ex-ample of regression to the mean; they are simply unable to sustain extremely high performance levels year after year (in most cases). Usually the regression to the mean is a bigger concern in smaller samples, and researchers can attempt to recruit for their studies using inclusion and exclusion criteria that help to limit people with extreme scores.

- *Selection bias:* When groups are formed without random assignment, there is a possi-bility that groups will be biased on some or many characteristics. This can occur when participants volunteer to participate (e.g., men with cardiac arrhythmias who call to be involved in a sport study are likely more motivated to play sport or have a history of playing sports). The use of intact groups (e.g., teams, classes) can also inflate selection bias. Random assignment is the best way of addressing selection bias.

- *Experimental drop-out:* Also known as mortality, this threat relates to people dropping out or leaving the study for reasons such as boredom, sickness, injury, inconvenience, discomfort, or other unknown reasons. This attrition can occur in either the experi-mental or control group and affect the outcomes of the study. Experimental drop-out is less of a concern in studies with large samples because the impact of losing partici-pants from any one group is less than if there are small samples. Also, researchers can statistically compare the drop-outs from the participants who completed the study.

- *Placebo and Hawthorne effects:* Participants may react in a way they expect they should react when they are in an experimental study (placebo effect). Also, partici-pants might react in favourable ways just because they are being observed (Hawthorne effect). Blinding of participants to the experimental condition can help limit placebo effects. Also, researchers often try to be as hands-off as possible in the study to limit participants' perceptions that they are being observed.

Threats to external validity

External validity refers to the ability to generalize the research findings, such that the results of the study can be appropriately used among other people, settings, or time. The greater the ability to generalize the results of a study, the higher the degree of external validity. External validity can be threatened by interactions arising from timing, sample, and setting character-istics and treatment manipulation:

- *Selection and treatment interaction:* When the unique characteristics of participants involved in the study makes the treatment effective only for them, researchers cannot generalize to individuals who do not have the same characteristics as the participants. For example, a researcher might be attempting to conduct a high-intensity interval training intervention in schools, and the researcher contacts the 15 schools in the local district. However, only one school accepts the invitation. As it turns out, the school that accepts the intervention is a specialized school that targets athletes and is therefore unique in that all students are attending that particular school to train for their sport. As a result, the sample in the study is not representative of other schools in the district; as a consequence the intervention might function differently in a different school (e.g., the researcher might be able to change the level of physical activity for only the students in their study since they are already competent in sport). To limit the selection and treatment interaction, researchers should conduct the experiment with groups that have different characteristics whenever possible.

- *Setting and treatment interaction:* When studies are conducted in highly controlled environments, it is challenging to know if the same outcomes would be found in real world settings. We presented an example of the setting and treatment interaction in the example of the exercise drug. It would be ideal to conduct the experiment in new settings/environments to ensure the findings are not a result of a highly controlled setting that could also increase the possibility of Hawthorne effects.

- *History and treatment interaction:* Given that the results of an experiment are dependent on the timing of implementation, the findings cannot necessarily be generalized to past or future settings. For example, sociology of sport researchers who examined the effects of media portrayals of women in sport in the 1970s would have very different sport media to examine in 2018 given the advancements in the number of sport opportunities and experiences for women in the last few decades. Similarly, conducting an analysis of the functional movements (and attire!) in a 1980s Jane Fonda workout video would likely have limited contribution to current knowledge and action. In sport and exercise contexts, technology and equipment change rapidly, and research conducted with athletes a decade ago is almost certain to be based on the use of different equipment than what we would use now (e.g., wooden hockey sticks that might have been used in a slap shot biomechanical analysis in a prior research study would now be replaced by a Kevlar hockey stick for the same analysis). Ideally, studies would be replicated over time to ensure that any findings are not time dependent.

If we revisit our important questions pertaining to the research elements of a quantitative study, one answer remains to be discussed: *What type of measures or observations are you going to use?* The same measurement or assessment tools can be used to collect data for experimental, quasi-experimental, and non-experimental studies. The key is to use **valid** (i.e., the degree to which a test measures what is intended to be measured) and **reliable** (i.e., the degree to which a test is consistent) instruments to collect data.

Measurement in Quantitative Research

For all quantitative studies, the type of measures that are used will result in data that are numerical and quantifiable. Specifically, the types of data collected in quantitative studies can be described as discrete or continuous and as nominal, ordinal, interval, or ratio. **Discrete data** take on particular values that are either numerical (e.g., number of different exercises in a program) or categorical (e.g., blood pressure in categories of hypertension, hypotension, normal). Discrete data are further classified as nominal or ordinal data. **Continuous data** can take on any value and range (e.g., the weight of a mouse, a person's maximal energy expenditure, a gymnast's height).

Nominal data refer to categorically discrete and mutually exclusive data; such as the name of your favourite sports team, the colour of your hair, or the name of this book. This type of data is important for descriptive purposes only in quantitative studies.

Ordinal data refer to quantities that have a natural ordering. The ranking of favourite sports or placement of runners finishing a race are both examples of ordinal data, as are measures on a rating scale (e.g., How happy are you right now while reading this book? Responses can be: 1 = not at all happy, 2 = somewhat happy, 3 = very happy). One of the defining features of ordinal data is that the intervals between each value may not be equal. For example, on a 3-point scale of happiness, the difference between a 1 (not at all happy) and a 2 (somewhat happy) is not necessarily the same difference as the difference between a 2 (somewhat happy) and a 3 (very happy).

Interval data are also ordered, but the intervals between each value are equal. For example, if we look at temperature in degrees Celsius we know that the difference between 10 and 11 degrees is the same magnitude as the difference between 84 and 85 degrees. Interval data provide information on the difference, direction of difference, and amount of difference in equal units.

Ratio data are interval data with a natural or absolute zero point. An absolute zero point means the absence of a trait, and also means that comparisons can be made with other scores. For example, 5 kilometres is half the distance of 10 kilometres, and 60 seconds is three times as long as 20 seconds.

The types of data and examples are presented in Figure 4.2.

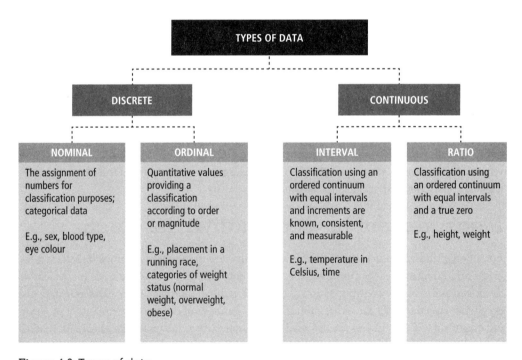

Figure 4.2 Types of data.

Taken together, the type of data is important to consider because it affects how the data are presented and the choice of the statistical analyses that will be needed to answer the research questions posed. The specific statistics that align with the type of data will be covered in Chapter 5. The types of data are a result of the inherent characteristics of the variables of interest (e.g., eye colour cannot be changed), as well as how variables are measured (e.g., blood pressure can be assessed as a continuous variable for systolic and diastolic pressure or categorized based on medical classifications for low, high, and normal blood pressure, making it a discrete variable). Tools used for the measurement of these data in kinesiology will be briefly discussed in the next section.

Data collection tools for quantitative studies

The main data collection tools measuring psychological and social variables, such as attitudes, beliefs, perceptions, affect, and emotions, include observation, structured interview, and self-report surveys. Briefly, **observation** involves visual and/or audio records and counts of particular behaviours, settings, or interactions and scoring what is seen and heard. For example, if a researcher is interested in knowing the brand name of the shoes represented in the university fitness centre, she or he could observe all students entering the centre and record the type of shoe worn; resulting in a frequency count of the number of people wearing Nike, Adidas, Asics, Reebok, Puma, Brooks, Saucony, and New Balance shoes, for example. Another example would be observing the play behaviours of children in school playgrounds. **Objectivity** is an important concern in observational data collections to ensure there is reliability or consistency of measurement between different researchers.

A **structured interview** is a data collection tool that is often used to facilitate responses to specific questions that have set answers (i.e., closed-ended). The structured interview is different from an open-ended or unstructured interview protocol that is often used to generate qualitative data. If you have ever answered the telephone and been asked to complete a survey, this is typically an example of a structured interview. Basically, it involves the researcher verbally requesting the responses to the questions and writing in the responses rather than having the participants complete the questions themselves on a paper or online survey. Statistics Canada uses a telephone-based structured interview to collect data on a number of topics, including health.

Surveys (or questionnaires) involve the use of paper-and-pencil or online-delivered questions, usually consisting of a mix of rating scales providing ordinal or interval data responses. Many questionnaires have been developed to assess a multitude of variables relevant to kinesiology research, including depression and anxiety symptoms, personality, use of imagery in sport, coach leadership behaviours, social identity on teams, injury, and physical activity preferences (and the list goes on and on).

Other common measurement tools in kinesiology include technologies and instruments used to assess variables such as time and intensity of physical activity (e.g., pedometers and accelerometers), time to complete tasks (e.g., stopwatch), body composition (e.g., skinfold calipers, waist circumference, weight scale), aerobic capacity and ventilator threshold (e.g., metabolic cart and gas exchange), heart rate and function (e.g., monitors, electrocardiogram), and muscular strength (e.g., 1 Repeated Maximum, hand dynamometer). This is not an exhaustive list, but one thing to point out is that these measures are typically considered to be more objective than the observation, interview, and survey measures.

Writing Exercise

Revisit the research purpose that you identified in Chapter 2 (or come up with a new one). Design (a) an experimental and (b) a non-experimental study that can address the purpose. Write out the procedures that you will use to design your study, and identify the measures that you will collect for your dependent variable (and perhaps your independent variable). Make sure to answer the questions that have been discussed throughout this chapter (e.g., Are the people in your study assigned to groups? How many measurements are you going to do? What type of measures or observations are you going to use? Are you interested in generalizing the findings to others? Can you conclude that the findings are based on the independent variable?). Justify your responses.

You might still be asking, *"Why does it matter what measurement tool we use?"* The short answer is that without appropriate and strong measures of variables, the findings from research studies will be of little use. Because of its importance, specific examples of the role of measurement and construct validity will be covered in Chapter 6. However, now that we have identified quantitative study designs, presented strategies to help improve the quality of the study, and listed various measures that can be used in collecting quantitative data, we are missing one key piece to our quantitative study discussion: *"Who are we studying and how do we find them?"* To answer this question, we need to talk about the sample.

Sampling for Quantitative Studies

The **sample** represents a group of participants (or organizations, teams, schools, etc.) selected to be in a study. The specific members of a sample are ideally chosen as representation of a **population** to whom we are interested in generalizing our findings. Thus, the sample is drawn from the population, or at least the population that is accessible to the researcher. For example, if we are interested in generalizing the findings of our exercise drug study to older adult men and women, our ideal population includes all men and women in Canada who are over the age of 80 years. However, it is not likely that we will have access to all of these older adults in Canada, so our population that is accessible might be limited to those living in our city or general geographical area. This is called our **sampling frame** because it is the group of people we can connect with about our study. Researchers always identify their specific study sample (i.e., the people selected for the study) from the sampling frame.

But how do we get the people involved in our study? The two main strategies for sampling include probability and non-probability protocols. **Probability sampling** is any method that ensures that the different units in the population have equal probabilities of being chosen. Examples of probability sampling include random selection, stratified random sampling, and systematic sampling. The use of probability sampling is important for generalization of the study results to a larger group or population. This practice of generalizability is called **inference**. If the sample represents a larger group, then the findings can be generalized or inferred to the larger group. Alternatively, **non-probability sampling** is any method that does not use random selection. The sample identified using non-probability methods *might* be representative of the population, but it is unlikely. Non-probability sampling increases the chances of selection bias (one of the threats to internal validity). Examples of non-probability sampling include convenience or purposive sampling methods.

Random selection

Random selection is a process that ensures that every unit (e.g., person, team, organization) in the population has an equal probability of being selected for the sample. The sample can be randomly selected from the larger sampling frame or population using procedures like a random numbers table, computer programs, or even pulling names/numbers "out of a hat." The key to random selection is that the sample is representative of the population to which it is being generalized.

Stratified random sampling

If the population (or sampling frame) is divided and grouped on a characteristic before random selection takes place, researchers are using **stratified random sampling**. This approach to sampling can be particularly important if there is a certain characteristic that needs to be represented in the sample. For example, if we are interested in studying the exercise habits of university undergraduate students, we would want to understand these habits among students who are in various years of university (especially with the known challenges of healthy behaviours among first-year students!). As such, we would stratify our population into first-, second-, third-, and fourth-year (and possibly beyond fourth-year) undergraduate students. Then we would randomly select students from each stratum to ensure representation across all years.

Systematic sampling

If the population is very large, random selection and stratified random sampling methods will be very time consuming. **Systematic sampling** is a process whereby researchers use lists or inventories of units in a population (e.g., telephone book, index of registered members) to identify (select) every Nth entry for the sample, such as every 10th or 100th person. Of course, there are some concerns with the use of lists since they have a characteristic in common (e.g., anyone in the member directory for a fitness club will have paid to have access to that club) and might have inherent biases (e.g., alphabetical lists by last name might inherently order or cluster people of certain ethnicities in certain locations in the list).

Convenience sampling

Drawing a sample from groups of people that are familiar or convenient is a common non-probability method of sampling. For example, it is common practice that psychology programs offer course credit for participation in research studies. Clinicians might ask patients to participate in their studies, whereas kinesiology professors might ask students, coaches, and teams. In general, this method of sampling is simply asking people to volunteer.

Purposive sampling

As the name implies, **purposive sampling** involves identifying units (e.g., people, organizations, teams) that represent a characteristic of interest; as such, the sample is identified with that purpose in mind. There are several different methods of purposive sampling, such as **snowball sampling** (e.g., identify one person with the characteristic of interest, and have that person connect with others in their own network; for example, a woman with breast cancer might ask all the members of her survivorship group at the hospital to participate in a study), **quota sampling** (e.g., identifying a certain number or representation needed for the study and then sampling up to that number; for example, needing 10 women to complete a fitness test), and **expert sampling** (e.g., identifying people with known experience and expertise in an area of interest; for example, asking all heart surgeons from a local hospital to complete a survey).

Case Study

An graduated with a Bachelor's degree in physical and health education from Nipissing University and went on to become a registered kinesiologist in Ontario. She now works as a personal trainer and owns a gym where she has a booming fitness clientele. One of the questions she frequently gets asked by her clients is "Which exercise program is most beneficial for weight loss?" To accurately answer this question, An designed a research study looking at changes in body weight after a six-week exercise regime. She collaborated with a researcher at a local university, they applied for ethics and received approval from the research ethics board, and now An has recruited 40 participants who will be randomly assigned into four groups of 10 people. Each group will receive a different exercise program: Condition 1 will receive a three-day/week Crossfit training program to do at home, Condition 2 will receive a three-day/week yoga program at a local yoga studio, Condition 3 will take part in three group exercise sessions a week at the local gym, and Condition 4 will be the control group and will not participate in exercise during the six weeks of the study.

Discussion Questions

1. What kind of study would this be considered?
2. What are the benefits of randomly assigning participants to the conditions?
3. Identify some ways to ensure random assignment to the conditions.
4. What is the purpose of the control group?
5. Identify the independent and dependent variable(s), and write out null and alternative hypotheses.
6. Based on your knowledge of study design, when should An measure the outcomes of her study? How might An measure her main study variables?
7. Identify other possible study designs that could be used to answer An's research question.

Summary

Chapter 4 focused on the ways in which researchers can design and implement quantitative studies. Working within a postpositivist philosophical worldview, quantitative designs include experimental, quasi-experimental, and non-experimental research designs. Questions pertaining to the methods of assessment and tools and instruments were presented and discussed, as were factors that need to be considered when implementing a research design, such as threats to internal validity and external validity. Sampling was discussed as it pertains to the quantitative research designs, and statistical inference was described. With the use of the chapter writing exercises, the design strategies were linked back to the purpose and research questions to demonstrate the fluidity needed between what is intended and what is designed. The design strategies are also critical to understanding the methods of quantitative data analysis (i.e., statistics) that will be covered in Chapter 5.

Discussion Questions

1. What are key similarities and differences among experimental, quasi-experimental, and non-experimental study designs?
2. What are three examples from kinesiology for each of nominal, ordinal, interval, and ratio data types?
3. How do you define stratified random sampling?
4. What are three purposive sampling strategies that could be used to identify a sample?
5. You are interested in studying the effects of exercising in the cold on energy expenditure among males and females (e.g., "Does exercising in the cold relate to higher energy expenditure?"). How would you describe the possible threats to internal and external validity that you will consider in this study?
6. Think back to your main interests in kinesiology and identify one main outcome that you could measure as a dependent variable in a study. How would you measure it? What are the strengths and limitations of your measure?

Recommended Readings

Courneya, K. S., Sellar, C. M., Trinh, L., Forbes, C. C., Stevinson, C., McNeely, M. L., . . . Reiman, T. (2012). A randomized trial of aerobic exercise and sleep quality in lymphoma patients receiving chemotherapy or no treatments. *Cancer Epidemiology, Biomarkers & Prevention, 21*, 887–94. doi:10.1158/1055-9965.EPI-12-0075

Creswell, J. W. (2014). *Research design: Qualitative, quantitative, and mixed methods approaches* (4th ed.). Thousand Oaks, CA: Sage.

Field, A., & Hole, G. (2003). *How to design and report experiments*. London, England: Sage.

5 Data Analysis in Quantitative Studies

Learning Outcomes

By the end of this chapter, you should be able to:

- Discuss the importance of statistics.
- Apply appropriate statistical analyses to various types of research questions.
- Identify appropriate measures of central tendency and variability.
- Describe the process of hypothesis testing.

Introduction to Data Analysis

After a study has been designed and data have been collected, it is time for researchers to re-visit their research questions and hypotheses and see if they found what they thought they were going to find. This means they need to look at and analyze the collected quantitative data, interpret them, and make conclusions based on their findings. The design of the study (which was informed by the research purpose) offers a foundation for the type of statistics that are needed to analyze the data. Thinking back to the types of research problems that we identified in Chapter 2, **statistics** are objective ways of interpreting observations used to help researchers address questions related to description, prediction and association, and explanation of differences.

The most appropriate analysis for each research question depends on the type of research design that was used to conduct the study. The number of people in the sample, the number of conditions or manipulations, and the distribution and type of the data are also important factors to consider when choosing statistical analysis. Researchers' hypotheses are also integral to determining the type of statistical analysis. In fact, hypothesis tests are one of the most important statistical procedures because they inform the decisions that researchers make about the outcomes of their study. These and other factors will be presented throughout this chapter.

Descriptive Statistics

Remember from Chapter 4, *nominal data* refers to categorically discrete and mutually exclusive data, *ordinal data* refers to quantities that have a natural ordering or rank, *interval data* are also ordered with the intervals between each value being equal, and *ratio data* are interval data with a natural or absolute zero point. These data types allow researchers to decide how they will describe and depict their data graphically (as appropriate) as well as inform the type of analyses that are suitable to use with the collected data.

One of the critical considerations in a research study is what the data look like. Researchers need to have a way of summarizing data to describe and identify patterns, direct further analyses, and explain their results. Researchers often create and examine graphs or tables for this purpose.

The simplest graph is called a **frequency distribution** or **histogram** and involves plotting how many times each score occurs. In an example of imagery use among athletes, we could count how many times each of 20 athletes in the study practised imagery. Researchers could gather the scores and then count how many times each possible response occurred (i.e., the frequency). When doing this by hand (a good way to learn statistics is doing them by hand), it is easiest to arrange the scores in either ascending or descending order. The number of times each score of imagery use is reported can then be plotted on a graph, with the number of imagery uses on the horizontal axis (also called the *x*-axis) and the frequency on the vertical axis (also called the *y*-axis). An example of a histogram is depicted in Figure 5.1.

One thing immediately noticeable in Figure 5.1 is that most athletes report 4 or more imagery uses, because the bars on the right side (i.e., for 4, 5, and 6+ number of imagery uses) are higher than the bars on the left side (i.e., for 1, 2, and 3 number of imagery uses) of the graph. Also, it is easy to identify that the most frequent imagery use score was 5, since that bar is the tallest. So then, what is the least frequent imagery use score? Just look for the lowest bar in the graph, and you can identify that a score of 1 is the least reported among our sample of 20 athletes. Another feature of the frequency distribution graph is that the total number of athletes in our sample can be identified by adding up or summing the frequencies (i.e., moving from left to right on the *x*-axis, there is one athlete with a score of 1, two athletes with a score of 2,

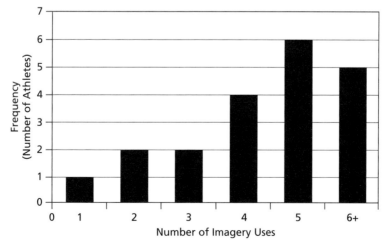

Figure 5.1 A sample histogram of data from 20 athletes reporting on their imagery use.

another two athletes with a score of 3, four athletes with a score of 4, six athletes with a score of 5, and five athletes with a score of 6+; therefore, $1 + 2 + 2 + 4 + 6 + 5 = 20$ athletes total in the study).

Statistics Exercise

Mateo is a physical education teacher who has noticed that his students seem tired all the time, which is affecting their performance on the activities during class time. The students in his class tell him that they sleep an average number of hours per night. These data are presented in Table 5.1.

Table 5.1 Data on number of hours of sleep for all students in Mateo's class.

STUDENT	NUMBER OF HOURS OF SLEEP
1	6
2	8
3	6
4	4
5	7
6	8
7	4
8	7
9	5
10	8
11	9
12	9
13	9
14	7
15	5
16	8
17	6
18	8
19	7
20	5
21	7
22	9
23	8
24	4
25	8

Based on this information, create a histogram and answer the following questions:

1. What is the most common or frequent sleep response?
2. What is the least common sleep response?

Here are some hints to ensure that you are on the right track. Make sure that you put the data in either ascending or descending order. Ordering will help you make an accurate count of the sleep scores. You can also compare the total number of students listed to the sum of the frequencies in your graph (i.e., you should get the same answer both ways).

Histograms are valuable for quickly examining the data distribution and shape. Another type of graph is called a **frequency polygon**, where the frequency of scores is represented by dots that are connected by a line. Using the data from the imagery use in athletes example, the line can be straight and angled (see Figure 5.2) or more smoothed out and curved.

As can be seen from the histogram (Figure 5.1) and polygon graph (Figure 5.2), all types of graphs can be useful in visually depicting and describing the data distribution. There are also various shapes to the data that can be described based on the amplitude (or peak) and direction of the distribution of the data.

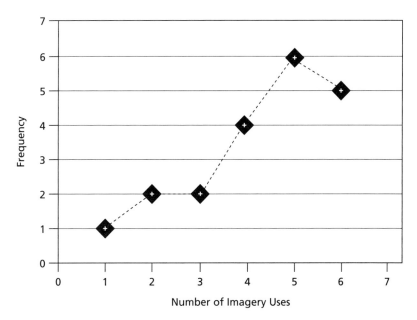

Figure 5.2 A sample frequency polygon of data from 20 athletes reporting on their imagery use.

Research Highlight

Many researchers use tables or figures to present descriptive data. In *Health Reports*, which is a Statistics Canada research outlet, there are often graphical representations of health data collected in regions in Canada. For example, a report by Garriguet, Tremblay, and Colley (2015) was published with data comparing physical activity collected using two self-report questionnaires and an accelerometer. The main purpose was to test the validity of a newly developed measure to assess adult physical activity (Physical Activity for Adults Questionnaire). Essentially, the researchers wanted to know if their newly developed measure was sensitive to the assessment of physical activity in a comparable way to the objective data collected using an accelerometer (e.g., the gold standard). Based on the results, moderate-to-vigorous physical activity measured by accelerometer had a higher correlation with data from the Physical Activity for Adults Questionnaire ($r = .44$) than with data from the more common self-report questionnaire called the International Physical Activity Questionnaire ($r = .20$). These values will be more meaningful by the end of this chapter, but basically higher values infer stronger relationships, and this means more evidence of validity for the new measure compared to the International Physical Activity Questionnaire. In this report, there is also a figure presenting the difference in minutes of moderate-to-vigorous physical activity measured by each self-report measure and the accelerometer. As presented in the figure, the differences were greater for the number of minutes spent in physical activity self-reported on the International Physical Activity Questionnaire than those self-reported on the Physical Activity for Adults Questionnaire when compared to the accelerometer data. Also, the percentages of participants meeting the Canadian Physical Activity Guidelines were 90% based on self-reported International Physical Activity Questionnaire minutes, 70% based on all accelerometer-measured physical activity minutes, and 61% based on self-reported Physical Activity for Adults Questionnaire minutes.

Further Reading

Garriguet, D., Tremblay, S., & Colley, R. (2015). Comparison of Physical Activity Adult Questionnaire results with accelerometer data. *Health Reports, 26*, 11–17.

Types of distributions

There are a number of different distributions that can be observed in data sets. Ideally, researchers want to see a symmetrical data distribution around a centre of scores, which is called a **normal distribution**. If you were to see a normal distribution, basically the highest bar in the graph (the centre of the scores) would be in the middle, and the rest of the bars would decrease in height on either side at approximately the same level. The height of the bars would gradually decrease to the points furthest away from the centre, where you would ultimately see the lowest/smallest (and eventually zero) bar height. Data that are normally distributed meet a key assumption (or underlying necessary criteria) in many statistical analyses.

Skewed distributions deviate from the symmetry seen in the normal distribution. Specifically, if the most frequent scores are at the low end of the scale (i.e., the highest frequency bar is closest to the *y*-axis and the lowest frequency of scores is at the far right of the graph), then the data are representing a **positively skewed** distribution. An example of a positively skewed distribution might be class grades on an extremely difficult biomechanics test whereby most of the students are represented at the lower end of the scale (e.g., C and D grades) and few students are represented at the top end of the range, or the A's. In contrast, if the lowest frequency of scores cluster closest to the *y*-axis and the highest frequency of scores are at the far right of the distribution, this is called a **negatively skewed** distribution. For example, the birth weight of babies might be represented by a negatively skewed graph, because few babies are born below 1.8 kilograms and the majority of babies are born around 3 to 3.5 kilograms. The point of the frequency graph where the scores trail off or become less frequent is called the "tail"; so the tail in the positively skewed graph is at the right and the tail in the negatively skewed graph is at the left.

When the tails of distribution have a clustering of scores, the peak of the distribution can be affected (the degree to which the peak of the distribution is flat or pointy). This is called **kurtosis**, and there are two main kurtosis characteristics that affect distributions. A flat distribution is called **platykurtic** (maybe remember it as "flat"ykurtic) and is defined by having more scores equally distributed across the entire distribution (including more scores in each of the tails). In a **leptokurtic** distribution there are few high and low scores and more scores near the centre creating a pointy distribution (although requiring perhaps a bit more imagination, maybe remember it as "leap"tokurtic). A **mesokurtic** graph basically represents a normal distribution. The skewness and kurtosis distributions are depicted in Figure 5.3.

A final distributional characteristic of data is called **modality**, which is the number of peaks (number of high bars in the histogram) and each represents an area of score clusters. Each peak is called a **mode**, which is defined as the most frequently occurring or most common score in a data set. A distribution with one mode is **unimodal**, whereas a distribution with two peaks or modes is **bimodal** (think: "Alice the camel has two humps, Alice the camel has two humps . . .") and a curve with three peaks is referred to as **trimodal**. It is very rare to see a distribution of scores with three or more common scores.

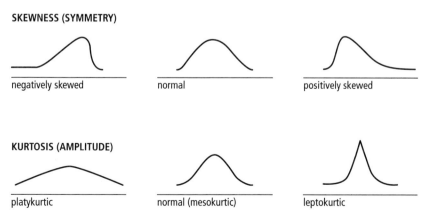

Figure 5.3 Frequency distribution examples demonstrating skewness (top line of graphs) and kurtosis (bottom line of graphs).

In addition to the skewness, kurtosis, and modality of the distributions; central tendency and variability of scores are also important descriptive characteristics of a data set.

Central tendency

Central tendency represents how scores in a distribution most commonly cluster together (i.e., if you had to choose one number that best represents a group of numbers as a whole, measures of central tendency provide you that number). There are three main measures of central tendency: the mode, median, and mean. As already described, the **mode** is the most frequently occurring score. It is calculated by placing all scores in ascending order and then counting how many times each score occurs. Since it is a count of scores, the mode can be used to describe nominal data as well as ordinal, interval, and ratio data. In fact, it is the only central tendency measure that is appropriate for nominal data.

The **median** is the middle score of a distribution when the scores are ordered in magnitude. In a data set with an odd number of scores, the median is simple to identify (i.e., the middle score); however, when there is an even number of scores, the median is calculated as the average of the two middle points. The median is not affected by extreme scores (e.g., if one of the students in Mateo's physical education class, from our previous example, reported 15 hours of sleep, she or he would still have the highest score, but that score would not affect the median score), and it is also less affected than the mean when scores are in the tails of a distribution (skewed). The median can be used as a measure of central tendency for ordinal, interval, or ratio data and is often the best choice as an indicator of central tendency for a distribution that has a small number of scores, extreme or atypical values (called **outliers**), or is skewed.

The **mean** (or average) is the sum of all scores divided by the total number of scores. The mean offers a better understanding of the actual data scores than the mode and median in most situations, yet it can be influenced by extreme values as well as by the skewness of the distribution. Specifically, in a negatively skewed distribution the mean value will be less than the median because the mean is pulled towards the outlying scores in the tail of the distribution (the median will also be lower than the mode in this case). In a positively skewed distribution, the mean will be higher than the median (which will be a bigger value than the mode).

The difference in these measures of central tendency will be greater with increasing skewness in the distribution. But in a normal distribution, the mean, median, and mode will be the same value (interesting statistics fact #1). As a final point, the mean (which is often denoted as M) should only be calculated for interval and ratio data (interesting statistics fact #2).

Statistics Exercise

A number of graphs were presented in Figure 5.3. Re-draw the top three graphs from Figure 5.3 and identify an estimated location of the mode, median, and mean on each graph using different colours or different lines. After you have identified these measures of central tendency, identify an example of a data set that might be represented by each of these graphs.

Measures of variability

The measures of central tendency offer insight into where the scores tend to cluster (similarity of scores), whereas **variability** of the scores is an index of how the scores vary or disperse (the spread of scores). As such, variability also tells the researchers something about the shape of the distribution of scores. Common measures of variability include the range, interquartile range, variance, and standard deviation. The **range** is the distance between the most extreme scores (lowest and highest) in a distribution. However, the range is sensitive to the value of the extreme scores and is determined only from those two values. The range is not overly telling of the distribution of scores within the extreme values but can be used to offer insight into the scores that fall within certain percentiles of the distribution. For example, the **interquartile range** identifies the scores that are the boundaries of the lowest and highest of the distribution, or the middle 50 percent of the scores in a distribution (or 25th to 75th percentile). If we re-visit Mateo's class data on hours of sleep, the range is the score of 9 (the highest data point) minus the score of 4 (the lowest data point), which equals 5. What does a score of 5 tell us? It means that the difference between the student with the least amount of sleep and the student with the most amount of sleep is 5 hours. In these same data, the interquartile range is equal to 2.5. How did we get that value? Look back to Table 5.1 and place all values for the number of hours of sleep in ascending order. You should have three 4s, three 5s, three 6s, five 7s, seven 8s, and four 9s. The median (mid-point) of these data is 7 (remember the median tells us that the mid-point of all the values is 7 hours of sleep). If we take the median of the scores that fall below the median and the median of the scores that fall above the median value we get 5.5 and 8, respectively. The interquartile range is thus 8 minus 5.5, which is a value of 2.5. The interquartile range is often depicted as a **boxplot** (also called a box-and-whisker diagram), which is a standard way of displaying the distribution of data based on the minimum and maximum scores, the first and third quartile, and the median. A sample boxplot for the data from Mateo's class is presented in Figure 5.4.

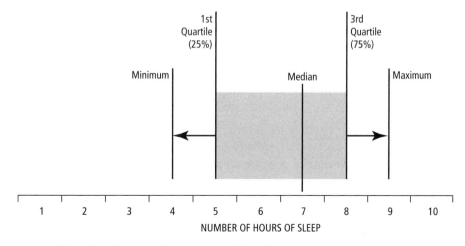

Figure 5.4 A boxplot diagram depicting the data from Mateo's class data on number of hours of sleep the students report.

Standard deviation and **variance** are intertwined measures of dispersion of scores within a distribution and offer insight into the differences among scores within a distribution as well as the differences or deviation between the scores from the mean of the distribution. The variance is the square of the standard deviation and is represented in units squared, which makes it harder to interpret than the standard deviation. But how does one interpret even the standard deviation (often indicated as *SD*)? A larger standard deviation represents a greater spread of scores than does a smaller *SD,* the latter of which suggests the scores are more similar and closer together. Without getting into the details of the calculation of *SD*, it is important to note that the mathematical calculation of *SD* cannot result in a negative value and therefore ranges from 0 upwards (a *SD* score of zero means that all scores in the distribution are the same; hence, zero deviation). However, SD is *interpreted* as being the spread of scores both above and below the mean (and hence *can* have a negative value).

For example, researchers collect maximum aerobic capacity (VO_2) data from a group of master track-and-field athletes and marathon runners over the age of 70 years. The mean VO_2 is relatively similar in both groups (46 millilitres of oxygen per kilogram of body weight per minute or ml/kg per min), but the *SD* is 9.8 ml/kg per min for the track-and-field athletes and is 3.7 ml/kg per min for the marathon runners. If you think practically about this, it makes sense that track and field athletes have more variation in their scores since the possible competitive events within the sport vary in their energy demands (e.g., shot put versus high jump versus sprinting) compared to the marathon demands of endurance running. Mathematically, and assuming a normal distribution, the *SD* values suggest that scores vary around the mean of the distribution of scores, such that the majority of scores fall between 36.2 and 55.8 ml/kg per min (46 minus and plus 9.8) for the track athletes and 42.3 and 49.7 ml/kg per min (46 minus and plus 3.7) for the marathon runners. The use of *SD* has a number of applications that are beyond the scope of this chapter, but readers are encouraged to review material related to the normal curve, confidence intervals, and *z*-scores in most statistics textbooks. For kinesiology-specific material, refer to Vincent and Weir (2012) and Thomas, Nelson, and Silverman (2015) for some great examples, equations, and more advanced statistical procedures.

With more experience, you might notice that most descriptive statistics are primarily used for *interval* or *ratio* data. When data are measured at interval or ratio levels, the mean is the most appropriate measure of central tendency, and the statistics are called **parametric tests**. For parametric tests, the data must be normally distributed; if the research question involves a comparison of means across groups or conditions, then the variances between these groups need to be relatively similar. Alternatively, **percentages** of responses or scores (frequencies) are used as the main descriptive statistic for *nominal* and *ordinal* data. The statistical tests used for nominal and ordinal data are generally called **non-parametric** tests. Overall, the main goals of the parametric and non-parametric tests are the same (e.g., a parametric test could be used to examine group mean differences, and the corresponding non-parametric test could be used to examine group differences in frequencies); however, the data used in the analysis have different distributional properties.

As a summary, the measures of central tendency and variability provide descriptive information about the data in your study, including (a) the most common score, (b) the highest and lowest score, (c) the middle score, (d) the average score, (e) the number of scores falling above and below any point in the distribution, (f) the spread of scores, and (g) the deviation of the scores from the average. So if the research question was really just to describe data, researchers could stop here. But where is the fun in that?! Plus, most of the research questions in kinesiology are founded on understanding prediction/association (e.g., relationship between variables) or explanation and group differences (e.g., comparing group means).

Matching Research Questions to Statistical Analyses

A decision tree will help follow the appropriate statistical analyses for the types of questions that are of interest to kinesiology researchers (see Figure 5.5).

Research questions focused on group differences

Let's start with the right side of the decision tree in Figure 5.5. If the research question is to compare means, three main questions are critical to the type of statistical test that would be appropriate. The first question is whether the comparison is between *two* different groups *OR* between the same people measured over *two* time points or within two conditions. If the

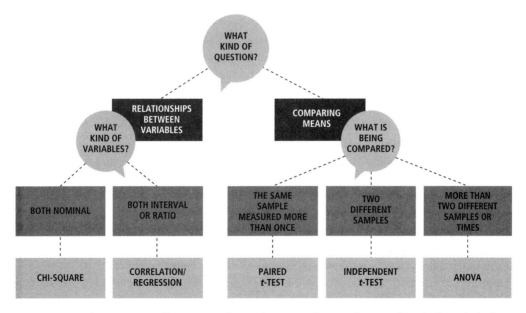

Figure 5.5 A decision tree illustrating the main research questions and logical statistical analyses associated with the questions.

comparisons are focused on two groups (regardless of whether they are different groups or the same people measured twice), the appropriate statistic is called a **t-test**. Generally, a t-test tests the difference between group means, while considering the extent to which the means would differ by chance. Two main types of t-tests are used in the comparison of two means, as represented in Figure 5.5, which are independent and dependent (paired) t-tests. Yet the convention of reporting the t-test is the same across all types of t-tests. Specifically, a t-test is a reflection of the difference in the means between the two groups, conditions, or time points on the numerator divided by the standard error of the differences. The main difference in the two types of t-tests is simply how the standard error is calculated to reflect the research design.

The **standard error** is a measure of how well the sample represents the population. For example, think about how researchers could conduct an experiment to look at how many cups of coffee are needed to stay up all night studying for a kinesiology exam. Researchers could not possibly include all kinesiology students across Canada (which would be the population) so they would need to identify a sample. If the researchers recruit 10 students from each of 10 university kinesiology programs to participate and subsequently study how many cups of coffee each of the 10 students from the different universities consume to stay awake all night, each program might have the following mean number of cups (called a **sample mean**): Students at the University of Ottawa need on average 11 cups, students at the University of Calgary need 9 cups, students at the University of Prince Edward Island need 10 cups (and so on). The average of all these sample means is the population mean (a mean that represents the consumption of cups of coffee among kinesiology students in general), and the standard deviation of the sampling means is an indication of the accuracy of averages. A high standard deviation of the sampling means suggests the scores deviate quite a bit from each other (for example the coffee consumption from the University of Ottawa, Calgary, and Prince Edward Island is quite different). High standard deviation of the sample means shows that the samples are not representative of the population. A smaller standard deviation of the sampling means suggest the scores are quite similar.

The standard deviation of the sampling means is called the **standard error of the mean**. In practice, researchers don't need to collect all kinds of different "sub-samples" to find a standard error of the mean, because this would not be feasible. Instead, there are ways of calculating the standard error using the sample standard deviation and the sample size (the specifics are beyond the scope of this textbook but are clearly described in kinesiology statistics textbooks, such as Vincent and Weir's [2012] *Statistics in kinesiology* textbook).

Now that you have an understanding about the standard error of the mean, which is the denominator in all t-tests, we can return to the discussion about the different types of t-tests. An **independent t-test** is used when the study has two groups of different participants (each participant contributes one score to the data). The name "independent" identifies that the groups are separate from each other. An independent t-test can be used for experimental (if participants are randomly assigned to these groups) and quasi-experimental (if the two groups are convenient or intact) designs.

Writing Exercise

Identify three research questions that would require an independent *t*-test. Specifically, your questions need to reflect having two manipulations (for example, a comparison of treatment condition and a control group, or a comparison of kinesiology students and engineering students). Once you have identified your research questions, do an online search of scholarly material for three articles that have been published that have addressed similar research questions. Look at the study purpose, hypotheses, sample description, measures used, and statistical analysis. Identify the finding resulting from the *t*-test and reflect on the authors' interpretations of the findings.

You might notice that the reporting of a *t*-test result looks something like this: $t (8) = 6.50$. Any *t*-test will be presented this way. The value of the *t*-test statistic is the calculation of the ratio of the group mean differences and the standard error of the differences (in the arbitrary example above, the value is 6.50). This value would then be compared to a critical value obtained from a table during hypothesis testing (presented later in the chapter) to make conclusions. The number in brackets (in this example, 8) is called the **degrees of freedom**. The degrees of freedom are the number of observations that are free to vary, and in an independent *t*-test this number is equal to the sample size (number of participants) of each group minus 2 (because there are always two groups when we use this type of analysis). In conventional statistics notation, the sample size is indicated by an "*N*" and sub-samples are indicated by "*n*." For example, if researchers have a sample of kinesiology students, they could report the sample size as $N = 250$; and then the students split up into recreation and physical education disciplinary areas (sub-samples) could be represented as $n = 100$ and $n = 150$, respectively.

As a quick analogy of degrees of freedom, think of a team-picking situation. Two students are nominated as captains, one for Team Blue and one for Team Red; each then get to pick the players on their team (remember that dreaded feeling of worry for being picked last?). If there are a total of 10 students to be picked for each team, the captains go back and forth picking their teams until two students are left standing. The captain who picked first now gets the chance to basically pick for both teams because her or his decision will identify one player for Team Blue and one player for Team Red. In this example, the number of players that were "free to vary" was eighteen (total team size of 10 individuals minus one for Team Red + total team size of 10 individuals minus one for Team Blue).

When two data points are collected over time (e.g., a pre- and post-test design) or when participants are exposed to the two experimental conditions, a **dependent (or paired) *t*-test** is used. The term "dependent" implies that the data points are related to one another because they are provided by the same people. In this case, each participant contributes two data points; since there is only one sample, the degrees of freedom are equal to the sample size minus one. An example of a research question involving a dependent *t*-test is any question involving a difference in means for two conditions in which all participants are exposed (e.g., "Do individuals

Professional Highlight

Dr Martin J. Gibala, Professor, Department of Kinesiology, McMaster University

....

Profile: Dr Gibala's research is focused on the regulation of skeletal muscle energy production with a particular focus on exercise and nutrition factors associated with metabolic adaptations in skeletal muscle. Dr Gibala conducts research studies examining acute versus chronic differences in metabolic adaptations to different volumes and intensities of exercise training. Most recently, Dr Gibala has been studying the metabolic effects of high-intensity interval training (HIIT). This type of exercise training (small doses of exercise over short periods of time) has garnered attention internationally because of the practical benefits of shorter exercise session durations that are found to have impressive health benefits. The benefits of HIIT training are often examined compared to other types of training at different intensities, and these differences are tested using *t*-tests and ANOVA statistics.

Further Readings

Cochran, A. J. C., Little, J. P., Tarnopolsky, M. A., & Gibala, M. J. (2010). Carbohydrate feeding during recovery alters the skeletal muscle metabolic response to repeated sessions of high-intensity interval exercise in humans. *Journal of Applied Physiology, 108,* 628–36. doi:10.1152/japplphysiol.00659.2009

Gibala, M. J., Little, J. P., MacDonald, M. J., & Hawley, J. A. (2012). Physiological adaptations to low-volume, high-intensity interval training in health and disease. *Journal of Physiology, 590,* 1077–84. doi:10.1113/jphysiol.2011.224725

Tjønna, A. E., Leinan, I. M., Bartnes, A. T., Jenssen, B. M., Gibala, M. J., Winett, R. A., & Wisløff, U. (2013). Low- and high-volume of intensive endurance training significantly improves maximal oxygen uptake after 10-weeks of training in healthy men. *PLoS ONE, 8,* e65382. doi:10.1371/journal.pone.0065382

report higher stress while exercising on a bicycle or on a treadmill"?) or there is an examination of difference/change in means over two time points (e.g., "Do individuals report more stress before or after they run on a treadmill"?). To answer these types of questions, thereby making a dependent *t*-test appropriate, the same participants would need to report stress on both a bike and a treadmill, or complete measures before and after a run.

Going back to Figure 5.5, and looking at the far right of the decision tree, if the research questions involve two or more groups (and many derivatives of this), researchers could use multiple *t*-tests; but it is more appropriate to use a test called an **Analysis of Variance** or **ANOVA**. For example, in Dr Gibala's research, if HIIT training were being compared to one other exercise program (e.g., moderate-intensity interval training) then a *t*-test would be appropriate to compare the means on performance outcomes. However, if HIIT training were being compared to two or more other types of training (e.g., moderate-intensity interval training and high-volume low intensity endurance training), there would be three comparisons to be tested: (a) mean of performance outcome for HIIT training group compared to the mean of performance outcome for moderate-intensity interval training group, (b) the mean of performance outcome for HIIT training group compared to the mean of performance outcome for high-volume low intensity endurance training, and (c) the mean of performance outcome for high-volume low intensity endurance training compared to the mean of performance outcome for the moderate-intensity interval training group. And if there were a control group, this would be an additional three comparisons. All said, the more comparisons that are made, the more chances for error (Type I and Type II errors will be discussed later in this chapter). To avoid this, ANOVA tests allow researchers to compare two or more groups in one test rather than across several separate tests.

As another example, let's consider walking distances of dog owners. Researchers might be interested in comparing the walking distances of pet owners who have teacup chihuahuas (group 1), Labrador retrievers (group 2), and great danes (group 3). If they did an independent *t*-test comparing chihuahua and Labrador retriever owners' distances walked per day, that would not give them the whole story. The researchers would have to do two more *t*-tests to compare Labrador retriever and great dane owners' distances walked per day and chihuahua and great dane owners' distances walked per day. With an ANOVA, researchers compare the three groups at once with what is called an omnibus test (gives a general understanding of whether there are significant differences, but does not specify precisely where those differences are). If the omnibus test (ANOVA) is significant, researchers can then conduct **post-hoc** testing or **planned comparisons** to see where the mean differences are between the groups. As the names imply, post-hoc tests are done after the main analyses to explore where there are group differences (e.g., is the difference in walking distance between owners of chihuahuas and great danes? Labrador retrievers and great danes?). Planned comparisons are proposed and identified before the omnibus test, are based on the alternative hypotheses, and should be limited to a small number (no more than the number of groups minus one; for example, in the walking-distance example no more than two planned comparisons should be done).

Similar to the convention of reporting *t*-tests, the ANOVA is conventionally presented as an *F*-statistic such as $F(2, 147) = 6.50$. In this fictitious example, the numbers in the brackets $(2, 147)$ are the degrees of freedom, the value of the *F*-test (6.50) provides an indication of whether there are differences among the two or more groups. In ANOVA models, there are always two degrees of freedom values reported. While the convention of these values changes depending on the type of ANOVA model, they basically represent degrees of freedom related to the number of groups (denoted as a k) minus one, and sample size minus number of groups $(N - k)$. In the example above, you could use the degrees of freedom to identify the following characteristics of the study. First, the "2" is $k - 1$ (number of groups minus one), which indicates that there were three groups. Second, the "147" is the "$N - k$" part (sample size minus number of groups); so if $k = 3$, then the sample size is $3 + 147 = 150$. Therefore, based only on the degrees of freedom, we already know that there were three groups and 150 people in the sample.

Different types of ANOVA models can be tested. If more than one independent variable is manipulated, we use a **factorial ANOVA**. This is quite common in kinesiology research because the questions are usually more complicated than a simple group difference. If we manipulated sex of the dog owner in our above example, we would need to use factorial ANOVA because we would have type of dog (which has three groups or levels) and sex (which has two groups or levels). In notation, our study would be a 3 (dog type) × 2 (sex) factorial ANOVA. Within this type of model, there are two **main effects** (mean differences in walking distance between owners of each dog type and mean difference in walking distance between men and women). There is also an **interaction** that is important (does walking distance depend on the sex of the dog owner and the type of dog?). In fact, the interaction is of primary interest in this type of design. Often, it is easiest to visualize this type of model. In Figure 5.6, you can see the data we are discussing in a visual 3 × 2 diagram.

Without going into details on the underlying math involved in calculating the *F*-statistic, there are a few interesting observations to make about the data presented in Figure 5.6. If you calculate the mean distance travelled for males, you would use the data (1.0 + 8.0 + 1.5) ÷ 3 = 3.5; for females it would be (1.5 + 10.0 + 2.0) ÷ 3 = 4.5. Visually, you can see there is a difference in walking distance between males and females, with females walking, on average, 1.0 units more than males (but without calculating the main effect, we don't know if this difference is statistically significant). You can also look at the mean walking distance for the different dog breeds (means = 1.25, 9, and 1.75, respectively for chihuahuas, Labrador retrievers, and great danes). Again, these simple calculations show you a little bit about the data because individuals who own Labrador retrievers walk further than those with great danes, who walk a little further than those with chihuahuas. The actual calculations to explore these differences would be done, compared to the critical value in the statistical table, and then decisions on the hypotheses would be made (but learning the actual statistics is beyond the scope of this text).

Other types of ANOVA models include **Repeated Measures ANOVA**, which is a statistical analysis to use when researchers have two or more time points (e.g., the same people measured a few or more times, such as a baseline assessment, post-intervention, and a follow-up). **Analysis of Covariance** (ANCOVA) is used when researchers have control variables that they have identified as important in the analysis. For example, if the researchers wanted to control for the age of their participants in the study on walking distance of dog owners, they would use an ANCOVA model that statistically equals out the distance walked across age so that they can look at dog type irrespective of the age of their participants. Multivariate ANOVA (i.e., MANOVA),

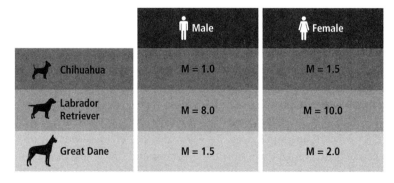

Figure 5.6 A fictitious example of a 3 × 2 Factorial ANOVA Model.

Dog illustrations: © iStock/Counterfeit_ua; People icons: © iStock/Sudowoodo

Statistics Exercise

Identify a research purpose and related hypotheses that would match the following statistical analyses:

1. Independent *t*-test
2. Dependent *t*-test
3. ANOVA
4. Factorial ANOVA
5. Repeated Measures ANOVA
6. ANCOVA

which is well beyond the scope of this chapter, simply means that the effects on more than one *dependent* variable are considered simultaneously as a collective set in the ANOVA analysis. Of course, all of these models can get very complicated with multiple levels of the independent variable, multiple independent and dependent variables, and multiple measurements or data collection time points!

A final type of group differences analysis needs to be discussed for data that are nominal or ordinal (i.e., non-parametric tests of differences). In this instance, researchers are interested in understanding and testing the difference in frequencies or numbers of responses and making comparisons to expected outcomes. A **chi-square test** (denoted as χ^2) is used to examine the discrepancy in frequencies between groups or a comparison between the frequency data outcome and what would be expected by chance. To use a chi-square analysis, the observations need to be independent and the categories need to be mutually exclusive (e.g., the data from the same person cannot be represented in more than one category). For example, researchers might be interested in knowing how many kinesiology students and arts and science students have a grade point average of a B+ or better in the first year of university. Each student in this example would fit into one of four categories: (a) kinesiology major and a grade less than B+, (b) kinesiology major and a grade of B+ or better, (c) arts and science major and a grade less than B+, or (d) arts and science major and a grade of B+ or better. A common practice in chi-square analysis is to report the data in a **contingency table** (i.e., a classification system in which two or more groups respond on two or more categories or outcomes). In our example, we would have both the number of students who are kinesiology majors and the number of students who are arts and science majors, and then from these two groups we would next need to identify how many students have a B+ average or better and how many students have a grade less than B+. The result is a 2 × 2 table shown in Table 5.2. Comparisons could be made in the actual number of students in these categories (indicated by a "$n = $" in Table 5.2) and the expected outcome (calculated as the number of students represented in each of the four groups divided by the total number of students in the sample). This statistical procedure is called the chi-square test and once calculated can be used in hypothesis testing to make decisions on whether there are differences in the grade frequencies of students in these majors.

Table 5.2 A 2 × 2 contingency table.

	GRADES	
	< B+	≥ B+
Major: Kinesiology	$n =$	$n =$
Major: Arts & Science	$n =$	$n =$

Other examples of kinesiology-related questions that might utilize a chi-square test include: How many varsity athletes continue to engage in competitive sports after university? How many women who weight train take protein supplements? How many individuals who suffer from a heart attack engage in running, cycling, or swimming exercise?

A number of additional tests could be used that are analogous to the parametric tests (e.g., Mann-Whitney *U*, Kruskal-Wallis) when the data are rank ordered. The key interpretations are similar, and at this point it is merely important to understand that different tests are used when the data are parametric or non-parametric.

Case Study

Teagan and Maya are Ph.D. students in two different kinesiology research laboratories at Acadia University. In her thesis work, Teagan has found that her participants experience fewer injuries in their sports during times when they are reporting the lowest levels of stress. Maya has results from her thesis research participants showing that higher levels of stress are related to lower academic performance in some classes. Based on their mutual interests, Teagan and Maya want to conduct a research project that combines their independent interests to look at the effects of stress in sport and academic performance.

Discussion Questions

1. Both researchers measured stress using a self-report questionnaire and salivary cortisol. If Teagan and Maya wanted to first compare the stress levels of their current participants, what type of analysis would they use?
2. Help Teagan and Maya design a study to examine changes in stress over time among student athletes. What would the study design look like? What would the research hypothesis be? Identify an appropriate measure of stress, and list any possible covariates or confounding variables in the study. Identify the appropriate analysis to answer this research question.
3. If the study were now designed to compare students and athletes, how would the analysis plan change?
4. After reading the next sections in the chapter, design a study based on the general topic of stress and performance involving a question that would be answered using correlation analysis.

In summary, various techniques can be used for conditions in which the primary interest is centred on differences among groups. The key is to understand why a certain type of analysis is appropriate. The best way to understand these concepts is to read research papers on the topics in kinesiology that interest you. Pay attention to the statistical analysis and results sections rather than jumping to the punch line in the discussion. The more you read, the more these concepts will become clear.

Research questions focused on relationships between variables

Go back to the decision tree in Figure 5.5. If the research questions pertain to associations between variables or prediction (the left side of the figure), the type of analysis is focused on correlation and regression. **Correlation** is a statistical technique that allows a researcher to determine the relationship between two or more variables. For example, what is the relationship between skating speed and number of injuries? Between height and weight? Between step count and fitness level? Correlations can be calculated between more than two variables as well, such as the relationship between number of years of sport participation and mental health outcomes including depression, anxiety, stress, and affect. In the language of correlation study designs, the dependent variable may be called the **criterion** and the independent variable(s) may be labelled as **predictor** variable(s).

The **correlation coefficient** can range from 0.0 to 1.0 in either a negative or positive direction. The closer the value is to 1.0, the stronger the association between the variables, whereas the closer to 0.0 means there is little to no relationship. In principle, a **positive correlation** exists when large values of one variable are associated with large values of another variable (e.g., the more steps a person takes per day is usually associated with a greater distance travelled) or small values on one variable are associated with small values on another (e.g., if an individual reports no symptoms of depression and also low stress). A **negative correlation** exists when large values for one variable are related to lower values on another variable or vice versa. For example, higher fat mass is associated with a lower number of chin-ups completed. Several different variations of correlations are depicted in Figure 5.7. The two top graphs depict positive relationships, the middle graphs visualize negative correlations, and the bottom image is a graphical representation of a null or no correlation. When you look at these graphs, do the ones on the left or the right depict stronger relationships?

To orient you on the graphs, the x-axis (the horizontal axis) represents one variable and the vertical or y-axis represents a second variable. As you can see in the figures on the left (both the positive correlation depicted at the top and negative correlation depicted in the middle), the diagonal lines representing the relationship between the variables are almost at perfect 45-degree angles. These graphs are representations of perfect or near-perfect correlations, and the coefficients would be close to +1 and –1, respectively. The graphs to the right of these (near) perfect associations represent relationships that are still generally positive or negative but not as strong as their counterparts to the left (yet still stronger than the bottom association). The coefficients would be somewhere between 0 and +1 (top right graph) and –1 and 0 (middle right graph).

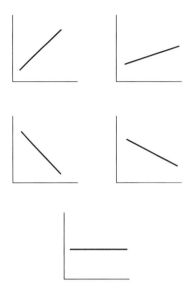

Figure 5.7 Graphical representations of positive (top two graphs), negative (middle two graphs), and no (bottom graph) correlation among two variables.

When a correlation coefficient is calculated between one criterion (dependent) and one predictor or correlate (independent) variable and both variables are interval or ratio data types, it is called a **Pearson product moment correlation coefficient** and is denoted by the symbol *r*. In this case, every person has provided a score on the measure of the criterion variable and a score on the measure of the predictor variable. For example, you would measure every person's body fat mass in your sample and have every person complete a chin-up performance test. Pearson correlation coefficients are often used to examine validity evidence in measures used in kinesiology research. The foundation of a correlation is essential to measurement validity and reliability such that you ideally want higher associations between your measures purporting to assess similar variables (e.g., skinfold thickness and waist circumference), which would provide evidence of construct validity (i.e., evidence that you are measuring what you think you are measuring). Remember, in the research highlight presented earlier in this chapter, positive correlations of $r = .20$ and $r = .44$ were provided as validity evidence comparing accelerometer data to the International Physical Activity Questionnaire and the Physical Activity for Adults Questionnaire. Based on these values, what self-report measure of physical activity would you choose when studying a large sample of adults? The higher correlation coefficient equates to higher validity evidence, and as such is the better measure. Also, you want higher associations between scores of the same test measured twice (e.g., reliability) to show consistency. Reliability might be assessed if the Physical Activity for Adults Questionnaire was completed twice in one day and the scores were compared, with higher values indicating better consistency. Construct validity will be described in more detail in Chapter 6.

When ordinal or rank-ordered data are collected, the association between these data is called a **Spearman Rank correlation coefficient**, denoted by *rho*. For example, if researchers were interested in knowing if the number of letters in a person's surname was related to their ranking in a running race, they would calculate a Spearman Rank correlation coefficient. This analysis would *likely* lead to a minimal relationship and small coefficient close to zero, although it could happen that surnames are ethnically and/or culturally bound; so it might happen that people with longer surnames run faster or slower than people with shorter surnames. We offer no hypothesis on this matter, this is an example of why correlation does not equal causation (e.g., even if surname length is correlated with running speed, changing someone's surname is probably not the most effective way to help them run faster!). In summary, when the research question is focused on associations, the statistical technique is to calculate a correlation coefficient. Now go back to the case study presented earlier (remember Teagan and Maya studying stress and performance) and answer the last question involving the design of a research study using correlation as the main analytical plan.

If researchers are interested in prediction (a concept related to correlation), **regression analysis** is used. Using regression analysis, researchers might be interested in understanding whether knowing an individual's fitness level (measured as maximal aerobic capacity) would predict their cycling speed in a long-distance race (i.e., can you identify, within a margin of error of course, whether someone will be faster or slower in a cycling race by knowing their fitness?). Regression analysis is based on the line of best fit and the foundational properties of a straight line (where the line intersects the *y*-axis [the intercept], and the slope or angle of the line). Essentially, the stronger the correlation between two variables, the better the prediction.

Research questions focused on summarizing findings

So far in this text we have presented the elements of a research study that flow logically from the identification of the problem, literature search that is foundational to focusing on a topic and purpose, and methodologies that fit with the purpose. However, a more detailed literature review (called a **research synthesis**) can also stand alone as a research publication, if the research question involves an evaluation and integration of published literature.

A common and emerging technique for research synthesis in kinesiology is called a **meta-analysis**, which involves the identification of a problem to address, a methodology that explains decisions for the literature review and analysis, and an analysis that integrates findings from a number of studies to quantify the findings in a standard metric called an **effect size**. Using an effect size, researchers can compare the findings from different studies that have used different designs, data collection methods and tools, and statistical analyses by examining the meaningfulness of group differences in the studies under review. In this way, experimental group means and control group means from different studies can be compared and summarized in a common metric that can be analyzed using the techniques described throughout this chapter (e.g., *t*-tests, ANOVA, chi-square, regression). For example, Oscar is interested in whether or not there are differences in the effects of hydrotherapy on joint pain for older versus younger individuals. He searches the literature and finds eight experimental studies examining hydrotherapy among adults over 75 years of age and another 12 studies examining the same treatment for adults under the age of 60 years. He calculates the effect size for each of the 20 studies, and then calculates the mean and standard deviation of the effect sizes for the studies focused on older adults and younger adults separately. Once he has these mean (and standard deviation) effect sizes, these values are then used in an additional statistical analysis, such as a *t*-test, to compare the effects of hydrotherapy on joint pain for older and younger individuals.

In their handbook of research synthesis and meta-analysis, Cooper, Hedges, and Valentine (2009) describe the various methods of meta-analysis in detail. Based on their recommendations, the following is a summary of the key steps that can be followed when conducting a meta-analysis:

1. Identify a problem.
2. Perform a literature search using specified criteria.
3. Review identified research publications to determine eligibility (i.e., do they fit with the purpose? Should they be included or excluded from the meta-analysis?).
4. Read and evaluate the studies to describe and code important characteristics.
5. Calculate an effect size.
6. Use appropriate statistical analyses to make conclusions.
7. Report all decisions and steps in the research publication.

Related to the last step, there is a well-documented reporting system for research syntheses and meta-analyses called the Preferred Reporting Items for Systematic Reviews and Meta-Analyses (PRISMA). The PRISMA represents an evidence-based minimum criteria for reporting this type of research. There are published guidelines, a chart, and flow diagram to help researchers appropriately report the steps involved in a meta-analysis with the goal of improving how these data and findings are published. See Figure 5.8 for a sample PRISMA flow chart published by Moher, Liberati, Tetzlaff, Altman, and The PRISMA Group (2009).

Given that meta-analysis uses a statistical technique to integrate results from multiple studies, this approach improves power over individual studies, improves the estimates of the size of the effect, and helps clarify if there is disagreement among individual study findings. Since this technique is an integration of various study findings, the results can be generalized in a way that fosters external validity. Although there are methods for identifying publication bias during the meta-analysis process, publication bias nonetheless can be a weakness of meta-analysis. Specifically, publication bias refers to the reliance on available, published studies in meta-analysis that might lead to exaggerated findings, and it often results from negative or non-significant findings not being published. In addition, a meta-analysis of poorly designed studies cannot correct for weak study designs, so an effective meta-analysis relies heavily on well-designed research studies. Finally, some meta-analyses might be driven by political, social, or economic agendas, which can also lead to biased outcomes.

Overall, meta-analysis is of increasing interest among kinesiology researchers, and there are even journals dedicated to reviews and syntheses in the field (e.g., *Exercise and Sport Science Review; Exercise Immunology Review; International Review of Sport and Exercise Psychology*). Many other journals also publish synthesis research, in particular when it

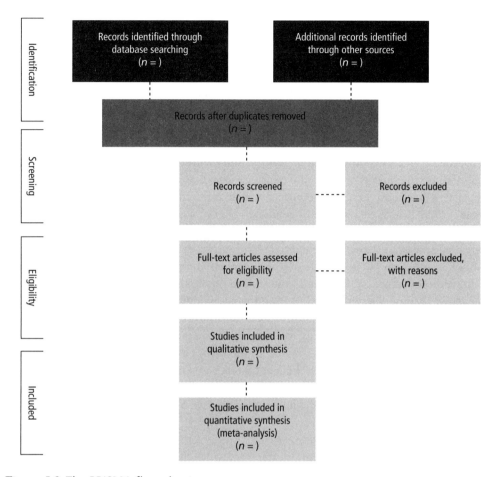

Figure 5.8 The PRISMA flow chart.

Source: Moher et al., 2009.

follows appropriate steps and guidelines (e.g., PRISMA). The augmented use and need for meta-analysis in kinesiology research is likely due to the importance of this technique for theory testing, building evidence-based guidelines, and making important decisions on key topics of relevance to kinesiology researchers and practitioners.

A Brief Primer on Hypothesis Testing

We have alluded to hypothesis testing throughout this chapter. As defined in Chapter 2, a hypothesis is the scientific guess that a researcher has about the study. The **null** (e.g., there is no difference between groups or relationship between variables) and **alternative** (e.g., directional difference or relationship) hypotheses are identified, and statistical procedures based on probability statistics are used to determine if they hold true (remember "reject the null hypothesis" and "fail to reject the null hypothesis"?). Statistics can also give researchers an indication of the amount of error in their decision. Remember that the hypotheses are stated in a way that only one or the other can be true (not both) and that the outcome of hypothesis testing includes a likelihood or chance of this decision being right or wrong.

Probability of error in statistics is usually depicted as a "*p*-value," and it should be of no surprise that researchers want to reduce the chances of error as much as possible. However, it is (nearly) impossible for researchers to conduct a study with *no* error. A *p*-value of .05 equates to there being 5% room for error or chance, which is equivalent to being 95% confident that the results are genuine and not a chance finding. If the probability of a finding is less than or equal to .05, then the null hypothesis can be rejected and the researchers can conclude that there is a significant relationship or mean difference (Fisher, 1956). This level of confidence is quite standard in kinesiology research practice; however, researchers also commonly use *p* less than or equal to .01 (which equates to 99% confident) or even *p* less than or equal to .001 (meaning 99.9% confident). The smaller the *p*-value the less error there is in the decision . . . but also the more precise one has to be and the more rare the outcome.

For example, the purpose of a group of researchers' quasi-experimental study might be to examine the difference between males and females on the amount of sweat they produce when exercising. Their null hypothesis (H_0) is that there is no difference between males and females on their amount of sweat when exercising. The alternative hypothesis (H_1) is that males sweat more than females when exercising. It is ideal to have a justification for alternative hypotheses, and usually this justification is based on theory or empirical evidence. In this example, the researchers have come up with this hypothesis based on physiological explanations that suggest males are "made" to sweat more (see Ichinose-Kuwahara et al. [2010] for an experimental test of this proposition). The null and alternative hypotheses can be described using conventional notation:

H_0: males sweat = females sweat
H_1: males sweat > females sweat

In our hypothetical example, the researchers' design has males and females exercising at 55% of their maximum oxygen consumption on a bicycle for 25 minutes in a laboratory. All participants have their exercise scheduled on the same day, with the room temperature held constant for all participants. Data are collected on sweat (as measured by absorption paper), and then the values for males and females are compared. Remember that the key question is: Do males and females sweat differently? There are two possibilities: First, there is an actual difference between males and females (due to physiological, biological, or other reasons); or, second, being male or female has no impact at all on sweating during exercise. Using conventional statistical procedures for hypothesis testing, the researchers would test their hypotheses with a *p*-value of .05, meaning that they would be 95% confident that the outcome of the hypothesis testing is genuine and not due to error.

Next, in the process of hypothesis testing, the researchers would calculate a statistic based on their data and compare that statistic to comparator statistics listed in **critical value tables** in most statistics textbooks. In a critical value table, the researchers can locate the *p*-value or level of confidence that they want to set for their research study, find the value that they need to achieve in order to have a statistically significant outcome, and compare their actual calculated value to this critical value. If their calculated value is equal to or larger than the critical value, they can claim statistical significance at the p-value they have chosen (in the example above, at $p = .05$). Think of this as a high jump analogy. The critical value at a corresponding p-value is the height of the bar and is the value identified in the critical value table. If researchers want to be 95% confident that their decision is not due to error, the bar would be set at a certain height; whereas if they wanted to be 99% confident (p-value of equal to or less than .01), they would need to set the bar higher. Their calculated statistic (the performer in the high jump) needs to be at least as high as the bar in order to claim that there is a statistically significant outcome and that they can reject the null hypothesis (e.g., if they clear the high jump bar, victory!). In principle, critical values are higher as the p-values get smaller.

Using this practice of hypothesis testing, the researchers in our sweating study example would reject the null hypothesis that there is no difference between males and females on the amount of sweat if the critical value at the corresponding p-value is less than their calculated value. The researchers would fail to reject the null hypothesis if the critical value is larger than their calculated value. However, even with only a 5% likelihood that the results occur by chance, there is still a small chance (or two) that the researchers made the wrong decision. These errors in decision are labelled Type I and Type II error.

A **Type I error** happens when researchers make the decision that a manipulation or treatment has been successful when in fact it has not been. This could arise when the samples are different for some reason other than the manipulation. Maybe the men in the previous example all used the sauna in the change room before the experiment and started with higher core temperatures; thus, the men in their study might sweat more simply because they started to sweat faster or earlier in their exercise than the females. A **Type II error** happens when researchers make the decision that the manipulation has failed, when in reality it actually did work. In other words, the researcher fails to reject the null hypothesis, when it actually should be rejected.

There is an obvious trade-off between Type I and II errors, since if we lower the probability of accepting an effect as genuine or true then we will inevitably inflate the probability that we will reject an effect that does not genuinely exist. As such, it is impossible to equally reduce the chances of making both errors, because making one type of error is always more probable than the other. Type I and II errors are often presented in the form of a truth table (see Table 5.3).

At this point in the chapter, we have addressed the steps in hypothesis testing to include stating the null and alternative hypotheses, setting a level of confidence or significance about the chance of making a Type I or Type II error, and then deciding whether to reject or fail to reject the null hypothesis. We have also discussed the actual analysis needed to make our "fail to reject" or "reject" decisions based on the hypotheses. While we have not

Table 5.3 The decision table for errors associated with hypothesis testing.

	NULL HYPOTHESIS IS TRUE	NULL HYPOTHESIS IS FALSE
Rejecting null hypothesis	Error Type I	Correct Outcome
Accepting null hypothesis	Correct Outcome	Error Type II

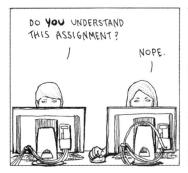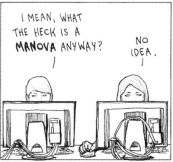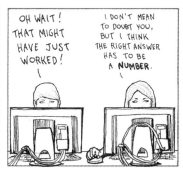

gone into the details on how to calculate specific statistics, it is important to mention that all of the statistics and related outcomes can be completed using computer software. Some of the analyses can be done in Microsoft Excel, including many of the ways of presenting the data. However, powerful statistical software packages that are commonly used in kinesiology research include the Statistical Package for the Social Sciences (SPSS), R, and SAS. These programs provide ways of visualizing data, testing assumptions, setting hypotheses and critical values, and running analyses that test the types of research questions illustrated in this chapter (and much more).

Statistical Significance versus Practical Significance

Remember the earlier example of dog type and walking distance in which we explored the mean distance travelled between male and female dog owners (and dog types)? We alluded to the idea that while the scores "looked" different, they might not be statistically different. In order to formally test the hypotheses, researchers need to make decisions based on the statistical outcome of their tests. These tests are essentially a comparison of the data they have collected to the critical values printed in statistical tables (including critical values for t, F, χ^2, r statistics, among others). Remember though that any decision based on the comparison of calculated and critical values is a *statistical* decision. However, this statistical significance (rejecting the null hypothesis with some level of confidence, usually 95%, which was discussed earlier as represented by $p = .05$) does not always correspond to meaningful decisions, especially in cases where the sample size is too small (or too large).

Practical significance or meaningfulness of the findings can be described as the effect sizes in research. A number of different coefficients are used for indicators of meaningfulness of the findings, but the general principle suggests that higher values infer greater effect sizes and are often reported as small, moderate, and strong effects (Cohen, 1988). These effect sizes are used to represent *practical* decisions. The idea of practical significance is often described in the context of data from clinical trials, where a study design might preclude large effects being seen but in which any observed effects are extremely valuable, such as the difference between life or death, or the difference between the experience of symptoms or not.

For example, researchers developed a drug that basically encapsulated all of the physical and emotional effects of exercise and tested the effects (remember this hypothetical example from Chapter 4?). They found only 10 people who were willing to try the new drug prior to further health and safety checks, but 6 out of the 10 people self-reported great benefits and improvements on physical measures related to cardiovascular health and weight. Since there were only 10 people, the findings of all the tests did not reach statistical significance (e.g., the calculated values of the dependent sample *t*-tests comparing pre- and post-test scores on measures of affect, mood, cardiovascular fitness, and body composition were smaller than the critical values at a *p*-value of .05). But despite the statistics being non-significant, the differences observed were still deemed to be quite meaningful (e.g., moderate effect sizes and an observation that the results were all in the direction that would be expected for beneficial effects of the drug). If the decisions were based solely on statistics, the researchers might have stopped their testing and concluded that there is no way of developing an "exercise" drug. However, the meaningfulness of the findings suggests that more research is needed before making final decisions. Maybe it is a good point in the experimental process to seek out some funding from the *Dragons' Den* investors and find more people to test the drug's effects.

In general, practical or meaningful decisions are more subjective and based on the reasons for conducting the research in the first place. If researchers want to develop new programs, make changes to course content, develop new tests, etc., their decisions might not always be hinged on statistically significant findings.

Summary

In this chapter, the different types of statistical techniques used in kinesiology research were discussed. There was an overview of hypothesis testing. There was a description of the match between the research question and design with the appropriate analysis focused on questions of description (measures of central tendency and variability), group difference (*t*-test, ANOVA), and relationships (correlation), or prediction (regression). An overview of measures of central tendency and variability was provided. Finally, statistical and practical relevance of findings in kinesiology research were briefly discussed.

Discussion Questions

1. Why are statistics important? (Identify as many answers to this question as you can.)
2. Can you identify the appropriate statistical technique for the following research examples? Hint: it might be useful to identify the number of groups, and number and type of measurement of the independent variables.
    a. Subha is interested in studying improvements in balance among older adults after a virtual reality intervention.
    b. Martine wants to examine the difference in time spent on a running wheel for mice exposed to a carbohydrate-only diet, a protein-only diet, or a fat-only diet.

    c.   Lyle will look at whether grades in university predict average lifetime income.

    d.   Ryan is interested in knowing whether her new running shoe design reduces ankle injuries in soccer players. She has access to a group of recreational and competitive athletes, so she randomly provides all the athletes with either her own shoe design or a competitor prototype model to examine the number of injuries in the athletes.

    e.   Ryan's brother Nafis wants to follow up with her study and looks at the differences in injuries based on the shoe type and the status of the athlete (recreational or competitive).

3.   How do you define the mode, median, and mean? How do you identify types of research problems and data types when these measures of central tendency are appropriate?

4.   Can you draw a histogram with a large standard deviation? What about a histogram with a small standard deviation?

Recommended Readings

Cooper, H., Hedges, L. V., & Valentine, J. C. (2009). *The handbook of research synthesis and meta-analysis* (2nd ed.). New York, NY: Russell Sage.

Thomas, J., Nelson, J., & Silverman, S. (2015). *Research methods in physical activity* (7th ed.). Champaign, IL: Human Kinetics.

Vincent, W., & Weir, J. (2012). *Statistics in kinesiology* (4th ed.). Champaign, IL: Human Kinetics.

6 Evaluating the Merits of Quantitative Research Studies in Kinesiology

Learning Outcomes

By the end of this chapter, you should be able to:

- Apply the standard of validity to evaluate the merits of quantitative research studies in kinesiology.

- Discuss why researchers are left to make judgments on the merits of a study based only on logical validity and construct validity in non-experimental designs.

- Discuss the strengths of experimental designs.

- Provide kinesiology examples of logical validity, construct validity, internal validity, and external validity.

A Brief Primer on Validity as a Standard for Evaluating Quantitative Research

A quote commonly attributed to Albert Einstein is, "If we knew what we were doing, it wouldn't be called research." High-quality research is very hard to conduct and often hard to identify—and although low-quality research might be easier to do, it can sometimes be equally hard to identify! As a result, one of the most challenging things about reading kinesiology research, especially for someone relatively new to research, is being able to evaluate whether or not a study is "good." Therefore, knowing *how* to critique the research you hear and read about is a necessary skill. It enables you to understand the merits of researchers' research questions, their justifications provided for the research, their choice in methods, their conclusions made, and the potential implications and application of the findings to professionals and the real world. An understanding of the concept of validity, which you were introduced to in Chapter 4, is essential in this effort.

Logical validity refers to the quality of researchers' arguments, their application of theory to support the needs for the study, and the appropriate interpretation of results based on the data. In other words, in assessing the logical validity of a study we want to ask the following question: Have the researchers provided a convincing justification for all aspects of the research project? There is obviously no single way to evaluate logical validity, since each study will have many unique elements. In addition, there can often be great debate among researchers over the logical validity of a study, because not everyone agrees on what a convincing argument entails. This is one reason why there are multiple theories of the same phenomenon in many areas of kinesiology research. What might be considered a meritorious argument from one perspective might be considered faulty from another perspective. Hence, the most effective way to adequately evaluate the logical validity of a study is to become knowledgeable about both kinesiology content and about research methods themselves . . . as well as to utilize strong critical thinking skills in the evaluation process.

Construct validity refers to whether the measures used by researchers do indeed measure what they intended to measure, and it is a bit more concrete to evaluate than logical validity. Measurement is at the heart of quantitative research, and without strong measures of variables of interest the research will be of little use. In other words, researchers need measures that are both consistent (reliable) and accurate (valid), which is why construct validity is a main focus of most research methods texts. Construct validity is critical to all research studies that measure variables. For example, if we are interested in studying the leisure-time physical activity levels of children using accelerometers, but the accelerometers can't be used in water without being destroyed (e.g., when swimming), their validity as a measurement tool to assess children's leisure-time physical activity will be limited. Also limited would be any subsequent conclusions we make as to how leisure-time physical activity is related to other variables (e.g., television watching).

One of the reasons experimental designs are held in such high regard as a quantitative research method is that there are simply more types of validity relevant to experimental designs compared to other types of quantitative research (e.g., cross-sectional or other non-experimental designs). Recall that **internal validity** specifically refers to researchers' abilities to claim that any change in an outcome is the result of a treatment or intervention and not a result of other factors (e.g., maturation, a change in the weather, social desirability). For example, if we are conducting a study on chiropractic spinal manipulation, we want to have confidence that patient improvement is indeed due to the spinal manipulation and not due to other factors such as change in activity level, natural healing processes, or other modalities. Otherwise the claims we make about the effectiveness of spinal manipulation might be inaccurate. However, regardless of the effectiveness of a treatment or intervention, the main point is that in order to make a judgment about internal validity, there *needs* to be a treatment or intervention, which is the hallmark of experimental designs.

Likewise, the concept of **external validity** refers to researchers' abilities to see similar successes of the treatment or intervention with other populations, in other contexts, and across time. If the effects of a particular treatment or intervention do not generalize to other people, places, and time, then the causal claims that are made become a lot more questionable. For example, if we are conducting a study on the effectiveness of ingestion of a particular protein supplement on soccer players' performances, but the benefits only occur in very tightly controlled laboratory settings and are specific to the players in our sample, any general claim that the protein is effective for soccer players' performances is likely not warranted (or weak at best). But again, because a judgment of external validity requires a treatment or intervention, it too is a standard of evaluation that we can only adequately make in the context of experimental designs.

In other words, in order to evaluate the internal validity and external validity of a study, a manipulation of an independent variable (as a result of a treatment or intervention) is required.

In the absence of a manipulation of the independent variable, as is the case in cross-sectional studies, researchers are left to make judgments on the merits of a study based only on logical validity and construct validity.

Experimental studies are one form of quantitative research. Four criteria, logical validity, construct validity, internal validity, and external validity, are used to evaluate the merits of experimental studies. Evidence of all four types of validity provide confidence in causal claims made by experimental researchers. Only two of those criteria, logical validity and construct validity, can be used to evaluate the merits of non-experimental quantitative studies.

This does not mean that experimental studies are always better than other types of studies (that depends on many factors). In addition, questions of *generalizability* (which you were introduced to in Chapter 4) are still important to non-experimental research, because a goal of most researchers who conduct quantitative studies is to be able to generalize their findings to a population beyond the specific sample included in their research, regardless of the design.

One of the most widely used guidelines to assist both researchers and readers of randomized control trial (RCT) research designs, often considered the "gold standard" of experimental research, are the Consolidated Standards of Reporting Trials (CONSORT) statements that were originally developed in 1996 and subsequently updated in 2001 and 2010 (Schultz et al., 2010). The most recent version, the CONSORT 2010 statement, includes a 25-item checklist and flow diagram outlining the types of information that should be included by researchers when reporting RCTs, more specifically RCTs with random assignment to two groups (Moher et al., 2010; Schultz et al., 2010). Examples of the types of things researchers should report include any changes to the methods after the trial began, specific methods used for random assignment of participants to groups, dates that define the period from recruitment to follow-up, any harms or unintended effects in each group, and sources of funding. In fact, many journals now require authors to explain how the CONSORT guidelines have been addressed in their submitted manuscripts (Schultz et al., 2010). The CONSORT 2010 statement is available for free at the website http://www.annals.org (the easiest way to find it is to type "CONSORT 2010" into the search engine on the website and download the "CONSORT *2010 Statement: Updated Guidelines for Reporting Parallel Group Randomized Trials*" article). These guidelines are relevant to kinesiology because many RCTs in our field use a two-group, randomized design, and are particularly useful guidelines for training studies in which there is random assignment of participants to either a training group

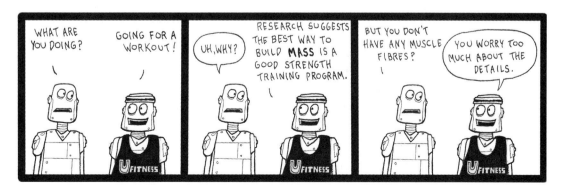

(e.g., high intensity interval training) or control group. However, despite the usefulness and widespread appeal of the CONSORT 2010 statement, it is simply meant to serve as a guide for what researchers *should* report, as opposed to an instrument that should be used to assess the quality of a research design (Schultz et al., 2010).

Another challenge that researchers face is that *all* studies have limitations. So rather than holding research to a standard of perfection using absolutes of "good" or "bad," it is best to consider the merits of any research study on a continuum ranging from high quality to low quality. As evidence of a particular claim shows up consistently across a number of high-quality studies (e.g., that strength training results in muscle hypertrophy), we can begin to have increased confidence that the findings are true. (Ascertaining truth is, ultimately, the goal of quantitative researchers who operate within a postpositivist philosophical worldview, as discussed in Chapter 4).

The remainder of this chapter provides a more specific focus on whether and how we might apply the standards of logical validity, construct validity, internal validity, and external validity to real-world examples of research in kinesiology. As a quick summary, Table 6.1 provides an overview of the types of evidence that can be used to evaluate the merits of experimental and non-experimental research.

Case Study

Juan is a consultant working for Sport Canada and has recently taken on a professional golfer as a client. His client says that she's struggling to hit her tee shots long enough to qualify for major championship tournaments. As a result, and in an effort to learn more about the technical aspects of the golf swing, Juan registers for a professional conference at which one of the advertised symposium topics is on "how to play better golf." During one of the talks at the symposium, Dr Watson refers to some of his "experiments" in which he claims to have discovered that when golfers use a driver with a shorter shaft length, they are able to hit much farther tee shots. Juan's immediate thought is that Dr Watson's "finding" has much relevance to his client. Unfortunately, Dr Watson doesn't go into the details of his experiment, and although intrigued, Juan wonders whether Dr Watson is correct in his claim and is hesitant to utilize this information in his work with his client until he has more confidence in Dr Watson's results.

Discussion Questions

1. What questions might Juan ask Dr Watson to help him make a judgment on the validity of Dr Watson's "experiment" and his claim that a shorter driver shaft length leads to longer tee shots? Specifically, think of questions related to:

    *   Logical validity
    *   Construct validity
    *   Internal validity
    *   External validity

2. How might Dr Watson's apparent knowledge of research methods impact Juan's reaction to (and confidence in) his answer?

Table 6.1 The types of validity evidence that can be used to evaluate the merits of experimental and non-experimental research studies.

	CAN THE TYPE OF VALIDITY BE USED AS CRITERIA FOR EVALUATION? (YES/NO)	
TYPE OF VALIDITY	**EXPERIMENTAL DESIGNS**	**NON-EXPERIMENTAL DESIGNS**
Logical validity	Yes	Yes
Construct validity	Yes	Yes
Internal validity	Yes	No
External validity	Yes	No (but generalizability is still important)

Application of Logical Validity

To assess the logical validity of a study, we must examine the logical flow of researchers' arguments and decision-making from the beginning to the end of their research. To do this, we need to read and critically evaluate the entire research report (typically presented as a journal article). Otherwise, we are unable to piece together the entire puzzle of a research study, and we risk missing elements that might make the research study more or less meritorious.

For example, you might read two separate studies, each stating in their final conclusion that "hip flexibility increases athletes' speed." However, what if one study was conducted with a sample of sedentary older adults and the other conducted with Olympic athletes? Even without knowing any other detail of the two studies, the latter would seem to warrant more confidence in the logical validity of the research than the former simply because it studied athletes (thereby having a sample that more closely matches the population identified in the conclusion). There are, of course, many other aspects that could further support or refute the logical validity of each of these two studies beyond the participants' characteristics. In each instance we should ask ourselves, "Does this logically make sense, and has it been sufficiently justified by the researchers?" If so, logical validity is strengthened. If not, logical validity is weakened.

To further apply the criteria of logical validity, let's consider a study conducted by Hurtubise and her colleagues (2015) at York University, in which they reported on severe injuries by sex and sport among Canadian collegiate-level athletes. Important to any research project is providing a context for the research, including a logical flow from the introduction to a clearly stated purpose of the study. Hurtubise et al. accomplish this across a number of steps. First, they emphasize the importance of identifying the risks and rates of injury to both injury prevention and sport safety. Second, they point out that there is currently insufficient research evidence available on injury severity risks, including sex and sport comparisons. Third, they describe some of the general findings on sex differences in injuries, highlighting that females have a greater risk of injury than males. Fourth, they make the case that researchers have not focused sufficiently on a wide variety of sports at the collegiate level in Canada (which further highlights the need for their study). Fifth, they discuss the need to focus on concussion risk as a type of injury because of the increased number of concussions reported by athletes in recent years. Sixth, they conclude the literature review with a clear statement of the study purpose (i.e., "The purpose of our study is to determine if difference in injury severity risk exists between males and females in sex-matched sports at the collegiate level," p. 45) and a presentation of the research hypothesis (i.e., "We hypothesize that females will have a higher percentage of severe injuries and a greater percentage of reported concussions," p. 45). Hence, the purpose statement and hypothesis flow naturally from the preceding context that they developed. Through these six steps the logical validity of their study is enhanced; important aspects of the study are covered in the literature review and there are no "surprises" for the reader in the content of the study purpose and hypothesis.

An evaluation of logical validity does not end at the study purpose and hypothesis. It is important to next consider the research methods, which can further support (or refute) the logical validity of a study because researchers use this section of their written work to describe how the study purpose will be addressed and how the study hypothesis will be tested. Many journal articles have commonly labelled sections (e.g., study design, participants, measures, data analysis) that allow readers insight into the methodological decisions researchers make. We look to these same sections as part of our evaluation of the logical validity of the Hurtibuse et al. (2015) study.

Hurtubise et al. (2015) identify their design as a "descriptive epidemiological study using previously collected data from York University's Gorman/Short Sport Injury Clinic sport injury database" (p. 45). Further aiding our understanding of their design choice (and supporting logical validity), they specifically identify the outcome variables of interest as injury severity and concussion. This would be expected based on what was presented in the literature review section. Also supporting the logical validity of the study is their choice to focus on injuries sustained in university sport competition by student athletes on the York University Lions' teams from a range of sports including soccer, ice hockey, volleyball, basketball, cross-country running, track and field, and football/rugby. Next, injury is defined as "any physical complaint sustained by an athlete during competition or training, which required medical attention by an athletic therapist or medical doctor" (p. 45), which again makes logical sense given the focus of their research. Finally, the methods section concludes with the identification of chi-square analyses and logistic regression as the primary strategies of data analysis. Remember from Chapter 5, these statistics are appropriate given the researchers' goal to compare percentages of injuries sustained across both sex and sport type and to quantify relations among sex, severe injury, and concussion. Similar to the literature review, all of these decisions are well-justified based on their study purpose and focus of their research, thereby further supporting the logical validity of their study.

The final conclusion presented by Hurtubise et al. (2015) is that "females, when compared with males, have higher odds of incurring a severe injury, as well as higher odds of sustaining a concussion in collegiate sport participation" (p. 50). Further supporting logical validity, their conclusion is based directly on the findings presented in the results. For example, 17.7% of females reported severe injuries compared to 13.3% of males, which was a significant difference based on the chi-square analysis (i.e., chi-square = 5.40, $p < .05$; see Chapter 5 in this text for further discussion of chi-square analysis). The main omission (and threat to logical validity) is that Hurtubise et al. make no mention of sport differences in their final conclusion section, which was a bit unexpected given the focus on sport differences identified earlier. However, in sum, the Hurtubise et al. study presents a good example of strong logical validity. Their literature review flowed naturally from the identification of the research problem to the study purpose and hypothesis, their methods were well-justified as a way to test their hypothesis, and their conclusions stayed within the boundaries of what the results had to offer.

In essence, to support the logical validity of a study, the entire study needs to flow logically from the introduction through to the final conclusions. And because every study is unique, the intent of presenting the example by Hurtubise and colleagues (2015) discussed above is just that, to provide *an example* of the types of evidence one might consider when evaluating the logical validity of a study. Based on the detail we provided above, it should be evident that there is no short-cut to doing so. You need to read the study from beginning to end, carefully assessing how each of the pieces fit (or do not fit) together, and ultimately making a reasoned decision as to the logical validity of a study.

Another way to support the logical validity of a study is to ensure that previous research in the field of study is being cited appropriately by the authors. It might be surprising, but quite often researchers do *not* cite existing research and literature properly when they write up their own research manuscripts. Knudson, Elliott, and Ackland (2012) provide an overview of principles that can be used to accurately cite research evidence, specifically as a way to justify and design applied research in kinesiology. The following is a verbatim (i.e., directly quoted) list of some of their principles (Knudson, Elliott, & Ackland, p. 132), which we feel serve as recommendations for authors conducting a wide range of research studies in kinesiology:

- Read and critically evaluate all literature to be cited (do not misrepresent/over-generalize findings, ignore flaws, copy references, or assume articles in top journals are of high-quality)
- Clearly note the kind of evidence claimed for each citation (e.g., anecdotal, hypothesis, descriptive, experimental data, or consensus of experimental evidence)
- Clearly summarize the size of experimental effects in the cited references
- Critically present all sides and consensus through citation of original research or via a review paper when appropriate
- Emphasize the most reliable sources and original evidence (avoid "empty references," sources without data, out-of-date data, and non-refereed publications)
- Strive for perfection in referencing details to support future work by verifying bibliometric data from original sources

We find the suggestions provided by Knudson et al. (2012) to be extremely useful (which is why we presented them verbatim), as many researchers often overlook the importance of ensuring previous literature is cited properly. Just as important, many people *reading* articles overestimate the accuracy of researchers' reporting of previous research and literature in the studies they read. If previous research and literature is not cited accurately by researchers, the logical validity of their research is severely compromised.

Logical Validity Exercise

Find two quantitative journal articles in your area of interest. Carefully read each article and make an evaluation on the logical validity of the studies. The types of questions that you can use to evaluate the logical validity of a research study are identified in Table 6.2.

Table 6.2 Types of questions used to evaluate logical validity.

TYPES OF QUESTIONS NEEDED TO EVALUATE THE LOGICAL VALIDITY OF RESEARCH STUDIES
Is the research issue/problem/question clearly identified?
Have all important variables been identified and discussed?
Is the research design appropriate to address the research purpose?
Are the participants chosen useful/appropriate for answering the research question?
Have all of the important variables been measured?
Is the data analysis appropriate to the study design?
Do the discussion and conclusion directly represent the results of the study and stay within the limitations of the research design?

You might even create a matrix to record notes related to each question as you go.

Remember that the question of logical validity does not have a yes/no answer. Rather, logical validity ranges on a continuum. As such, assign a value ranging from 0 ("poor") to 100 ("exceptional") to represent the logical validity of each of the two studies you selected. If you found any difference in ratings that you assigned the two studies, what was your key rationale for the difference?

Application of Construct Validity

When establishing the construct validity of a measure used in a study, the goal for researchers is to develop a web of evidence describing how that measure should be related to other measures of different constructs and behaviours. Messick (1989) referred to this process as developing a **nomological network**, a term often seen in the literature when discussing construct validity. This web of evidence is used to justify researchers' choices to use particular measures, as well as support that the measures are indeed measuring what they intend to measure (i.e., construct validity).

For example, if we wanted to evaluate the construct validity of a tool that measures body fat percentage, there are a number of things we might look at to make that determination. First, we might have the tool reviewed by experts in the field of body composition and as part of that process have them rate and provide feedback on the degree to which they think the tool measures body fat percentage adequately. Second, we could take multiple measurements on the same person using the tool, with the expectation that each measurement would result in approximately the same result (i.e., if there were no consistency in the scores, it wouldn't be a very good measure). Third, we could compare groups that are known to have different body fat percentages (e.g., marathon runners versus sumo wrestlers), with construct validity being supported if the tool was able to detect that known group difference. Fourth, the body fat percentage values found using the tool should be highly correlated with body fat percentages found using other measures (on the same person) that already have well-established construct validity evidence (e.g., dual-energy X-ray absorptiometry). Fifth, we could test how sensitive the tool is in differentiating between fat percentage and muscle percentage to ensure that it is only measuring the properties of the body that it intends. We could conduct many other tests to further develop a web of evidence needed to adequately evaluate the construct validity of our tool and give us confidence that we could use it to accurately measure body fat percentage. However, as with logical validity, we could do all of that and not have a clear "yes/no" answer. The evidence for and against construct validity will range on a continuum, ultimately requiring a judgement call by researchers as to whether the instrument is adequate for their purposes.

A good example applying the criteria of construct validity comes from the validation of the Physical Activity Questionnaire for Older Children (PAQ-C; Kowalski, Crocker, & Faulkner, 1997). The PAQ-C is a 9-item questionnaire developed to assess levels of moderate to vigorous physical activity in children from Grade 4 and above. A mean of all nine items on the PAQ-C is calculated, resulting in an overall physical activity score ranging from 1 (low physical activity) to 5 (high physical activity). Across two studies, Kowalski, Crocker, and Faulkner (1997) considered a range of evidence to evaluate the construct validity of the PAQ-C. Figure 6.1 presents the web of evidence or nomological network that they considered, which focused on relationships between the PAQ-C and other existing physical activity measures, as well as relationships between the PAQ-C and other related constructs. To provide a working example of construct validity, the following paragraphs of this section discuss each type of evidence in more detail (the upcoming discussion also provides more applied examples of some of the statistics covered in Chapter 5).

One of the best ways to establish the construct validity of a new measure is to test its relation with other existing measures of that same construct. In the case of the PAQ-C, Kowalski, Crocker, and Faulkner (1997) tested the PAQ-C against a number of other physical activity measures, including recall questionnaires (i.e., a single-item Activity Rating; a Moderate to Vigorous Physical Activity Questionnaire; the Godin Leisure Time Physical Activity Questionnaire), a teacher's rating of physical activity, a Caltrac accelerometer (i.e., motion sensor), and a physical activity recall one-on-one interview. Each of these are listed as "Other Physical Activity Measures" in Figure 6.1, with the correlation between scores on each of those measures and the PAQ-C listed. More than one correlation value is reported for some of the measures in Figure 6.1 for a couple of reasons. First, more than one total score can sometimes be calculated from different items on the same measure. Second, the same measure might have been used in more than one study. You will also notice that two different types of correlations are reported in Figure 6.1. The first one, r, represents a Pearson Correlation; whereas the other one, ρ, represents a Spearman Rank Order Correlation. Recall from Chapter 5 that the latter is used when there is either a non-normal distribution or it is a categorical measure (as is the case with the second Godin Leisure Time Physical Activity Questionnaire score reported in Figure 6.1).

As can be seen in Figure 6.1, correlations between the PAQ-C and other physical activity measures ranged from .39 to .63 in the Kowalski, Crocker, and Faulkner (1997) research studies. The question then becomes: Are these correlations of sufficient magnitude to support the construct validity of the PAQ-C? As with most questions regarding construct validity, the

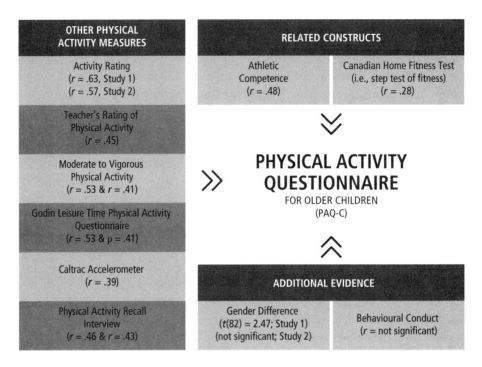

Figure 6.1 Web of evidence used to evaluate the construct validity of the Physical Activity Questionnaire for Older Children (PAQ-C). *Correlations (r and ρ) represent relationships with the PAQ-C; whereas t-tests represent tests of difference on the PAQ-C between groups.*

Source: Kowalski, K. C., Crocker, P. R. E., & Faulkner, R. A. (1997). Validation of the Physical Activity Questionnaire for Older Children. *Pediatric Exercise Science, 9,* 174–86.

answer is "it depends." Because there was no gold standard (i.e., "perfect" measure) of physical activity included to compare the PAQ-C scores against, the likelihood of finding correlations nearing $r = 1.00$ (or $ρ = 1.00$) with any of the other physical activity measures would be unexpected. In many areas of study there isn't a gold-standard measure available, and the challenge with not having a gold standard to compare scores against is that researchers never know whether lower correlations are the result of the measure they are validating or a result of limitations with the comparison measure. For example, although a correlation of $r = .39$ might not seem very high, as is the case between the PAQ-C and the Caltrac accelerometer (see Figure 6.1), it is important to consider that the Caltrac accelerometer cannot be used in water (e.g., when swimming) and doesn't do a very good job at detecting activity where there isn't a lot of vertical acceleration (e.g., when cycling). Therefore, even if the PAQ-C itself were a gold-standard measure of physical activity, it would still have limited correlational strength with the Caltrac due to limitations in the Caltrac. When *both* measures have limitations, the meaning of specific correlation values can be extremely challenging to determine. In the case of the PAQ-C, finding significant relationships with a wide range of other physical activity measures does provide initial support for construct validity.

A similar body of evidence is sought out when comparing scores on a measure that we wish to validate with scores on measures of related constructs. In the case of the PAQ-C studies, Kowalski, Crocker, and Faulkner (1997) looked to the relationship between physical activity and both athletic competence and physical fitness as providing additional construct validity evidence. As shown in Figure 6.1, both relationships were significant, further supporting the construct validity of the PAQ-C. Particularly noteworthy, when testing construct validity we would expect higher correlations between measures of similar constructs (e.g., two separate measures of physical activity) than between measures of different constructs (e.g., physical activity and physical fitness). This was the case for the PAQ-C evidence, in that the correlation with physical fitness ($r = .28$) was lower than that found with any of the physical activity measures. However, the correlation with athletic competence ($r = .48$) was *higher* than some of the relationships between the PAQ-C and some of the physical activity measures. Because athletic competence is also a recall measure, this magnitude of correlation in comparison to some of the correlations between the PAQ-C and other non-recall physical activity measures (e.g., accelerometer) might suggest that there is some error in the measurement of physical activity introduced by its reliance on retrospective recall (which really isn't all that surprising given that limitations of recall are well known). This would be a piece of evidence *against* the construct validity of the PAQ-C.

Additional construct validity evidence considered by Kowalski, Crocker, and Faulkner (1997) were tests of gender differences on the PAQ-C and the relationship between the PAQ-C and a measure of behavioural conduct (i.e., how children generally behave in the classroom). These two pieces of evidence are a bit unique compared to others described earlier because they do not involve similar or related constructs. Instead, they rely on discriminating between groups and unrelated constructs as additional evidence. For example, boys are typically found to be higher in physical activity levels than girls in both Canada and the United States in studies using objective measurement devices like accelerometers (e.g., Colley et al., 2011; Troiano et al., 2008). Therefore, evidence that would support the use of the PAQ-C is its ability to detect gender differences in physical activity. You'll notice that a gender difference was found in only *one* of the two Kowalski et al. studies, as reported in Figure 6.1 (also note that the gender difference was tested using the *t*-test statistic you were introduced to in Chapter 5). This inconsistency in results provides partial support for construct validity and is the best indication yet that at least some aspects of the PAQ-C might make it limited as a physical activity measure. However, the evidence that the PAQ-C is not related to behavioural conduct provides support that the PAQ-C can discriminate itself from constructs that it should *not* be related to but that share a similar method of assessment.

Taken together, the web of evidence described in the Kowalski, Crocker, and Faulkner (1997) validation research article is a good example of how, as with logical validity, construct validity evidence ranges on a continuum. The task for researchers is to carefully examine the construct validity evidence that is available and make a decision as to whether or not a measure would be sufficient for use in their own research. It is then those researchers' responsibility to describe the measure that they used in their own research report, along with a description of some of the construct validity evidence that led them to choose that particular measure in the first place.

It should be noted, however, that in some cases researchers use measures that do not have a body of construct validity evidence to judge against. In those cases, the research needs to be interpreted with particular caution because the question of whether the measure really measures

Construct Validity Exercise

Find two quantitative journal articles in your area of interest. Read the authors' descriptions of the measures that they used in their research. Is enough detail presented to allow you the opportunity to make a judgment on the construct validity of the measures that they used? If not, what type of information is missing that would be useful for you to evaluate the construct validity of their measures? Subsequently, for one of the measures used by the authors, try to find three to four other articles that use a different measure of a similar construct. What are some of the strengths and limitations of the authors' choice compared to those alternatives?

Professional Highlight

Dr Phillip Wilson, Associate Professor, Applied Health Sciences—Kinesiology, Brock University

Profile: Dr Wilson has a reputation as an expert in statistics and instrument development. His work in validating the Behavioural Regulation in Exercise Questionnaire (BREQ) in particular has had a significant impact on research exploring motivational processes in exercise and physical activity both within Canada and internationally. His research also provides an example of how establishing the construct validity of a measure is an ongoing process. The BREQ was originally developed by Mullan, Markland, and Ingledew (1997), but has subsequently undergone two revisions (i.e., BREQ-2 and BREQ-3)and extensive validation testing since its original development as it evolves to most accurately measure the full spectrum of the self-determination continuum across a range of populations. Dr Wilson and his colleagues have played a crucial role in the evolution of the instrument. In particular, their research relies heavily on the evaluation of construct validity evidence as a way to guide other researchers in their choices as to whether or not to use the BREQ in their own work on exercise and physical activity motivation.

Further Readings

Mullan, E., Markland, D., & Ingledew, D. K. (1997). A graded conceptualization of self-determination in the regulation of exercise behavior: Development of a measure using confirmatory factor analysis procedures. *Personality and Individual Differences, 23*, 745–52. doi:10.1016/S0191-8869(97)00107-4

Wilson, P. M., Rodgers, W. M., Loitz, C. C., & Scime, G. (2006). "It's who I am . . . really!" The importance of integrated regulation in exercise contexts. *Journal of Applied Biobehavioral Research, 11*, 79–104. doi:10.1111/j.1751-9861.2006.tb00021.x

Wilson, P. M., Sabiston, C. M., Mack, D. E., & Blanchard, C. M. (2012). On the nature and function of scoring protocols used in exercise motivation research: An empirical study of the behavioral regulation in exercise questionnaire. *Psychology of Sport and Exercise, 13*, 614–22. doi:10.1016/j.psychsport.2012.03.009

what it intends to measure cannot be adequately answered. Regardless of whether new or existing measures are used, construct validation is always an ongoing process. This is one reason why, in addition to the Kowalski, Crocker, and Faulkner (1997) research studies, additional validation studies have been conducted on PAQ-C since its original publication (e.g., Moore et al., 2007).

Application of Internal Validity

To apply the criteria of internal validity, we next look to the research by Skelly and her colleagues (2014) at McMaster University. Their research team was interested in finding out whether high-intensity interval training has the same energy expenditure 24 hours following exercise as continuous moderate-intensity training. Recall that internal validity refers to the merits of researchers' claims that any change in an outcome is a result of their intervention and not the result of other factors. Therefore, if we want to evaluate the internal validity of Skelly et al.'s study, we need to be confident that any change in energy expenditure 24 hours post-exercise is indeed a result of high-intensity interval training and not the result of other factors.

To increase confidence in their findings, and internal validity more specifically, Skelly et al. (2014) utilized a number of strategies. First, they had all of the participants participate in a control condition, consisting of no exercise, in addition to participating in a high-intensity interval training condition and a continuous moderate-intensity training condition. Because of the inclusion of a control condition, the authors were better able to rule out a number of potential threats to internal validity, such as history or maturation. In other words, finding a difference in 24-hour energy expenditure between the control condition and both the exercise conditions strengthens the case that it is indeed their exercise training that is causing the differences in energy expenditure 24 hours later. Second, the order of participation in the three conditions was *randomized*, such that each of the participants might complete the high-intensity interval training either first, second, or third. This randomization helps us to have confidence that their results are not simply due to additional threats to internal validity, such as testing learning effects or instrument calibration drift.

Having a control group and random assignment in particular are important features of true experimental designs and a key characteristic that make experimental designs so powerful in detecting causal relationships. Skelly et al. (2014) included both a control group and random assignment in their experimental design, and as such they significantly enhanced the internal validity of their research. But *just* having a control group and random assignment are not sufficient to protect against all threats to internal validity. Therefore, in addition to including a control condition and randomization, they also (a) had a 10-hour overnight fast period for participants prior to each condition, (b) standardized meals across the 24-hour data collection period for all conditions, (c) removed the first 10 minutes of data collection each time to "avoid using data influenced by the initial application of the equipment" (p. 2), and (d) ensured that there was a consistent total time (i.e., 60 minutes) during the "treatment" (i.e., exercise or control) for all conditions. The use of these four procedures provided additional protection against threats to internal validity because they all strengthen the standardization of their procedures. Standardization of procedures allows researchers the opportunity to rule out many threats to internal validity. For example, had Skelly et al. not standardized the meals prior to exercise, the

24-hour energy expenditure results might have been unduly influenced by differences in what the participants ate, making it more difficult for the researchers to know what changes were the result of their intervention and which were simply the result of fluctuations in diet.

A challenge that researchers of exercise training studies in particular often face is that it is hard to blind participants to the condition that they are in (i.e., it would be pretty difficult to set up a design in which the participant didn't know if she or he were doing no exercise, high-intensity interval training, or continuous moderate-intensity training). This lack of blinding can introduce potential threats to internal validity, such as participants working harder in certain conditions to try to please the researchers. However, it should be evident in reading this text that there is no perfect study, and researchers need to proceed making the best decisions they can, trying to rule out as many threats to internal validity as possible. The study by Skelly and colleagues (2014) is a good example of the types of decisions that can be made to strengthen internal validity, while recognizing that it is impossible to control for all threats to internal validity. Another reason we chose to highlight the Skelly et al. research study is that it is a good example of the type of high-quality research being led by undergraduate students in kinesiology programs in Canada (i.e., the lead author, Lauren Skelly, was an undergraduate student when the research took place!).

Internal Validity Exercise

Choose a topic of interest within kinesiology and select an outcome variable that you think might be a target of intervention. What intervention might you use to influence that outcome variable? Think about what factors could influence your outcome variable other than your intervention, and then identify five specific research design strategies that you could implement to give you more confidence that any observed change in your outcome variable is a result of your intervention and not a result of some of the other factors you identified. In other words, what design strategies could you implement to increase the internal validity of your study?

Research Highlight

The Behavioural Medicine (BMED) lab, led by Director Ryan Rhodes, within the School of Exercise Science, Physical and Health Education at the University of Victoria uses intervention designs across a wide range of research areas within kinesiology. As just a few examples, they have tested the effectiveness of a school-based fruit and vegetable nutrition program (Naylor et al., 2014a), a text messaging intervention aimed at action planning for physical activity (Mistry et al., 2015), a children's screen-time family-focused intervention (Naylor et al., 2014b), and a dog-walking intervention for inactive dog owners (Rhodes et al., 2012). Critical to their research is the attempt to design high-quality research with strong internal validity to minimize the threat that findings are due to factors other than the inter ventions they are testing. As such, methods to strengthen the likelihood of equivalence among comparison groups prior to their interventions (e.g., randomization, matching, fixed assignment, clear inclusion criteria) are often used within their research program.

Further Readings

Mistry, C. D., Sweet, S. N., Rhodes, R. E., & Latimer-Cheung, A. E. (2015). Text2Plan: Exploring changes in the quantity and quality of action plans and physical activity in a text messaging intervention. *Psychology & Health, 30*, 839–56. doi:10.1080/08870446.2014.997731

Naylor, P.-J., McConnell, J., Rhodes, R. E., Barr, S. I., Ghement, I., & Scott, J. (2014a). Efficacy of a minimal dose school fruit and vegetable snack intervention. *Journal of Food & Nutritional Disorders, 3*, 4. doi:10.4172/2324-9323.1000147

Naylor, P.-J., Tomlin, D., Rhodes, R., & McConnell, J. (2014b). Screen Smart: Evaluation of a brief school facilitated and family focused intervention to encourage children to manage their screen-time. *Child & Adolescent Behavior, 2*, 1. doi: 10.4172/jcalb.1000124

Rhodes, R. E., Murray, H., Temple, V. A., Tuokko, H., & Higgins, J. W. (2012). Pilot study of a dog walking randomized intervention: Effects of a focus on canine exercise. *Preventive Medicine, 54*, 309–12. doi:10.1016/j.ypmed.2012.02.014

Application of External Validity

The fourth main type of validity that researchers use to evaluate the merits of quantitative research is external validity (i.e., the generalization of the intervention to other people, contexts, or time). For example, if a particular exercise training intervention only works with a very specific sample under very specific laboratory conditions, the external validity would be very low. On the other hand, if the exercise training intervention is subsequently shown to be effective across a number of different samples and populations, researchers have increased confidence that their intervention "works" in the ways they claim it does, and hence the external validity of the study would be high. The key then to external validity is ensuring that the sample chosen for a study is representative of the populations that researchers wish to generalize their results to. Another factor supporting external validity is the extent to which the conditions of the experiment reflect the real world in which an intervention is likely to take place.

A strategy that many researchers implement to enhance external validity is to clearly identify inclusion criteria specifying who can and cannot be part of the sample studied. For example, in order to be eligible to participate in the Alberta Diabetes and Physical Activity Trial (ADAPT; Plotnikoff et al., 2010) participants needed to (a) be 18 years or older, (b) have been diagnosed with type II diabetes mellitus, (c) have regular access to a telephone, (d) be able to read and understand English, and (e) be deemed safe to start a physical activity program by their doctor. Having this type of selection criteria helps researchers to enhance the external validity of their findings to other groups of people with similar characteristics (but note this choice to identify strict inclusion criteria also has the potential to *decrease* the external validity of their findings, if their intent is to generalize their results to others not sharing those characteristics).

External Validity Exercise

The Alberta Diabetes and Physical Activity Trial (ADAPT; Plotnikoff et al., 2010) was designed to test the effectiveness of three intervention strategies, including (a) standard printed physical activity education materials; (b) standard printed physical activity education materials plus pedometers, a log-book, and physical activity information tailored to each individual; and (c) tailored physical activity counselling over the telephone plus the materials provided to the other two groups. Although the selection criteria used by Plotnikoff et al. (2010), as discussed above, was included to enhance the external validity of their study findings to others with similar characteristics, what types of limitations do these choices impose on their ability to generalize the effectiveness of a physical activity intervention to people *without* those characteristics? For example, would there be a difference in the effectiveness of their three types of interventions in English versus non-English language groups or for those with versus without regular access to a telephone?

One challenge that limits the external validity of most studies conducted in kinesiology is the reliance on non-random selection of participants for studies. In other words, most researchers in the field rely on *volunteers* for their studies. There are a number of reasons why this is the case (e.g., time, resources, limited access to the entire population), but most paramount among them is ethics. Because the ethical principle of autonomy (i.e., freedom to make one's own choices; see Chapter 3) is key to ethical conduct of research in Canada, human participants have a choice whether to participate or not. Thus, although ethically necessary, this freedom of choice imposes a natural limitation on the external validity of research in kinesiology. For example, we already discussed how researchers make the assumption that if they find that their intervention is effective those findings should generalize to others with similar characteristics. However, whenever people have the autonomous choice to participate in research or not, there might be some characteristic (often unknown or not assessed) that might be impacting that choice.

In kinesiology research, particularly physical activity intervention studies, the people who volunteer for studies might do so because they have an interest in physical activity, whereas the people who do not volunteer might not share that similar interest. In some ways, it is no different than the reasons why students might choose to enrol in kinesiology undergraduate programs. They likely have an increased interest in physical activity compared to most of the population on average. Put another way, people simply gravitate towards things that interest them, and signing up for research studies is no different. But this biasing towards the inclusion of people in research with an interest in physical activity might impact our findings. For example, if people with an interest in physical activity have a greater tendency to sign up for kinesiology research studies, we will systematically be missing important information on ways to get (and keep) other types of people active.

However, perhaps an even more systemic threat to external validity in general is whether the populations that researchers are including in their studies are well-suited to the broad claims that they intend to make. Henrich, Heine, and Norenzayan (2010) at the University of British Columbia discussed the concept of Western, educated, industrialized, rich, and democratic, or WEIRD, societies and the limitations that relying on data from WEIRD samples has on the generalizability of research findings. The intent of their argument is to make the case that although researchers often rely on WEIRD samples to conduct their research, especially when one looks globally, the WEIRD samples are actually outliers compared to other populations. If their argument is accepted, even though much research is conducted on WEIRD samples, the generalizability of those results is relatively low. Although Henrich, Heine, and Norenzayan were making their case in the context of human psychology and behaviour specifically, an important lesson to take away is that researchers have to be really careful as to whom they intend to generalize their results. Studies that make broad claims based on volunteer samples from WEIRD societies might need to be particularly cautious of threats to external validity.

Summary

Chapter 6 focused on evaluating the merits of a wide range of quantitative research designs used in kinesiology. The standards for quantitative research were applied to real-world examples of research in kinesiology. The specific focus of the chapter was on the application of logical validity, construct validity, internal validity, and external validity. An examination of internal validity and external validity requires the manipulation of an independent variable (e.g., as a result of a treatment or intervention), which is the hallmark of experimental designs. Thus, for non-experimental designs, researchers are left to make judgments on the merits of a study based only on logical validity and construct validity.

Discussion Questions

1. What types of evidence might you look for when trying to evaluate the logical validity of a research study?
2. What strategies could you utilize if asked to conduct a study designed to evaluate the construct validity of a questionnaire assessing calcium intake via self-reports (across 10 items) each day for a one-week period?
3. What makes internal validity and external validity specific to experimental research studies?
4. Why is there often a trade-off between internal validity and external validity (i.e., why as you try to reduce threats to one do threats to the other often increase)?
5. What are five key questions you might ask a researcher at a scientific conference to adequately evaluate the merits of her or his quantitative research study?

Recommended Readings

Henrich, J., Heine, S. J., & Norenzayan, A. (2010). The weirdest people in the world? *Behavioral and Brain Sciences, 33*, 61–83. doi:10.1017/S0140525X0999152X

Knudson, D., Elliott, B., & Ackland, T. (2012). Citation of evidence for research and application in kinesiology. *Kinesiology Review, 1*, 129–36.

Moher, D., Hopewell, S., Schulz, K. F., Montori, V., Gotzsche, P. C., Devereaux, P. J., . . . Altman, D. G. (2010). CONSORT 2010 explanation and elaboration: Updated guidelines for reporting parallel group randomized trials. *BMJ, 340*, c869. doi:10.1136/bmj.c869

Schultz, K. F., Altman, D. G., Moher, D., & CONSORT Group (2010). CONSORT 2010 statement: Updated guidelines for reporting parallel group randomized trials. *Annals of Internal Medicine, 152*, 726–32. doi:10.7326/0003-4819-152-11-201006010-00232

7 Qualitative Study Designs

Qualitative Strategies of Inquiry

You may hear nonsensical debates about which type of design, qualitative or quantitative, produces "better" research. However, recall from Chapter 2 that it is having a well-defined research question that informs the necessity to utilize either a qualitative or quantitative study design (or perhaps both). You will also remember from Chapter 1 that researchers' philosophical worldviews serve as a framework to guide the research process, including the formulation of research questions and the subsequent methods for generating, analyzing, and interpreting data. Researchers with a constructivist philosophical worldview, for example, will likely adopt a qualitative study design and can draw upon various strategies of inquiry. Each qualitative strategy of inquiry has defining features, as well as common processes for sampling participants and generating data.

Defining features of qualitative research

Various qualitative strategies of inquiry are described in this chapter, but it is first necessary to highlight some of the defining features of all qualitative studies that were briefly mentioned in Chapter 1. For instance, researchers using qualitative methods are *key instruments* in the research process, whereby they play integral roles in generating and/or collecting data. Rather than the term *data collection*, the term *data generation* is becoming more popular within qualitative research because such terminology emphasizes the important role that researchers play in working with participants to generate data. As well, data generated within qualitative research typically occur in a *natural setting*, rather than in a lab or controlled space. However, qualitative interviews are usually conducted in spaces that support confidentiality, and therefore could take place in a private lab setting. Qualitative research is also *emergent* in that the research questions and various phases of the research process (e.g., participant sampling) may need to change even after data generation has begun in the natural setting.

Despite the recognized need for *flexibility* within qualitative studies, researchers in kinesiology will typically identify one of many possible strategies of inquiry to guide their qualitative research. Although each strategy of inquiry is described as having unique features, you will notice that there are also similarities across the various approaches. As well, it *is* possible for researchers to use a combination of strategies of inquiry to engage in qualitative research, but for emerging researchers (and even more advanced researchers for that matter) it is useful to identify one strategy of inquiry that will subsequently guide the sampling, data generation, and data analysis strategies.

It would be nearly impossible to provide a detailed description of all qualitative strategies of inquiry, particularly since they are often described and classified differently depending on research disciplines or philosophical assumptions. For instance, Creswell (2013) typically refers to five qualitative strategies of inquiry: narrative, phenomenology, grounded theory, ethnography, and case study. Mayan (2009) also describes those outlined by Creswell, but adds a number of others including qualitative description, interpretive description, and collective biography. It is important to note that Mayan refers to such strategies of inquiry as research methods. We highlight this difference because you will notice that researchers may use different terminology, even though they are typically referring to the same thing. Within the context of this book, we refer to a qualitative study design as an overarching term that encompasses strategies of inquiry, philosophical worldviews, and methods (e.g., processes of data generation, data analysis). Within this chapter we provide an overview of common qualitative strategies of inquiry used by researchers in kinesiology including *narrative, ethnography, phenomenology, case study, qualitative description*, and *grounded theory*. Within each overview, the common methods are described.

Narrative

Narrative research focuses on the stories of individuals. When used as a strategy of inquiry, stories are used to bring understanding or meaning to the lived experiences of individuals. This strategy of inquiry is based on the idea that individual stories serve as a representation of broader social experiences. Within narrative research, stories can be analyzed in great depth or stand alone as a description of experience(s). Narrative, as a form of inquiry, originated in humanities disciplines and is increasingly being used by researchers in kinesiology. For instance, a narrative approach has been used to better understand the body, exercise, and food relationship for distance runners (Busanich, McGannon, & Schinke, 2012). Through in-depth unstructured (i.e., conversational) interviews, nine runners were asked to tell stories about their bodies as well as share their experiences as a runner. Specifically, participants were asked to "Imagine that the experiences you have had as a runner could be turned into a story; take as long as you'd like and relay that story to me" (p. 584). The researchers conducted an in-depth analysis of the content of the shared stories in an effort to explore how the stories were contextually positioned. The findings from their research suggest that when constructing meanings about the body, food, and exercise, participants drew upon one of two opposing narratives, which were referred to as "just do it" and "just do it better" (p. 585). Busanich and colleagues described how stories served as a medium to gain insight into athletes' complex meanings surrounding the body, food, and exercise, and also the runners' experiences of such meanings.

Researchers may choose to identify their strategy of inquiry simply as a narrative approach, or they may describe a more specific form of narrative inquiry. For instance, a **life history** may be used to depict the entire life of an individual such as an elite athlete. **Oral history** refers to a form of narrative inquiry that involves the collection of memories that hold historical significance. Such memories can be shared by one or multiple individuals. The use of oral history may be particularly salient for certain populations, including Indigenous peoples, who have traditionally used storytelling to teach current generations about the past.

Generally speaking, within narrative research the stories of individuals are typically generated through in-depth and unstructured interviews. You will remember from Busanich, McGannon, and Schinke's (2012) narrative study that unstructured or conversational interviews were used as an opportunity for runners to share their stories. Observations and participant journalling may also be used to construct stories, and researchers and participant(s) will often work together to construct the stories. We will talk more about these specific processes of data generation a bit later in this chapter.

Ethnography

With roots in anthropology, **ethnography** has been described as one of the oldest qualitative strategies of inquiry. Ethnographers are driven by questions that seek to understand cultures or a cultural group and, therefore, the concept of *culture* is foundational to ethnography. Using an ethnographic approach, researchers focus on describing and interpreting shared features of a cultural group, such as behaviours, values, and beliefs. Within anthropology, researchers have traditionally immersed themselves in "exotic" cultures to study those cultures that are vastly different from their own. More recently, researchers in kinesiology have used ethnographic approaches to study a variety of cultures and subcultures that exist within sport, exercise, physical activity, and health contexts.

Researchers may choose to employ one of the many specific forms of ethnography, such as critical ethnography or autoethnography. **Critical ethnography** includes a political agenda and some form of advocacy for underrepresented populations. **Autoethnography** is the study of one's own culture and is also a form of narrative inquiry, which is sometimes referred to as self-narrative. As such, autoethnography demonstrates the intersection between two qualitative strategies of inquiry (i.e., ethnography and narrative). Based on her graduate research in the College of Kinesiology at the University of Saskatchewan, Heather Kuttai (2010) published an autoethnography on her embodied experience of pregnancy, childbirth, and disability. Kuttai self-identifies as a woman with a spinal cord injury who uses a wheelchair and drew upon personal journals she had written over a 20-year period, particularly

Research Highlight

Michael Atkinson drew upon ethnographic data to "examine how triathletes learn to physically manage, socially perform and individually reflect upon the endurance sport of triathlon as a microcosm of the 'civilising process'" (Atkinson, 2008, p. 165). Canadian triathletes shared pain and suffering narratives that were analyzed alongside three years of ethnographic data that were generated in Ontario. Specifically, Dr Atkinson described how data were generated through participant observation with triathletes, which involved over 600 hours of training with athletes, socializing with athletes, and spending time at competitions. The data generated from participant observation was essential for developing an in-depth understanding of the context in which triathlon occurs. In addition to participant observation, 62 triathletes participated in semi-structured interviews that were designed to elicit narratives that described participants' backgrounds and experiences with triathlon. The results of this ethnography suggest that triathletes learn to come together as a "pain community" and learn to appreciate the mental and physical suffering in the sport. His research provides a detailed description of how ethnographers immerse themselves into a culture, such as the culture of triathlon, to generate in-depth data.

Further Reading

Atkinson, M. (2008). Triathlon, suffering and exciting significance. *Leisure Studies, 27*, 165–80. doi:10.1080/02614360801902216

the journals she wrote while pregnant. She described how an autoethnographic approach supported the sharing of her own personal experiences while at the same time supporting a more in-depth understanding of the broader culture of disability, pregnancy, and childbirth.

Regardless of whether one employs ethnography in general or in a more specific form (e.g., autoethnography), participant observation is typically the primary process used for data generation in ethnographic approaches. However, with the emergence of ethnography as a strategy of inquiry used by a variety of research disciplines, interviews and documents (e.g., poetry, art, personal journals) are also now used to generate data on the culture being studied.

Phenomenology

Phenomenology involves the study of a *phenomenon* or a concept through the exploration of lived experiences. Although all strategies of inquiry are informed by researchers' philosophical worldviews, phenomenology has particularly strong philosophical roots. Early phenomenologists were critical of the scientific method and the extent to which it assumes an objective reality. They argued that human consciousness and lived experiences provide an avenue for understanding the nature of social reality. Given the focus on understanding lived experiences, phenomenology can be understood as a philosophy *and* a qualitative strategy of inquiry.

Phenomenological studies can take a variety of forms. **Interpretative phenomenological analysis** (IPA) stems from a phenomenological tradition and is gaining increased attention in kinesiology research. This strategy of inquiry is focused on understanding how experiences of the phenomenon are *perceived* by participants and how people make sense of their social and personal world. For example, IPA has been used to explore the experiences of National Hockey League (NHL) players who retired as a result of concussions that were incurred during their hockey careers (Caron et al., 2013). Findings from Caron et al.'s research document how participants experience career-ending concussions, including a description of ongoing physical symptoms (e.g., headaches) that have affected their daily functioning.

Empirical phenomenology is a form of phenomenology that is particularly descriptive whereby a structural analysis of participants' experiences results in a description of the *essential structure(s)* of the phenomenon. This phenomenological approach has been used by researchers to explore body self-compassion among young adult women exercisers (Berry et al., 2010). Within their research, Berry et al. relied on the accounts of women exercisers to identify the essential structures or components of body self-compassion. The result was the identification of three essential structures (i.e., taking ownership of one's body, engaging in less social comparison, appreciating one's unique body) and one facilitating structure (i.e., the importance of others) of body self-compassion.

Researchers using a phenomenological approach seek to include multiple individuals who have experienced the phenomenon that is being explored. Data are typically generated through multiple in-depth interviews with participants but could also include other sources (e.g., personal diaries) that provide rich insight into the lived experiences of the phenomena. Phenomenological studies often include a process of **bracketing**, whereby researchers describe and record their own experiences of the phenomenon. This process of bracketing provides an opportunity for researchers to outwardly acknowledge and "set aside" their experiences so that their sole focus can be on those experiences shared by the study participants. The idea that an individual can indeed bracket her or his assumptions is a topic that has received great debate among qualitative researchers (e.g., LeVasseur, 2003). Such debate has likely occurred because different researchers are often informed by various philosophical worldviews that may or may not support the belief that bracketing is possible.

Case study

Case study is often referred to as a strategy of inquiry despite the contention by some researchers that this is an inappropriate conceptualization of case study (for further discussion see VanWynsberghe & Khan, 2007). Some would argue that case study simply identifies *what* is to be studied (i.e., a case), but not *how* it should be studied. Given the emergence of this approach within kinesiology research, we have included case study in our overview of commonly used strategies of inquiry. Case study is focused on studying the complexity and distinctiveness of a case within important circumstances. The **case** or "bounded system" is bound by time and place, and people are often cases of interest to researchers. In addition to people, a case of interest may also be a team, event, organization, or community.

Stake (1995) described how case studies often fit within one of three categories, including intrinsic, instrumental, and collective case study. An **intrinsic case study** is used when the focus is on understanding the *complexity of the case*, whereas an **instrumental case study** focuses on a specific case because it can provide insight into an *issue of interest*. **Collective case study** is essentially an instrumental case study that includes *several cases*. It is not necessary for researchers to describe their case study approach using the terminology or the categories provided by Stake. For instance, researchers from the University of Ottawa used a case study approach to study a high school ice hockey program that was designed to teach life skills and values to players (Camiré, Trudel, & Bernard, 2013). The intent of their case study was to understand the unique features of the program, or case, through the perspectives of players, coaches, parents, and administrators. In addition to interviews, document analysis (e.g., copy of the "player's handbook") and observations supported a detailed description of the case. Findings from Camiré, Trudel, and Bernard's research identified a number of the program's strengths (e.g., constant coach-player interactions) and challenges (e.g., compressed academic schedule), providing necessary understandings for the development of similar sports programs in school systems.

An essential feature of a case study approach is that it provides a detailed or in-depth description of the case(s). As such, data generation within case study research is extensive and involves various sources of information. Data are typically generated through interviews and often include observations and visual methods; it would be unusual for a case study to include only one form of data generation.

Qualitative description

Qualitative description is used as a strategy of inquiry by researchers who want to develop a *comprehensive description* and summary of a phenomenon or an event. Qualitative description involves relatively little interpretation in comparison to other strategies of inquiry (e.g., phenomenology), and it results in a description of the event or phenomenon in "everyday language." Qualitative description is arguably "one of the most frequently employed methodological approaches in the practice disciplines" (Sandelowski, 2000, p. 335). However, researchers do not always acknowledge that their study is indeed a qualitative description and, instead, try to justify their strategy of inquiry as one that may be deemed more rigorous or complex (e.g., phenomenology). Sandelowski argued that qualitative description should be considered the approach of choice when the intent of research is to provide a basic description of a phenomenon or an event.

A qualitative description was used by researchers in Edmonton, Alberta, to explore young Indigenous women's experiences of bullying in team sports (Kentel & McHugh, 2015). Given that relatively little research has explored bullying in sport contexts, they sought to provide a comprehensive description of such experiences. Eight young Indigenous women took part in semi-structured one-on-one interviews and a second follow-up phone interview. Data were analyzed using a content analysis, and the detailed descriptions shared by the participants were reported using "everyday terms." Findings from this research contribute to a more in-depth understanding of the broad range of bullying experiences that occurs in sport.

Qualitative description is a distinct strategy of inquiry but, similar to other qualitative strategies of inquiry, this approach can take on the "hues, tones, and textures" of other approaches (Sandelowski, 2000, p. 337). For instance, a qualitative description could take on the hues of a phenomenological approach; therefore, the sampling or processes of data generation could *feel* like a phenomenology. Generally speaking, qualitative description studies include participants who are purposefully selected because they are deemed to be particularly knowledgeable about the topic of study. Individual or group interviews are typically used to generate data in qualitative description studies. However, it is also possible to include observations or other visual methods such as photographs or drawings to understand the basic nature of the phenomenon or event.

Grounded theory

Grounded theory research is focused on the generation and analysis of data to construct a *theory* (Charmaz, 2014). Theory is typically conceptualized as a general explanation of an event, a process, an action, or a phenomenon. Iterative strategies or processes are often employed within grounded theory, whereby researchers use comparative methods to examine the data against each other in an effort to identify similarities and differences. The data can be compared with other data in the same study, or data can be compared with concepts or theories that currently exist in the research literature. The end product of this particular strategy of inquiry is a theory that are grounded in data that are generated by the views or experiences of participants.

Grounded theory research has a rich history that originated in sociology, and it has grown in popularity to become a commonly used strategy of inquiry across many academic disciplines. For instance, researchers have worked towards the development of a grounded theory of exercise imagery (Giacobbi et al., 2003) and a grounded theory of positive psychological growth based on breast cancer survivors' experiences in dragon boat programs (Sabiston, McDonough, & Crocker, 2007). Tamminen and Holt (2012) developed a grounded theory of the ways in which adolescent athletes learn about coping in sport. Within their research, semi-structured one-on-one interviews were conducted with 17 athletes, 10 parents, and seven coaches. Findings from Tamminen and Holt's research suggest that learning about coping is an experiential process that involves reflective practices, learning through trial and error, and coping outcomes (e.g., consistent performance). As well, within this experiential process, parents and coaches play a central role.

Regardless of the discipline, data within a grounded theory are typically generated via one-on-one interviews with participants. One of the greatest challenges of grounded theory research is determining when **data saturation** has been reached, and when a theory can be fully developed. To saturate the data means that no new information will surface; therefore, no additional data need to be generated. The topic of saturation has been of great debate among researchers who engage in qualitative research because, depending on one's philosophical worldview, it could be argued that saturation will never be reached!

Strategy of Inquiry Exercise

Applying your knowledge of the various qualitative strategies of inquiry, identify which strategy of inquiry was used (or could have been used) to guide each of the following studies:

1. Nine community organizations from across Canada were selected to participate in this study that focused on exploring the role of microgrants (i.e., small grant or sum of money) in enhancing physical activity opportunities for Canadian adolescents.

   Tamminen, K. A., Faulkner, G., Witcher, C. S., & Spence, J. C. (2014). A qualitative examination of the impact of microgrants to promote physical activity among adolescents. *BMC Public Health*, *14*, 1–26. doi:10.1186/1471-2458-14-1206

2. The purpose of this research was to understand the leisure experiences, and to understand the meaning given to those experiences, of older adults with and without impairments who attended a community-based senior citizens' recreation centre.

   Rossow-Kimball, B., & Goodwin, D. L. (2014). Inclusive leisure experiences of older adults with intellectual disabilities at a senior centre. *Leisure Studies*, *33*, 322–38. doi:10.1080/02614367.2013.768692

3. The purpose of this research was to provide a detailed description of the cultural factors that facilitate the participation of Canadian South Asians in cardiac rehabilitation.

   Banerjee, A. T., Grace, S. L., Thomas, S. G., & Faulkner, G. (2010). Cultural factors facilitating cardiac rehabilitation participation among Canadian South Asians: A qualitative study. *Heart & Lung: The Journal of Acute and Critical Care*, *39*, 494–503. doi:10.1016/j.hrtlng.2009.10.021

4. Using semi-structured interviews and focus groups with youth tennis players, ex-youth players, coaches, and parents, the purpose of this research was to develop a theory of optimal parental involvement in youth sport tennis.

   Knight, C. J., & Holt, N. L. (2014). Parenting in youth tennis: Understanding and enhancing children's experiences. *Psychology of Sport and Exercise, 15*, 155–64. doi:10.1016/j.psychsport.2013.10.010

To see if your answers correspond with the strategy of inquiry identified in each study, use the references provided to find each study and check your answers.

Role of Theory in Qualitative Research

We ended our discussion of strategies of inquiry by providing a general description of grounded theory, and clearly theory plays a central role in grounded theory. What about the role of theory in other strategies of inquiry? Recall from Chapter 2 that theory can be used in a variety of ways within quantitative and qualitative research studies. We briefly described how theory could be used in qualitative research to inform the research problem and purpose, or that theory may be an outcome of the research (as is the case in grounded theory).

Professional Highlight

Dr Audrey Giles, Professor, School of Human Kinetics, Faculty of Health Sciences, University of Ottawa

....

Profile: Dr Giles is well-known for her qualitative research expertise. Her program of research is focused on the intersections among gender, ethnicity, injury prevention, and health promotion. She has extensive experience working with Indigenous populations in Northern Alberta, Northwest Territories, and Nunavut. Her research has explored Dene Games, Arctic Winter Games, and Northwest Territories aquatic programs using community-based participatory research approaches and various qualitative strategies of inquiry, including ethnography. For instance, in one community-based study, Giles and her colleagues (Giles et al., 2010) used participant observation, semi-structured interviews, and archival research of government documents and northern newspapers to better understand why residents of Tuktoyaktuk, Northwest Territories, rarely wear lifejackets. Giles and her colleague (Rousell & Giles, 2012) also drew upon participant observation, semi-structured interviews, and focus groups in a case study that examined the ways in which leadership styles used by lifeguards influenced Indigenous peoples' experiences at a Northern Canadian aquatic facility. Her qualitative research expertise is demonstrated in her publication record, which documents the use of various qualitative strategies of inquiry and processes of data generation.

Further Readings

Giles, A. R., Castleden, H., & Baker, A. C. (2010). "We listen to our Elders. You live longer that way": Examining aquatic risk communication and water safety practices in Canada's North. *Health and Place, 16,* 1–9. doi:10.1016/j.healthplace.2009.05.007

Giles, A. R., & Darroch, F. E. (2014). The need for culturally safe physical activity promotion programs. *Canadian Journal of Public Health, 105*(4), e317–e319.

Thus, it should be clear that theory *could* be used in a number of different ways within qualitative research. For instance, theory can be used as a **theoretical lens** or perspective to guide a qualitative study, whereby a theory helps to shape the research question(s), participant selection, data generation, and data analysis. Theory can also be used as an **interpretive framework**, whereby a specific theory is drawn upon to interpret or make sense of the research findings. It is also possible for some qualitative studies not to employ any explicit theory. In the latter case, researchers instead focus on constructing a detailed description of, for example, the phenomenon being studied. Although some researchers may not articulate the specific use of theory in their research, Sandelowski (1993) argued that "it is naïve to assume that any human project can ever be approached naively or atheoretically" (p. 215).

However, there are no strict guidelines to dictate *how* theory should (or should not) be used within qualitative studies. Drawing upon some examples from kinesiology research, we can see the various ways in which theory has been situated within qualitative studies. For example, Humbert et al. (2006) explored the factors that youth consider important for increasing physical activity participation among their peers, and they used an ecological model as a *theoretical lens* for their study. Humbert et al. stated that in order to understand the various factors that affect physical activity participation among youth, it is necessary to draw upon an ecological model that acknowledges various levels of influence (e.g., intrapersonal, social, environmental). Not only was an ecological model drawn upon at the outset of their study to guide their research question and shape their interview guide, but the model was also used as a framework for organizing results and interpreting findings. As another example, McHugh and her colleagues (2015) also drew upon an ecological model in their study, but it was used more as an *interpretative framework*. That is, McHugh et al. did not start with a specific theory, but used the Integrated Indigenous-Ecological Model as a framework for data analysis and the interpretation of findings. Their research was focused on better understanding the meanings of community, as it is understood within the context of sport, for urban Indigenous youth and adults. Participants were engaged in one-on-one interviews, and the findings or themes were organized and represented by the ecological leverage points that were identified by the Integrated Indigenous-Ecological Model.

Specific qualitative strategies of inquiry also draw upon theory in a variety of ways. For example, in a grounded theory approach, the theory is produced from the data and as such the theory is the *end* result in grounded theory. Ethnography, on the other hand, often *starts* with a strong theoretical lens. Researchers who use an ethnographic approach are often guided by a theory about the culture (e.g., beliefs, values, ideas) of the group they intend to include in their research. Qualitative description is arguably one of the least theoretical strategies of inquiry. Researchers using such a strategy of inquiry are committed to providing a detailed description of a specific phenomenon or event, and they are typically not committed to a specific theoretical understanding of the phenomenon or event. Researchers who employ a qualitative description approach may indeed begin with a specific theory as a framework for data generation, but the study may become less theoretical as the research progresses.

Sampling for Qualitative Studies

It is essential that researchers recruit a sample of participants that best enables them to answer their research question. Recall from Chapter 4 that a research **sample** can include individuals, organizations, teams, or schools. Qualitative research might also include documents, photographs, or any other information that can provide in-depth insight into the topic that is being explored. Some researchers will identify these other sources of data as part of their sample. For the purposes of this chapter, we will focus on samples that include people.

Purposeful sampling, sometimes referred to as purposive sampling (see Chapter 4), is a central feature of qualitative research. The intent of purposeful sampling is to recruit a sample of information-rich participants who will purposefully inform an understanding of the topic being studied. Typically, researchers identify a set of well-justified criteria that must be met by participants for inclusion in their study. For instance, the purpose of a study might be to explore adolescent women's experiences of social physique anxiety. The criteria for inclusion in the study could state that the participants must be women between the ages of 12 and 18 years who have had in-depth experience with the phenomenon of interest (i.e., social physique anxiety). Participants who fit such criteria will then be invited to participate in the research.

Table 7.1 Select types of purposeful sampling strategies that can be used in qualitative research.

SELECT TYPES OF PURPOSEFUL SAMPLING	DESCRIPTION	EXAMPLE
Extreme case	Identifying participants who are unusual or represent extremes; also called deviant cases	Selecting kinesiology professors who are rated as the best and worst instructors
Maximum variation	Seeking heterogeneity in people, experiences, places, perspectives, etc.; participants represent diversity	Sampling rehabilitation centre programs in urban and rural areas in different parts of Canada (diversity in location)
Snowball	Participants identifying other potential participants who are deemed fitting to the research purpose	Asking recruited recreation program managers to identify event coordinators, administrative support staff, and consumers

Many researchers will indicate that they have used the broad process of purposeful sampling, whereas others may choose to identify a specific form of purposeful sampling. Patton (2002) provided a detailed list of 16 specific types of purposeful sampling. For example, researchers might use **extreme case sampling**, whereby they sample participants who are deemed outliers to the topic of study. Alternatively, researchers might choose to engage in **maximum variation sampling** and identify individuals who represent a wide range of experiences or perspectives with respect to the topic of study. **Snowball sampling** is a commonly used process in which one individual or case identifies other individuals or cases that are deemed fitting to the purpose statement. However, these examples, which are represented in Table 7.1, are just three possibilities of the various types of purposeful sampling strategies that researchers might employ.

Case Study

Yves has been provided with a wonderful opportunity to lead an undergraduate research study while completing his Bachelor of Kinesiology at Memorial University of Newfoundland. Not only will he identify a research topic that he is passionate about, but he will also get to conduct the study! After months of preparation, Yves has finally identified the following research purpose (if you don't remember how he did this, go back and review Chapter 2): *The purpose of this phenomenological study is to better understand experiences of "choking under pressure" among elite athletes.* To provide in-depth insight into this phenomenon, Yves will need to purposefully sample his participants. Write down your answers to the following questions:

1. What are the *criteria* that Yves will use to purposefully select participants?
2. How do such criteria contribute to an information-rich sample?
3. How could Yves use extreme case sampling in his study?
4. How could Yves use maximum variation sampling in his study?

Sample size

Sample size is a hotly debated topic within the qualitative research literature. In Chapter 1 we discussed that the intent of qualitative research is not to generalize findings to a broad range of people (which is often the case for quantitative research), but instead to provide in-depth detail and understanding about the topic being studied. As such, there is general consensus that qualitative research samples should be relatively small compared to sample sizes in most quantitative studies. Saturation is often used to justify sample size, whereby researchers recruit participants until no (or very little) new information is being uncovered through data generation. Janice Morse, the founding Director and Scientific Director of the International Institute for Qualitative Methodology, outlined a number of considerations for reaching saturation and ultimately determining sample size (Morse, 2000). Some of the factors to consider include:

1. *Scope of the study*: Studies with topics that have a broad focus will likely take longer to reach saturation than studies with narrowly focused topics, and, therefore, will likely need to include more participants.
2. *Nature of the topic*: The extent to which the topic is obvious and clear will also impact saturation. A phenomenon, for example, may be very intriguing, but it might be challenging for participants to articulate or share their experiences because many phenomena are both abstract and complex (e.g., embodiment). As such, larger sample sizes might be needed to reach saturation in these cases.
3. *Quality of the data*: Some participants will be able to share their knowledge and experiences in great detail, yet others may not be able or willing to share the same level of detail about their experiences. If the quality of the data lacks depth, it may be necessary to include more participants.
4. *Number of interviews per participant*: Studies that involve multiple interviews per participant, rather than single interviews, will likely produce more data. Therefore, studies with multiple interviews might have fewer participants than studies with single interviews.
5. *Study designs*: Study designs that focus on multiple people in an organization or family (e.g., an intergenerational study that explored experiences of active transportation among a child, mother, and grandmother) will likely produce more data than studies that include a single interview with a participant.

Although there are many factors to consider when determining sample size, there are some general guidelines about sample sizes for each type of strategy of inquiry. For instance, a *narrative* often includes one or two individuals, a *phenomenology* often includes five to eight participants, a *grounded theory* may include 30 to 50 participants, an *ethnography* may include a single group of people that share the same culture, and a *case study* could involve an in-depth exploration of a single case or four to five cases. Given that a *qualitative description* may take on the hues of other strategies of inquiry, researchers may use sample sizes that are consistent with other strategies of inquiry.

Drawing upon examples from kinesiology, we can see how sample sizes often differ across different qualitative studies. For example, a *narrative* study by Sutherland et al. (2014) sought to explore six female athletes' experiences of emotional pain and self-compassion. Each participant took part in two semi-structured interviews, whereby one of the interviews included a reflexive photography task. Although a sample of six participants will likely not support the breadth of understanding that is sought in a study employing quantitative measures, the multiple processes of data generation employed within Sutherland et al.'s study contributed to the depth of this study. In other examples, qualitative study designs can include relatively large sample sizes. For instance, Holt and Dunn (2004) included a sample of 40 participants in their study that presented a *grounded theory* of factors associated with soccer success. Within their study, data were generated primarily through one-on-one interviews. Despite the general guidelines for sample sizes of various qualitative strategies of inquiry, it is important to remember that these are indeed just guidelines and the number of participants needed for a study will depend on a variety of factors (e.g., nature of the topic, quality of the data).

Data Generation in Qualitative Research

Data generation within qualitative research is varied. Interviews are notably the most common method for generating data in qualitative research, but with the surge of qualitative research studies being conducted across numerous disciplines, new or refined processes of data generation are continuously being published in the research literature. For instance, in kinesiology research, one-on-one interviews can be used to better understand participants' motivation to engage in extreme sports; group interviews might be used to explore the facilitators and barriers of cardiac rehabilitation programs; and observations may be used to better understand specific contexts, such as public exercise facilities or youth sport environments. In addition, qualitative studies often include more than one form of data generation. Some of the most commonly used processes are described in this section, including *interviews, observations, written documents*, and *visual data*. Table 7.2 summarizes common methods of data generation in qualitative studies.

Table 7.2 Common methods of data generation in qualitative studies.

INTERVIEWS	OBSERVATION	WRITTEN DOCUMENTS	VISUAL AND AUDIO SOURCES
One-on-one	Complete participant	Public	Art objects
	Participant as observer		Photographs
Group	Observer as participant	Private	Music
	Complete observer		Videos/ Film

Interviews

Interviews are often thought to be synonymous with qualitative research. Understanding the experiences of participants, and the meanings participants make of such experiences, are foundational to conducting interviews. Interviews conducted with a single person are referred to as **one-on-one interviews**, while **group interviews** include focus groups, sharing circles, and talking circles. One-on-one interviews might be used when research is focused on a sensitive topic (e.g., abuse experienced in sport), when individual participants reside in different geographical areas, or when participants do not know each other and a group interview may not be a comfortable environment for discussing the research topic. Group interviews might be used because the interaction among the group (e.g., teammates on a wheelchair basketball team) may result in a more information-rich and dynamic discussion. Group interviews can range in size, but researchers should typically consider having a group size of 6 to 10 participants to ensure that all participants are provided relatively equal opportunity to share their experiences (Patton, 2002). In addition to the size of the group interview, researchers should consider whether they want to include participants who are familiar with each other or new to each other. As well, grouping of participants might depend on other factors that are important to the topic of study, such as participants' age, gender, or ethnicity.

Regardless of whether the interview is one-on-one or group, it is essential to consider the relational nature of interviews. Researchers and participant(s) work together to generate data. Researchers must pose questions that are clear, relevant, and respectful; the participant strives to use words to articulate her or his experiences. Researchers do not simply *collect* the words or knowledge of participants. Instead, researchers and participant(s) work together to *generate* data to address the research topic.

Given the relational nature of interviews, it is necessary that researchers build **rapport** with the participant(s) in their studies. Rapport suggests that a harmonious relationship has been established whereby researchers and participant(s) can easily communicate because they understand the others' ideas and feelings. There is no set amount of time that is required to establish rapport. In some studies, particularly ethnographic studies, researchers might spend prolonged time (e.g., weeks/months/years) in the field to establish rapport. In other studies, rapport might be developed within the first few minutes of meeting participants. Especially in situations where the rapport phase is relatively brief, researchers and participants might engage in "everyday conversation" to become comfortable with one another prior to beginning data generation via one-on-one interviews, or do some sort of ice-breaker activity in a group interview setting. Remember, participants are recruited in qualitative research because they are deemed information-rich and the experts of their everyday lives and experiences. As such, it is necessary for researchers to create an environment whereby participants feel respected and that their knowledge and experiences are important. Assuming that the researchers conducting the study have had little or no contact with participants prior to the interview, they will likely strive to establish rapport during the introduction of the study and then work to maintain such rapport throughout.

Qualitative interviews typically comprise three main phases, including the introduction, questioning, and closing.

1. *Introduction:* The participants are introduced to the researcher and, if unfamiliar to one another, the focus of the introduction is on building rapport and creating a comfortable space for discussion. The researcher also provides a general introduction to the research topic and important information about ethical procedures, including obtaining informed consent and the voluntary nature of the study.

2. *Questioning:* This main phase of the interview process is typically shaped by an interview guide for semi-structured and structured interviews. The phase usually begins with questions that are relatively easy to answer and progresses towards more challenging or sensitive questions.

3. *Closing*: The closing phase of the interview comprises a number of features. It is focused on regulating emotions so that the interview ends on a positive note, which is particularly important when the research is focused on sensitive topics. During this phase the researcher offers the participants the opportunity to share final thoughts on the questions or general research topic. The closing phase should also include an outline of next steps (e.g., Will participants be contacted to confirm findings and share interpretations of findings? Are there instructions for another phase of data generation that follows the interview?) and an opportunity to thank participants for sharing their knowledge.

Interviews might take place face to face, over the telephone, or through various computer software forums (as might be the case for groups in different geographical areas whose only option is to connect electronically). Research that was led by Dany MacDonald at the University of Prince Edward Island used telephone interviews to better understand how coaches of athletes with intellectual disabilities gain their coaching knowledge (MacDonald et al., 2015). Given that the 45 participants were coaches recruited from across Canada, telephone interviews provided an ideal method for generating data among this geographically dispersed sample. Interviews might also vary from **structured** (i.e., specific set of interview questions), to **semi-structured** (i.e., a short interview guide with room to discuss topics not included on the interview guide), to **unstructured** (i.e., no interview guide and just a guiding topic for a conversational discussion). Unstructured interviews are relatively common in *narrative research* where the focus of the research is on the stories of participants as told by participants. *Phenomenological* studies, on the other hand, seek to provide a common meaning for several participants on a specific phenomenon. As such, interviews are often semi-structured so that a similar set of questions about experiences of the specific phenomenon can be asked in all interviews. The questions also vary from **closed-ended** (i.e., participants must choose their answer from a list of defined answers) to **open-ended** (i.e., there are no defined answers to questions and participants answer the questions using their own terms).

It should not be surprising that the development of a strong interview guide is often central to the success of a research study. The **interview guide** lists the questions or topics to be explored in the interview, and the guide is used to ensure that the same (or similar) questions are asked to multiple participants. Generally speaking, a semi-structured interview guide will include 7 to 10 main questions related to the topic of study, each of which may be accompanied by follow-up questions. Main questions may seek to understand participants' behaviours, feelings, or opinions regarding the research topic. To clarify specific details and to gain deeper insight into a response, researchers will use follow-up or probing questions. To build discussion, researchers should also seek to generate open-ended questions for the interview guide. Such questions could start with *who, what, where,* and *when. Why* questions can also be included, but researchers should ensure that such questions are carefully posed so as to not come across as judgmental.

Writing Exercise

Think about a kinesiology-related phenomenon that you are particularly interested in learning more about. Imagine you are about to engage approximately 10 participants in your phenomenological study and that your data generation includes one-on-one semi-structured interviews. Write down your responses to the following questions:

1. What is the phenomenon to be studied?
2. What is your research question and purpose?
3. What are the criteria for the purposeful selection of your participants?
4. What are seven main questions that you could include in your interview guide?
5. What are one or two possible probing questions for each of your seven main questions?

It is common for researchers to audio-record interviews (with the consent of participants of course!). Many years ago, recording devices were large and cumbersome; however, nowadays, audio-recorders are discrete and typically do not distract from the flow of the interview. Thus, in most cases audio-recording is recommended. The biggest benefit is that audio-recorded interviews can then be transcribed verbatim (i.e., the interview is typed word for word) so that the interview data are in a format ready for further data analysis. You can imagine how challenging (and distracting) it would be for researchers to handwrite everything that is said during an interview. However, it is common for researchers to write brief notes during the interview to document particularly noteworthy statements, body language, and details regarding the interview location. Notes might also be used to record information (e.g., seating arrangement of participants) that could be useful when later trying to decipher who is talking when listening to an audio-recorded group interview or when participants do not want their

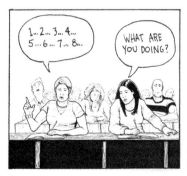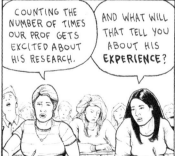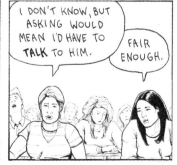

interviews formally recorded. But as another benefit, audio-recording provides researchers the opportunity to use direct quotations from participants' interviews in the final reporting of findings. Researchers might also want to consider using two audio-recorders for backup in case one does not work. The specific process of transcribing is critical to data analysis in many qualitative research studies and is, therefore, discussed in even more detail in Chapter 8.

Observation

In addition to interviews, observation is a key process for generating data in qualitative research. Observation can be used in most qualitative strategies of inquiry, but is particularly relevant to certain approaches. For example, ethnography often requires researchers to become immersed in the culture that is being studied, and observation is central to developing an in-depth understanding of a cultural-sharing group. **Observation** is a form of data generation that requires researchers to go into the field, or natural setting, to try to better understand the phenomenon or topic of study. Researchers use various senses, including sight, touch, and hearing, to study the phenomenon. Generally speaking, observation usually begins quite *broadly*, whereby researchers seek to develop an in-depth understanding of the context. For instance, a researcher interested in studying athlete-coach relationships in competitive swimming might attend a practice session to observe and record the sounds and sights of the pool, pool deck, spectators, and the sport facility structure. After these initial visits, she or he might then begin to have a more *specific* focus by observing the actual athlete-coach relationship. Of interest might be the number of times the coach and athlete interacted, the body language of the coach and athlete, the verbal tone used by the pair, as well as the type of information that was exchanged.

It is important to note that what one person observes in a particular context will be different from what another person observes. Researchers' philosophical worldviews, interests, and personal experiences inform their observations. For instance, researchers who have personal experiences in competitive swimming will likely have very different observations than researchers who have little to no personal experiences, in part because they will pay attention to different things. This is not to say that personal experience is a necessary component or that such experiences will make observations better. A person who has been involved in competitive swimming might not notice or observe the unique smells of the pool, the layout of the pool deck, or the constant chatter among coaches. These experiences might be so familiar that they don't seem particularly noteworthy. On the contrary, a person without competitive swimming experience might not notice a subtler, but particularly relevant, interaction between an athlete and a coach about a certain technical cue during a practice. Researchers should not worry about observing the "right thing" as it is clear that observations will differ from person to person based on their experiences.

Observation can take various forms. A researcher might be a **complete participant** and take part in the activity, event, or phenomenon under study. As such, she or he essentially becomes a participant, which is particularly useful in developing rapport with participants. It is also possible to engage in observation as the **participant as observer**. In this instance the researcher engages as both a participant *and* researcher. Her or his role as researcher is more obvious because active participation is combined with time taken to record observations. Another form of observation is **observer as participant**. In this case the researcher participates in the activity with participants, but participation is of secondary importance to actually recording observations. When acting as observer as participant, the researcher typically observes from a distance, but the participants are still aware that the researcher is present. Researchers who choose to engage in observation as **complete observer** have no interaction with the participants, and they are typically not noticed or seen by participants. It is also important to know that given the emergent and flexible nature of qualitative research, it is possible for researchers to shift their type of observation throughout the duration of the study.

Field notes are often used to record observations. Field notes describe what was observed through researchers' various senses. As well, field notes are used to record the feelings, hunches, and interpretations about what was observed. To ensure that such observations and reflections are easy to retrieve, field notes should be recorded when in the field (e.g., when acting as observer as participant) or as soon as possible, ideally within an hour after leaving the field (e.g., when acting as complete participant). Templates can be used to guide researchers' field notes (see Figure 7.1), or more advanced researchers might develop their own process for recording field notes.

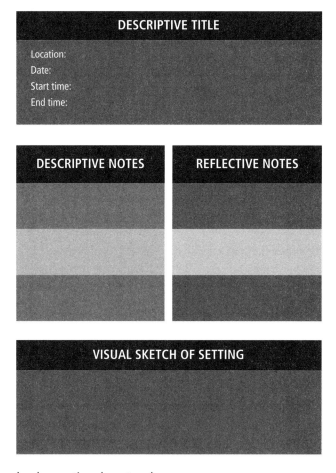

Figure 7.1 Sample observational protocol.

Creswell (2013) refers to such templates as an **observational protocol**, and he has suggested a number of features that should be included on the observational protocol:

- *Header:* This is a brief descriptive title about the observation session, including the length of the observation period.
- *Descriptive notes:* This section provides a space for summarizing and describing activities or phenomenon. Such descriptions are typically reported in chronological order, with specific times recorded.
- *Reflective notes:* This section, which is a column directly beside the descriptive notes, provides a space for the researcher to describe her or his feelings, reflections, or brief interpretations of the activities or phenomenon.
- *Visual sketch:* A visual depiction of the setting in which the observation took place may provide additional information that is useful for describing the context and the activity or phenomenon being studied.

Writing Exercise

You are interested in better understanding what motivates young men to access fitness facilities on campus. In addition to interviewing young men who are purposefully selected to participate in your research, you also acknowledge the importance of better understanding the context of fitness facilities on campus. As such, observation is used as another form of data generation in your study.

1. Take 20 minutes to engage in the process of "complete observation" at one of your university fitness facilities. Complete the *observational protocol* provided in Figure 7.1. Draw upon your senses (e.g., What did you *see*? What did you *hear*?) to describe and reflect upon information that you deem necessary for better understanding the fitness facility context.
2. Discuss with a classmate, or someone else who also engaged in this observational exercise, the differences in your observations. How were your descriptive notes similar or different? How were your reflective notes similar or different? Discuss the similarities and differences in your visual sketch of the setting.
3. If you were to do this observation again, what would you do differently?

Written documents

Various types of written documents can be used to generate data in qualitative research. For instance, researchers may choose to include public documents such as policies, newspaper articles, or historical archives. Researchers might also include written documents from participants, such as logbooks (e.g., exercise log), personal diaries or letters, or performance reports. Written documents are typically used in addition to other forms of data generation, such as one-on-one interviews, but they can also serve as the primary source of data generation. For instance, researchers from Dalhousie University (Huybers-Withers & Livingston, 2010) examined the discourses and images of a technology-focused mountain bike magazine and found that the magazine represents the gendered identities that are created through consumption practices. More specifically, Huybers-Withers and Livingston described how males are the main focus of the magazine and that mountain biking is portrayed as a male domain. In a different study, four major North American newspapers were the main source of data used to better understand how the mass media reports traumatic brain injuries in hockey (Cusimano et al., 2013). That research describes how newspaper articles portray violence and aggression as integral to hockey. As well, the newspaper articles also condemned violence and recognized the significance of traumatic brain injuries in hockey. The researchers argued that an understanding of reporting about traumatic brain injuries is necessary for determining whether media appropriately communicates the dangers of sport-related traumatic brain injuries. As demonstrated by the Cusimano et al. study, written documents can provide necessary insight into the study topic. In addition, written documents might also highlight more research questions or points of inquiry that could be subsequently explored in future research involving participants.

Visual data

Visual data might play a particularly valuable role in qualitative research. Researchers can draw upon photographs, drawings, mapping, diagrams, or videos to provide valuable insight into a phenomenon or an event. Researchers have used photographs to explore positive youth development in sport (Strachan & Davies, 2015) and to explore the impact of curling on the community life and health of rural women (Leipert, Scruby, & Meagher-Stewart, 2014). In both studies, the researchers demonstrated how photographs provided participants with opportunities to "show" their experiences. It is presumptuous of researchers to think that all participants express themselves comfortably through words; therefore, other processes of data generation (e.g., photographs) may be more relevant for certain populations. The strength of using visual data in qualitative research has been summarized by Mayan (2009), who said, "the visual can be so evocative and meaningful, it can entice and inspire people to draw on experiences and think about issues in ways that would otherwise be unavailable to them" (p. 83). For instance, mapping has been used by researchers to examine children's perceptions of places to play and be physically active (Holt et al., 2008). Children were asked to create maps, based on memory, that depict places in their neighbourhood where they can play and be physically active.

Summary

Chapter 7 outlined the defining features of qualitative research and provided a general overview of the qualitative strategies of inquiry that are commonly used in kinesiology. The various ways in which theory can be used in qualitative research was also discussed, and the use of theory within the context of specific qualitative strategies of inquiry was outlined. Given that people are often the main source of data in qualitative research, processes for purposeful sampling and identifying sample size were described. As well, various forms of data generation that are commonly used in qualitative research were also outlined. Interviews and observation were described as two of the most commonly used processes of data generation, and considerations for the development of interview guides and observation protocols were provided. This chapter ended with a brief discussion of the various types of written documents and visual data that have become more common as a source of data generation in qualitative research.

Discussion Questions

1. What are two defining features of qualitative research?
2. What are four qualitative strategies of inquiry commonly used by researchers in kinesiology?
3. How can theory be used in qualitative research?
4. Saturation is often used to determine sample size. What are three factors that should be considered by researchers as they strive to reach saturation?
5. What are the differences between an unstructured one-on-one interview and a structured talking circle?
6. What are three types of written documents that can be used to generate data in qualitative research?

Recommended Readings

Mayan, M. J. (2009). *Essentials of qualitative inquiry*. Walnut Creek, CA: Left Coast Press.

Morse, J. M. (2000). Determining sample size. *Qualitative Health Research, 10*, 3–5. doi:10.1080/ 15459624.2013.843780

Sandelowski, M. (1993). Theory unmasked: The uses and guises of theory in qualitative research. *Research in Nursing & Health, 16*, 213–18. doi:10.1002/nur.4770160308

8 Data Analysis in Qualitative Studies

Learning Outcomes

By the end of this chapter, you should be able to:

- Discuss various methods of qualitative data analysis.

- Apply the principles of qualitative data analysis to qualitative data.

- Identify strengths and challenges researchers often face in the qualitative data analysis process.

Introduction to Qualitative Data Analysis

As we discussed in Chapter 7, many different types of data can be generated within a qualitative research study. Although data resulting from interviews are probably the most common type within kinesiology research, data from observations and other visual methods (e.g., photographs) are often also part of the data-generation process in qualitative research studies. Appropriate analysis of these various sources of data is crucial to helping researchers answer their research questions, as well as to opening exciting new avenues for future research. Similar to quantitative analysis (i.e., statistics), a lack of thorough and proper qualitative analysis can lead to faulty interpretations and representations of participants' experiences and meanings.

An important starting point for all analysis is to realize that any one method of data generation can result in many different types of data analysis. For example, if researchers are interested in better understanding communication between athletes and coaches, one method to collect data might be via one-on-one interviews with both athletes and coaches. The resulting data set from those interviews could be used in different ways. On the one hand, the researchers might count the number of positively toned adjectives that athletes use to describe their coaches (and vice versa). In this case, because counting results in *numerical* data, *statistics* would be the appropriate analysis approach. Alternatively, the researchers might be interested in identifying general themes that best reflect both the athletes' and the coaches' experiences of communication with one another. As a result, rather than counting athletes' responses, the data might remain language-based, and a *qualitative data analysis* approach would be needed.

In essence, qualitative data analysis is used when researchers generate (and wish to analyze) non-numerical data. However, because data might include verbatim transcripts, field notes, documents, and audio-visual materials (to name just a few), it is probably no surprise that there are a wide range of qualitative data analysis methods to choose from.

In an attempt to overview some of the variety and choices researchers have when deciding on a data analysis strategy, Leech and Onweugbuzie (2008) provided a *compendium* of 18 qualitative analysis techniques. As they argue, "analysis of the data is one of the most important steps in the research process" (p. 587), but most researchers are not even aware of the variety of choices they have. Although developed specifically in the context of school psychology research, the types of data identified by Leech and Onweugbuzie (i.e., talk, observations, drawings/photographs/video, and documents) are similar to the types of data often generated by kinesiology researchers. A full review of Leech and Onweugbuzie's compendium is beyond the scope of this chapter; however, it is important to note that some of the data analysis techniques they discuss are more common (e.g., constant comparison analysis) than others and that some can be used with multiple sources of data (e.g., both transcripts and visual image data).

Identifying the goals of data analysis

In addition to considering the type of data when identifying an analysis approach, the specific goal of the qualitative analysis is also important. Bradley, Curry, and Devers (2007) encouraged researchers to think about the types of results they want from their analysis (e.g., taxonomy, themes, theory), keeping in mind that the types of results they seek should be informed by the goal, or purpose, of the research.

If a researcher's goal is to increase clarity in defining certain constructs (e.g., physical self worth) or to compare complex constructs (e.g., sports competence and physical strength), the result might be a **taxonomy**, which represents a formal system for classifying multi-faceted and complex phenomenon. For example, Kowalski and colleagues (2006) developed a taxonomy of coping based largely on adolescents' opened-ended written responses. Specific dimensions within their taxonomy ranged from acceptance, to behavioural avoidance, to seeking professional support; each dimension had a clearly defined conceptual description that can be used to disentangle the many ways adolescents cope with situations in which they experience body anxiety.

In other cases, the goal might be to develop **themes** from the data as a way to characterize the responses of participants and provide insight into the essential components of their experience. For example, semi-structured interview-based research conducted at the University of Toronto by Tjong and colleagues (2013) showed that three themes underlie the decision to return to sport following anterior cruciate ligament (ACL) reconstruction: fear, lifestyle priorities, and differences in personalities. As another example, O'Reilly, Tompkins, and Gallant (2001) from St. Francis Xavier University developed themes from their research that examined the word "fun" as it is conceptualized by seven female physical educators. Two themes represented their findings: (a) fun is not competition . . . or maybe it is, and (b) fun (and) games for life.

Alternatively, the goal might be to develop **theory**, or to develop a set of interlocking causal variables to explain some aspect of our personal, social, or physical realities.

Recalling our discussion in Chapter 7, the entire goal of grounded theory is to develop theory; however, theory can develop from many different types of qualitative data analysis approaches.

Inductive and deductive data analysis

Another general decision point in qualitative data analysis is whether to utilize inductive or deductive processes (recall Figure 2.2 in Chapter 2). In an **inductive data analysis**, researchers identify taxonomies, themes, or theory from the data generated in the research. There is no presumption on the main categories, and, as a result, the findings are grounded in the data that are generated. Alternatively, in a **deductive data analysis** process, there is an existing framework or starting list of categories by which researchers code the data. However, it is

Professional Highlight

Dr Fiona Moola, Assistant Professor, Faculty of Kinesiology and Recreation Management, University of Manitoba

....

Profile: Dr Moola has conducted a number of qualitative research studies, primarily focused on psychological well-being in people with chronic illnesses and disabilities. She is also known for her applied work with children and families in clinical settings and finding ways to use physical activity and exercise to improve mental health. She and her colleagues (Moola et al., 2015) conducted a qualitative interpretive phenomenological research project on the experience of children with congenital heart disease at Camp Woodland. Camp Woodland is based in Ontario and offers sick children, many of who are child survivors of chronic illness, opportunities to experience a variety of outdoor camp activities (e.g., swimming in the lake, hiking through forest trails, rock climbing). An important aspect of Camp Woodland is the philosophy of children's success being measured by a willingness to try, rather than the amount that they are able to accomplish. Their research is critical in showing how the children's pleasurable camp experiences can play an important role in helping the children build friendships and enhance their quality of life. Dr Moola and her colleagues have used a number of different qualitative data analysis strategies across their research studies. Their publications also include some excellent examples of the level of detail researchers are encouraged to provide when describing their qualitative data analysis process.

Further Readings

Moola, F. J., & Faulkner, G. E. J. (2014). "A tale of two cases": The health, illness, and physical activity stories of two children living with cystic fibrosis. *Clinical Child Psychology and Psychiatry, 19*, 24–42. doi:10.1177/1359104512465740

Moola, F. J., Faulkner, G., White, L., & Kirsh, J. (2015). Kids with special hearts: The experience of children with congenital heart disease at Camp Woodland. *Qualitative Research in Sport, Exercise, and Health, 7*, 271–93. doi:10.1080/2159676X.2014.926968 important to note that researchers conducting qualitative data analysis often use a *combination* of inductive and deductive processes. They might start with a theoretical framework but allow the data to form emergent categories that are unique to (and not bound by) existing theory. As such, qualitative data analysis can be very fluid and flexible and helps researchers answer research questions in a way that both acknowledges existing theory and rings true to the words and experiences of participants in the study. You will see mention of inductive and deductive processes again later in this chapter, as they have particularly important implications to the coding of qualitative data.

Qualitative Data Analysis as Immediate, Ongoing, and Spiral

When conducting a *quantitative* study, researchers eagerly await completion of the data collection process prior to running their statistics, and then they typically only do a re-analysis if an error or a new type of statistic emerges that can further inform their research questions (or they have different types of research questions that are based on different sub-sets of a larger data set). This is not the case for *qualitative* data analysis. Although the same data collection method can result in many different types of data, there are three prominent ways in which qualitative data analysis is fundamentally distinct from quantitative data analysis. Qualitative data analysis is immediate, ongoing, and spiral.

As described by Sparkes and Smith (2014), "qualitative data analysis is an artful and scientific interpretive process of meaning-making that begins at the outset of the investigation" (p. 115). We really like this description because it clearly highlights that qualitative analysis is both an art and a science; as such it begins *immediately* as part of the development of the research. But how can data analysis begin before data are generated? To answer this question it is important to recognize that within a qualitative research study, the *investigator* is the primary data collection instrument, such that all the other methods (e.g., interviews, observation) ultimately filter through the lens of the researcher. Hence, data analysis begins the moment the investigator begins thinking about her or his research. The combination of personal experience, theoretical and empirical knowledge, along with the data that results from data generation are all integrated together into an interpretive framework that informs the research question. Hence, to do justice to this process, researchers need to reflect on the role they play as part of the data analysis process from the beginning formulations of the research question through to the final representation of the results.

To say that qualitative data analysis is *ongoing* is to acknowledge that there isn't just one moment (or finite amount of time) when data analysis takes place. Rather, data analysis is something researchers engage in throughout the entire process of a research study. This is particularly evident as additional information that might challenge previous interpretations is generated from new participants. As a result, researchers should not treat their initial interpretations as precious; a reluctance to be flexible to new insights that might emerge can detract from the quality of the research. Embracing data analysis as an ongoing process from start to finish can add a level of depth and richness to the final interpretations. In many cases, researchers continue to think about their findings, and other possible interpretations, long after official publication

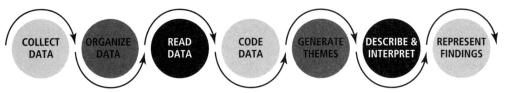

Figure 8.1 The data analysis spiral in qualitative research studies.

or presentation of their work. This is, in part, recognition that the insight resulting from high-quality qualitative research likely raises even more questions than it answers.

Not only is qualitative data analysis ongoing, but it is often considered a *spiral* process. Creswell (2013) outlines the data analysis spiral, which he uses to emphasize that data analysis in qualitative research is not a fixed linear approach. Rather, he talks about "analytic circles" that create a spiral from the beginning of data generation through to the final account of the findings. Researchers flow through the data analysis process, often returning to earlier steps in the analysis as new insights and reflections emerge. The fluidity of this process is at the heart of the art of qualitative inquiry, and without embracing the spiral nature of qualitative data analysis, much insight can be missed. Even though we discuss general steps to qualitative analysis in the next section, researchers need to keep in mind that these aren't necessarily discrete steps. Researchers can move between steps, often returning to earlier steps, as a way to build the most credible interpretation of the results possible. Qualitative data analysis is inherently complex and multifaceted. As researchers experience their data, they will always be thinking and re-thinking the meaning of the findings and how new information informs their prior interpretations. The data analysis spiral in qualitative research studies is depicted in Figure 8.1.

Steps in Qualitative Data Analysis

Based on the previous sections, clearly there is no one best way to conduct a qualitative data analysis. The ideal approach is one in which the steps in the data analysis match the goals of the research purpose and the strategy of inquiry. For example, if the goal is to conduct an ethnographic study on the culture of a youth sports team, the analysis will likely vary from the analysis of a study in which the goal is to construct a narrative of young women's experiences of body image. Hence, it is always best practice to consult key texts to identify specific data analysis strategies that might be particularly important within a particular strategy of inquiry (e.g., see Stake's, 1995, *The Art of Case Study Research* for case study analysis options). However, despite differences in analysis approaches across qualitative strategies of inquiry, a number of steps appear to be fairly common across a variety of approaches to qualitative data analysis. Creswell (2014) presents one of the most useful and practical overviews of data analysis in qualitative research by highlighting the following six steps in the data analysis process:

- Step 1: Organize and prepare the data.
- Step 2: Read or look at all the data.

- Step 3: Start coding all the data.
- Step 4: Generate descriptions or themes.
- Step 5: Decide how the findings will be represented.
- Step 6: Interpret the findings.

Step 1: Organize and prepare the data

In cases where data generation results in written text, **transcribing** is a key part of the organization and preparation process. Transcribing refers to the process of taking oral data and reproducing it as faithfully as possible as a written text (i.e., writing it out fully). For example, researchers might have conducted interviews with elderly exercisers to gain insight into their meanings of social support; however, at the end of the data collection phase, the participants' words might only exist within a digital audio file. While potentially useful in that format, transcribing the interviews verbatim (i.e., exactly what was said by the elderly exercisers) into written text is often a necessary step as a way to review the content of the interviews and to prepare it for the data-coding step. The end result of transcribing can be *a lot* of data. To give a bit of perspective, Sabiston et al. (2007) reported that they ended up with 1053 pages of *single*-spaced data transcripts from interviews with adolescent females. That's over a thousand pages of transcribing required prior to even beginning formal coding of the data!

While it might seem relatively straightforward (and time consuming), the process of transcribing itself is an art. First, no matter the quality of the equipment, certain portions of the audio file can be difficult to hear or make out what was said. In these cases, some notation might be needed on the transcripts to reflect that a portion of the interview was inaudible or that the transcriber is taking a best guess as to what was said. Second, there are many aspects of language that are nuanced and could be part of the transcription process. For example, were there pauses in speech? What about changes in voice and inflection? Was there excitement or agitation in the participant's response? Were multiple voices trying to be heard at the same time (as is often the case in a focus group)? What nonverbal communication could be captured? These are just a few questions that might be asked by a reader of a transcript. If the text is simply transcribed word for word, much information and insight can be lost. Because context is so important to qualitative data analysis, having extra layers of information in a transcription can often provide invaluable insight into a research question.

Blake Poland, a faculty member in the Dalla Lana School of Public Health at the University of Toronto, discusses a wide range of errors that can occur when preparing interview and focus group transcripts (Poland, 1995). Transcription errors can range from deliberate alterations of the data (e.g., the transcriber changing the text to correct participants' grammar), to accidental alterations of the data (e.g., the placement of the start and end of sentences; missing a section in the recording), to unavoidable alteration (e.g., translation of body language to written text). However, as Poland notes, transcription itself is an interpretive activity, so even the determination of what is an "error" in some cases is not straightforward. Poland also provides a number of concrete strategies for maximizing the quality of transcriptions, particularly through the use of syntax as part of written text. For example, brackets can be used to show an overlap in text, time elapsed in silence, or an inability to hear what was said; underscoring or capitalization can represent aspects of voice such as pitch or sound level; and colons can indicate prolonged sounds (e.g., O:kay).

As an example of how two transcriptions from the same interview might look very different from one another, take the following examples:

- *Example 1*: "My experience in soccer camp was great, but I really had to work hard to stay positive and keep up my self-confidence"
- *Example 2*: "Uh . . . hmmm . . . my experience in soccer camp was great (!), but I . . . like . . . re:::ally had to work hard to stay positive and like . . . uh . . . keep up my self-confidence (shy laugh)"

Both of the above transcriptions could come from the same audio file, but they read very differently. In the first case, the content is actually easier to follow because a lot of the "extras" have been deleted. In the second case, the added notation adds a great deal of depth to the content itself. Neither transcription is necessarily wrong, because both could be considered accurate from certain points of view. Their relative usefulness, however, will depend on the goals of the research and the intended focus of the remaining steps in the data analysis process.

Having an effective strategy to maximize the quality of transcripts is particularly important in cases where the researchers are not the ones actually doing the transcriptions. Although it is likely ideal for the researchers to also do the transcribing, in many cases doing so is not feasible. Hence, professional transcribers are often hired. When having someone else transcribe, it is recommended by Poland (1995) that researchers review the first set of transcriptions for accuracy and as a way to prevent systemic errors from occurring across the entire data set. However, it is important to note that having researchers themselves transcribe interviews doesn't necessarily mean that there will be less error. Chad Witcher, currently a faculty member in Public Health at the University of Lethbridge, discusses the concept of being a "relative insider" (i.e., familiar with the research context) and how a researcher's position can contribute to transcription quality (Witcher, 2010). It can be beneficial in helping to understand local dialect; however, close ties to community members can also result in participants' reluctance to reveal certain types of information to the interviewer. Hence, he argues that it is crucial for researchers to examine their own backgrounds and how those backgrounds can impact the data transcription process.

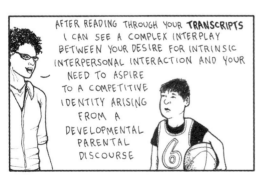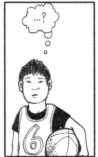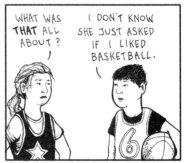

At this point in our chapter, it is important to remember that not all data requires transcription into written text . . . but non-written data also needs to be organized and prepared in a way that it is accessible and ready for subsequent data analysis steps. Often photographic data are generated as an electronic file on the memory card in a digital camera. However, this format is rarely most effective for subsequent steps in data analysis. Hence, researchers might print all photographs and lay them on the floor of a large room so that they can view them all at once, while at the same time having the ability to move the photos around as needed. Others might use electronic-based formats (e.g., publishing or digital illustration software) to organize the photographs.

The choice of format can have important implications. For example, the resolution of images (e.g., compare a 72dpi digital image to a 600dpi digital image), the colours represented (e.g., colours often look different on a computer than on a printed page), and even the amount of information viewable at any one time (e.g., because of cropping or screen size) can all be impacted. The choice of format made by researchers in turn can play a role in how the data are viewed, coded, and interpreted. Thus, regardless of the specific type of data, finding the most effective strategy to organize and prepare that data is essential to an effective qualitative data analysis process.

Transcription Exercise

Prepare a short interview guide (e.g., three or four questions) focused on a kinesiology-related topic of interest to you and framed around a qualitative research-based question (e.g., the meaning of physical activity; experiences in high school physical education; narrative of injury rehabilitation). Interview yourself using the guide that you created, audio-recording your responses (one option is the audio recorder on your smartphone), providing as much insight into each question as possible. Once the interview is complete, transcribe your interview (or a portion of the interview) using the guidelines presented in Table 2 (page 301) of Poland's (1995) article on transcription quality:

Poland, B. D. (1995). Transcription quality as an aspect of rigor in qualitative research. *Qualitative Inquiry, 1*, 290–310. doi:10.1177/107780049500100302

1. What were some of the biggest lessons learned in transcribing your interview responses?
   a. Were the guidelines offered by Poland (1995) useful?
   b. What information would be missing in the transcript if you had not followed his guidelines?
2. What information in your transcript would have been lost had the interview been transcribed by someone else?
   a. Were there parts of your responses that could have been misinterpreted by someone who read only the transcript?
3. How could you enhance the transcription quality, if you were to interview someone else (or perhaps even yourself again) in a subsequent research study on the topic?
4. What strategies could you use to ensure that the transcription was an accurate representation of the actual interview?

Step 2: Read or look at all the data

Whether it be transcripts, documents, or field notes, once the data are prepared and organized (i.e., Step 1), going through the data multiple times is the next important step in qualitative data analysis. While spending sufficient time reviewing data might seem like an obvious idea, researchers often get impatient in the data analysis process and rush going from preparation of the data (Step 1) to coding of the data (Step 3). In some cases there might be deadlines that need to be met (e.g., publication deadlines or thesis deadlines); in other cases it might be the result of a passionate quest to "know" the answer to a research question sooner rather than later. However, rushing from preparation of the data to coding of the data can lead to errors, particularly because themes might develop without adequate consideration of the entire context of the data set.

In essence, there are many benefits to reading or looking at all the data (particularly doing so multiple times). First, the more familiarity researchers have with their data, the less likely that something will be missed in the formal coding process that follows. For example, if you were intimately familiar with a set of interview transcripts, it would be much easier to remember content within the transcripts that might relate to the themes that begin to emerge. This could include aspects of the setting that were mentioned by the participants. It's sort of like reading or watching a good book or movie a few times—each time through it you'll notice different things, particularly layers of detail that were overlooked at the first reading or viewing.

Second, as we discussed earlier, because data analysis begins immediately and at the outset of the research project, resulting themes are typically in a state of flux throughout the research, shaping and changing as new insights emerge with time. Reading or looking at all of the data over and over simply takes time. Each pass through the data can shift researchers' thinking about the data, resulting in a more rich and insightful final interpretation. Without taking time with the data, the research can proceed too quickly and researchers can become tempted to accept their first insights as an end result. Often, allowing for weeks and even months to pass between reviews of the data can be a useful exercise, as it provides the opportunity for reflection, critical analysis, and new insights to emerge.

Third, and perhaps most importantly, it is critical that researchers not get lost in the minute details of a data set, thereby causing them to miss the larger picture the results are meant to represent. Thus, reading and looking at all the data multiple times allows researchers the opportunity to take a step back from the data. Sufficient time with the data allows for that bigger perspective and identification of a key thread (or threads) that run through it. For example, if we were doing an analysis of the entire *Star Wars* saga it might be easy to get lost in the vast amount of detail, resulting in a focus that would invariably differ across researchers. However, by watching the series of movies a number of times, prior to a specific analysis of component parts, you'll probably notice George Lucas' intent to tell a story that it is primarily about universal themes like mythology, religion, and compassion. With that lens, it's much easier to see how the collection of movies simply inform those main themes. Without that lens, the Star Wars saga might be interpreted simply as an adventure story about robots and outer space (which it is, but to miss the larger universal themes would be an oversight). There are similar implications for research in kinesiology. Researchers can lose sight of the context of someone's experience or the essence of a phenomenon or culture by simply focusing on the details.

It's easy to see when an artist rushes a drawing or a painting, and the same is true for qualitative data analysis. Without spending time with the data, the layer of richness in the final product is often missed. Without adequate time spent reading and looking at all of the data, researchers can miss an opportunity to answer their research questions in a way that best represents the data generated in their study.

Reading the Data Exercise

Read the following narrative passage, which is an excerpt from Rachel Donen's (2007) kinesiology graduate thesis exploring the inquiry processes of eight middle-aged women in a mindfulness program. This excerpt, reprinted with permission from Rachel Donen, is from her results section and serves the purpose of developing context for her main findings:

> I have been living in this house for over 25 years. Through the years my home has remained a place of stability, a place of support, and a place I feel centred in. My home is a very large home close to the end of the block. From the front grass you see a white cement house with gray trim around the windows, doors, and roofs. The cement at the bottom of the house is cracking and some of the gray trim is chipping.
>
> This house has a lot of charm. It is a two-level house with a basement, where the two upper levels from the outside are divided by trim that forms the shape of two sailor hats stacked one on top of each other. Around the house is a whitish picket fence; each section of the fence is leaning in somewhat different directions. The front grass is mainly coarse with patches of new growth that are moist and soft, and there are leaves scattered everywhere. A cool breeze is present, yet the sun is warm: it is spring!
>
> Every now and then I enjoy lying on the grass and taking naps in the shade. The front yard is flat and shaped like a long dining room table, and a brick walkway runs through the middle of the grass to the front door. The front door is on the south side of the house, as is a large lengthwise rectangular window. A large, smooth, rounded, gray stone sits on the ground at the left side of the front door. There is an outer and inner door: the outer door is mainly filled with glass windows, whereas the inner door is heavy wood that has been painted gray. A lion's head rests at the center of the door.
>
> The front entrance of my home is graced with different plants growing wildly on the right side, open space, and cool gray tiles line the floor. There is a large window on the right allowing the sunlight to fall in, and a glass hexagon light fixture hangs down from the tall prickly ceiling. There are prickly ceilings and walls throughout the house that look like various whitish stalactites. The front entrance is warm. From the front entrance, sunken from the rest of the house, you can see the entrance into the kitchen. White crown moulding lines this entrance. A closet with tall white doors stands straight ahead and blends into the whitish walls and ceiling. A winding staircase sits beside the closet and

Continued

overtop of the front entrance. Art hangs throughout the house: all of nature, framed in multiple colors of either metals or woods. The house is illuminated each day with the sunrise.

Everything is large in this house: large rectangular windows, endless hardwood floors, and oversized furniture. You must pass through a doorway on the left to enter the living room, where sometimes the glass door lining the doorway is open, which I enjoy.

At the front of the living room is a large bay window covering the entire front wall. You can almost see the entire block from here. A row of birch trees lines both sides of the street; and robins, chickadees, crows, cars, and people sporadically flow past the window.

I like to watch the birds from this window. Their movements are flowing, graceful, fearless, sharp, and bouncy. The robins have the most peculiar movements: hop, hop . . . scuttle, scuttle and repeated again and again. As I watch the birds for longer periods of time I start to notice the pauses between their movements, the stillness. It seems as though whenever the birds produce movement there is also stillness: stillness before, in the middle, or at the end of movement. The movement and stillness are one, connected. Watching the birds brings a smile to my face and a gentle depth to my breath.

At both bottom corners of the window are smaller wooden tables with glass tops. They both display oversized gray lamps with shades covered in gray chiffon. Pictures of the family are scattered on top of the tables, along with wooden and stone sculptures. Coming out from the window are two couches that are on outward diagonals to each other. There is room for two on a couch. One armrest on each of the couches holds a knitted blanket.

Sitting on the couch farthest from the entrance into the living room, I can see the large wooden coffee table with a glass top that rests in-between the couches. A plant sits on the table, along with a book and more wooden and stone sculptures. Despite the number of objects in the room, there is space to walk because each object has been organized like a gallery. The walls are covered with rows of framed art, almost museum-like in display, where overhanging lighting illuminates each nature scene. The room houses a black fireplace, and a wooden antique chair sits by the fireplace waiting for the warmth of the fire. There are numerous books lining a mahogany bookshelf. The books rarely see the light of day because they are overshadowed by the piano standing in the corner of the living room. The piano has a little bit of dust on it and is covered with various shaped vases and an oversized gray lamp that is identical to the others in the living room.

From the couch I can see the dining room at the back of the house. A few large, but tame plants sit on either side of the entrance to the dining room. The living room is quiet. All you can hear is the classical music coming from the kitchen (and the ticking of the clock over the main entrance into the dining room).

"Yes," I say to my friend Nadine who is sitting beside me on my living room couch. "Yes, time seems to pass so quickly in my adult life. Yet I can still recall, very clearly, some memories of when I was just 16 years old attending high school."

Nadine is 63 years old, tall, white haired, an athletic build. She sports an ageless face, is a mother of two daughters, and a wife. I met Nadine in passing at yoga a year ago, but we did not start socializing until last month. We always say how surprised we are at how open and trusting we are of one another, even though we have known each other for such a short time. Nadine suggests that perhaps it is our shared experience at yoga that provides this familiarity, this depth of relationship.

1. Write down as much detail as you can remember from the excerpt, as though you were trying to remember verbatim the details to share with someone else.
    a. What details stand out for you after reading the excerpt?
    b. What parts of the excerpt are particularly hard to remember?
2. Now read the excerpt a second time. After reading it again, is there any information that was particularly noteworthy that you missed in the first reading?
    a. How did reading the excerpt again inform the details you remembered after the first reading only?
3. Now read the excerpt a third time. Notice how your interpretation of the events and the narrator begins to shift as you read it multiple times, particularly as more of the excerpt becomes familiar to you.
4. How many times do you think you would need to read the excerpt to feel like you know it intimately?
    a. How would your understanding of the context be different had you just read one paragraph from the excerpt but not the whole thing?

Step 3: Start coding all the data

Coding is a key step in qualitative data analysis and represents a systematic organizing of the data into meaningful chunks that, once brought together into something shared, become the significant themes of the research. As Creswell (2014) describes, coding the data "involves taking text data or pictures gathered during data collection, segmenting sentences (or paragraphs) or images into categories, and labeling those categories with a term, often a term based in the actual language of the participant (called an *in vivo* term)" (p. 198). Coding is the step most people typically associate with qualitative data analysis.

There is certainly no one way to go about the coding process in qualitative data analysis, and the specific strategy chosen by researchers will depend largely on two things: (a) the type of data, and (b) the types of coding categories of interest. The type of data plays a major role in the specific coding strategy used. For example, the coding of an interview transcript will need to be very different from that for a visual image, because the data itself is very different (i.e., written versus visual). For written language, researchers might use sticky notes to highlight common words, use different colour highlighters to mark intersections in content within and across participants, or electronically group similar items in a spreadsheet, to name just a few options. For visual data, researchers might post all of the images on an office wall and use a coding system to identify themes related to the use of composition, balance, rhythm, and colour.

Research Highlight

Shaunna Taylor and her colleagues at the Universities of Ottawa and Calgary conducted a case study exploring the lifelong learning of a parasport coach (Taylor, Werthner, & Culver, 2014). This study provides a good example of the coding process. They conducted three interviews with an elite-level coach resulting in approximately 100 pages of double-spaced transcripts. Four additional interviews with four other individuals who collaborated with the coach to enhance his coaching and practice were also conducted, resulting in another 60 pages of double-spaced transcripts. Their coding of the data around the coach's life experiences and learning situations resulted in a number of themes related to how he used his formal education in his coach practice, how his interactions with others helped him learn within the parasport context, and what personal initiatives he invested to become a better coach. Specific examples of codes within the themes included things like early life experiences, types of formal and informal training, and technical adaptations. All told, the Taylor et al. research presents an example of how interviews become transcripts, how transcripts become a dataset to be coded, and how the coding process transforms into meaningful and interesting themes that inform the initial research question.

Further Reading

Taylor, S. L., Werthner, P., & Culver, D. (2014). A case study of a parasport coach and a life of learning. *International Sport Coaching Journal, 1*, 127–38. doi:10.1123/iscj.2013-0005

The important point is that regardless of the specific approach, researchers should select a strategy that keeps them well-organized and comprehensive in their coding of the data.

When thinking of how to code for different categories of interest, Creswell's (2014) approach is a useful one to consider. He describes codes as falling into one of three categories: *expected* codes, *surprising* codes, and *unusual* codes. Expected codes represent things one might expect to see based on previous literature and previous experience. For example, if researchers were conducting a study on young women's experience in physical education class, there might be a set of codes used to represent gendered language around femininity and masculinity. Alternatively, surprising codes include things that were not anticipated at the beginning of a study. For example, McArthur and colleagues (2014) interviewed 53 middle-aged women living in an urban Canadian city about the enablers and barriers influencing their adherence to regular exercise. They were surprised to find that climate was not a significant concern to the women in their study. Hence, when they were coding the data, any discussion around climate in the transcripts, especially information contradicting it as a barrier, could be part of a surprise category. The final coding category mentioned by Creswell, representing unusual codes, is meant to capture aspects of a transcript that might be of particular interest to someone reading about the research. For example, in a study on coaches' experiences in elite sport there might be some discussion related to a particular international event that was unique in some way (e.g., weather conditions; equipment malfunctions; political system).

An alternative approach to coding categories of interest is presented by Bradley, Curry, and Devers (2007), who recommend that researchers clarify *what* it is that they are coding. They talk about five different code types, including those that identify essential components of key conceptual domains (i.e., conceptual codes); those that identify links between concepts (i.e., relationship codes); those that identify whether participants are positive, negative, or neutral about a particular experience (i.e., participant perspective codes); those that identify descriptive characteristics of the participants (i.e., participant characteristics codes); and those that identify characteristics of the setting in which the data are generated (i.e., setting codes). Each of these code types has a different application or purpose and is more or less useful in developing taxonomies, themes, and/or theory.

Taken together, both key points made by Bradley, Curry, and Devers (2007; i.e., the needs to identify the types of results desired and to clarify what is being coded) are important to keep in mind when setting out to conduct qualitative data analysis in kinesiology research. These key points direct researchers towards aspects of the data that will best enable them to answer their research questions, which is important because it is easy to become overwhelmed by the amount and diversity of data that often result from qualitative data generation. Their key points can be summarized as follows:

- Types of *results* researchers want from their analysis
  - *Taxonomy*: A formal system for classifying phenomena
  - *Themes*: A characterization of components of experiences
  - *Theory*: A set of interlocking causal explanations
- Important to identify *what* is being coded
  - *Conceptual codes:* Essential components of a conceptual domain
  - *Relationship codes:* Links between concepts
  - *Participant perspective codes:* Direction (e.g., positive, negative, or neutral) of the experience
  - *Participant characteristic codes*: Descriptors of the participants
  - *Setting codes*: Descriptors of the setting

Additional insight into the coding of qualitative data can be gleaned from the literature on content analysis. As described by Elo and Kyngäs (2007), content analysis is useful when trying to describe a phenomenon in a conceptual form, and it is particularly appropriate for coding of textual data (Hsieh & Shannon, 2005). Hence, strategies used in content analysis are often useful across a number of different types of qualitative research studies conducted in kinesiology. Similar to Creswell (2014), in their discussion of content analysis Elo and Kyngäs emphasize both inductive and deductive approaches to coding of qualitative data. They describe that, in inductive content analysis specifically, the concept of **open coding** refers to writing notes and headings in a text as it is being read, with the goal to find a way to describe all aspects of the content. Once a list of categories is generated, the coded content is then grouped into higher-order themes as a way to describe the phenomenon as effectively and efficiently as possible (we discuss this process of theme generation further in Step 4). Alternatively, in deductive content analysis researchers use existing categories developed from previous theory and research, which Elo and Kyngäs refer to as a **categorization matrix**. The content of the text is then coded using the categorization matrix as a guide. Researchers might choose to only code content that can fit into the categorization matrix or create additional categories from the content that doesn't fit within the categorization matrix, in a manner similar to inductive content analysis. The notion of a categorization matrix is similar to Bradley, Curry, and Devers's (2007) taxonomy concept, in that both can serve as a pre-existing framework for coding qualitative data.

A consideration is whether researchers use qualitative data-analysis software (QDAS) as part of their data-analysis process, since it can be particularly useful when coding qualitative data. Two of the most commonly used QDAS programs in the health sciences are ATLAS.ti and NVivo (Woodset al., 2016). In their review of 763 articles published between 1994 and 2013 that reported using either ATLAS.ti or NVivo, Woods et al. showed that these two programs were most commonly used for analysis of interview data, focus group data, documents, observational field notes, and open-ended survey responses. However, they were also used with video or image data, conversational data, and online social media data, demonstrating a range of data sources that can be analyzed using QDAS. Perhaps of specific interest to us is that Canada was identified as having the fourth highest total number of researchers using QDAS (behind only the United States, the United Kingdom, and Australia) and that exercise science, sports, and kinesiology were listed among the subject disciplines of journals publishing ATLAS.ti or NVivo studies (with medicine most represented).

Although potentially attractive, QDAS is *optional* for most qualitative research and needs to be used with the goals of the research in mind. Áine Humble, a professor in the Department of Family Studies and Gerontology at Mount Saint Vincent University in Halifax, describes the growing use of QDAS in family-focused research journals (Humble, 2012). Among her recommendations is that researchers should be aware of the variety of software programs that exist for using QDAS as part of their data analysis process, as well as critically evaluate their chosen program's features (e.g., it is important to understand the ways in which an "auto-coding" option can influence the interpretative process). As is likely also the case in kinesiology more broadly, "Researchers appear to be increasingly using or interested in using qualitative data analysis software programs (QDAS) such as Atlas.ti, MAXQDA, and NVivo in their qualitative or mixed-methods research, yet training and understanding in this area lags behind such interest" (Humble, p. 122). Hence, QDAS, similar to any type of software, will be a tool that is most effective (and fitting) for knowledgeable, trained, and competent users.

In sum, there is no one approach to coding qualitative data. Researchers need to find an approach that is well-suited to their own competencies, is the best approach to answering their research questions, and is well-suited to their area of study. As such, deciding *how* to go about coding qualitative data can often be as challenging as actually coding the data. In addition, although we have provided an overview of some strategies that might be useful across a number of different types of qualitative research projects in kinesiology, it is important to note that each strategy of inquiry (e.g., phenomenology, case study, grounded theory) has a long tradition of data analysis that is wise to consider prior to beginning the coding process.

Coding Strategy Exercise

Find four to six qualitative research articles that the authors clearly identify as being conducted within *different* strategies of inquiry (i.e., narrative, ethnography, phenomenology, case study, qualitative description, grounded theory; see Chapter 7 for more details on these strategies of inquiry). Read the data analysis sections in each of the articles that you find, and consider the following questions:

1. What similarities and differences do you notice in the terms and strategies researchers use to describe the coding process across different strategies of inquiry?
2. Was the process used in each of the studies an *inductive* or a *deductive* coding of the data (or perhaps a *combination* of both inductive and deductive processes)?
3. What data analysis steps do the authors describe as *preceding* and *following* the coding process?

Step 4: Generate descriptions or themes

Once the data has been coded into categories, the next step is for researchers to generate descriptions or themes that best represent the data. This is perhaps the step most impacted by the philosophical worldview or theoretical lens a researcher brings to the data analysis process, because by its very nature it is a creative and integrative process. At this step, researchers look for organizing frameworks that tell the story of their data in a way that best informs their research question. Common categories might be grouped, isolated data points might be discarded, and unique elements might be highlighted. We can't stress enough that the goal at this point in the data analysis process is for researchers to tell the story that best represents the data, while at the same time recognizing that they themselves play a critical role in the construction of that story. If the descriptions or themes created do not resonate with the participants in the study, the merits of the research can be debatable. Hence, having participants review the generated descriptions or themes at this point in the data analysis process can be a useful strategy to employ (or perhaps even having participants play a role in the *generation* of the description or themes might be considered depending on the type of research).

As Creswell (2014) stated, descriptions focus on a detailed account of the people, places, and events in a setting; therefore, description is particularly important in narrative, case study, and ethnography. The length of description provided in a written report can vary substantially, ranging from a brief descriptive overview to an extensive depiction. The latter is meant to allow the reader direct entry into the setting of the research (as an example, see the level of detail provided in the Reading the Data Exercise Box presented under Step 2). In most cases, details about the setting are provided to offer context for the research findings and include a description of the researcher's role in the setting, as well as justification for that particular setting as appropriate for the research. The following is an example of a description from a participatory action research project in which the researchers worked directly with young Indigenous women in a school in Saskatoon, Saskatchewan to promote positive views of body image. This description is written in first-person perspective by the first author:

From the beginning of September 2006 until the end of June 2007, I was an active member of Nutana Collegiate, which is an urban high school in the city of Saskatoon. Saskatoon is the largest city in Saskatchewan, Canada and is geographically located along the banks of the South Saskatchewan River. The city of Saskatoon has a population of approximately 207,200, and about 10 percent of the population self-identifies as an Aboriginal person. Nutana was chosen as the site for this research project primarily because of some of the connections that I had established within Nutana during my previous research there. Ms. Phyllis Fowler, the director of Nutana's Integrated School-Linked Services (ISLS) program, was particularly enthusiastic about the goals of our research and helped to facilitate my integration into the school community by introducing me and my research goals to key school members (e.g. administrators, students, Aboriginal Elder). Nutana also has a large Aboriginal population (i.e. approximately 38% of the students self-identify as an Aboriginal person), which given the goals of this research project was an important factor in identifying it as an appropriate site. (McHugh & Kowalski, 2011, p. 224)

These types of descriptions are useful to readers to help them understand the context of the research, a step critical to the evaluation of the merits of a qualitative research study. Without a description of the specific setting of the research, qualitative research can fall dangerously close to impersonating the goals of generalizability in quantitative research (i.e., that the findings are meant to be generalizable across settings, time, and context). However, the goals of qualitative research are very different from those of quantitative research; as such, the description of the setting needs to be consistent with those goals.

Similar to the range and types of descriptions presented in different qualitative research studies, the types and numbers of themes can also vary widely. Here are a few examples of the types of themes that appear in the literature, which are specific to kinesiology within the Canadian context:

1. *Example 1:* Sean Horton at the University of Windsor and his colleagues conducted interviews with five people with multiple sclerosis (MS) and their spouses to better understand the exercise experiences of people with MS and the role of their spouses in those experiences (Horton et al., 2015). Three main themes emerged, including (a) maintaining independence, (b) overcoming isolation, and (c) negotiating if exercise is worth it.

2. *Example 2:* Fiona Webster at the University of Toronto and her colleagues conducted a longitudinal qualitative research study focused on why people do or do not participate in physical activities following hip or knee total joint replacement (Webster et al., 2015). A series of three interviews with 29 patients resulted in data organized around the following five themes: (a) losses due to osteoarthritis prior to surgery, (b) the experience of surgery as an intervention, (c) issues with multi-morbidity, including multiple painful joints and mental health problems, (d) socio-cultural context, and (e) fears around the new joint.

3. *Example 3*: Debbie Laliberte Rudman at the University of Western Ontario conducted a narrative study in which 30 participants ranging in age from 45 to 83 years were

each interviewed twice to gain insight into how they talk about their aging bodies as part of the retirement process (Laliberte Rudman, 2015). The data were represented as five themes, including (a) "oldness" as embodied: immobile, uncontrolled, and failed bodies; (b) distancing the self and one's body from "oldness": narrative and social strategies; (c) distancing the self and one's body from "oldness": the centrality of and responsibility of body work; (d) body work: practices of body monitoring, maintenance, and optimization; and (e) failures and limits of body work: self-blame, self-depreciation, tensions, and ambivalence.

Creswell (2014) suggests between five and seven themes as a general guideline to consider; however, it is not unusual to see fewer than five themes (e.g., *Example 1* above). Also, in many studies there are sub-themes within each main theme, in which case there might be fewer general themes, each with their own sub-themes (e.g., the second and third themes in *Example 3* above). This flexibility in both the number of themes and use of sub-themes gives researchers the opportunity to organize their coded data in a way that best represents the data and the experiences of participants in their research.

Step 5: Decide how the findings will be represented

There are many different ways researchers might choose to represent the findings of a qualitative research study. Journal articles are often considered to be synonymous with research, and many researchers do indeed choose to publish their qualitative findings in that form. There are a few reasons for this decision. First, journal articles have a long history within academia, so they are a "known" way for researchers to present their work. Second, journal articles typically require peer-review processes prior to publication, meaning that other experts in the field have reviewed the research and deemed it worthy of publication. As such, having research published in a peer-reviewed journal is considered one of the highest criteria of quality. Third, most researchers are trained within traditions that prioritize written documents as the final outcome of their work; hence, journal articles are often a natural fit for researchers' skills.

Although many qualitative research articles do end up as journal articles, others do not. The traditional journal article is limiting for many researchers who conduct qualitative studies for a few reasons. First, there are almost always page limitations on submitted articles, which severely limit researchers' opportunities to present their work in full, particularly if the work requires extensive description of the setting and themes. This is one reason why many qualitative research projects end up as books. Heather Kuttai's (2010) autoethnography *Maternity Rolls: Pregnancy, Childbirth, and Disability* (a study that was described in more detail in Chapter 7) is one such example. Second, there is sometimes a concern that the journal article format does not reach the intended audience. In many cases the audience that might benefit most from a research study is not the same audience that typically reads journal articles. Hence, other formats, such as a film documentary or web pages, might offer a more effective approach to reach the desired audience. Third, there might simply be no desire to write up the research as a journal article. Hence, other formats like ethnodrama, performance or visual art, or poem might be the desired final outcome of a research project.

Suffice it to say, journal articles are just *one* option for qualitative researchers. We'll address representation of findings across all types of research, including quantitative, qualitative, and mixed methods, when we introduce knowledge translation in Chapter 12.

Step 6: Interpret the findings

Qualitative research, as with other research, requires an interpretation of the findings within the context of existing theory and previous literature. This interpretation can occupy either a relatively minor or major role in the research project depending on the researchers' goals, type of study, and nature of the data. Interpretation of the findings can differ substantially depending on theoretical inclinations, knowledge of certain bodies of literature, and level of critical analysis. Hence, this is another illustration of how research is ultimately filtered through the lens of researchers. For example, how might interpretations of the excerpt presented in the Reading the Data Exercise Box presented under Step 2 differ depending on whether a reader's background was that of mindfulness instructor, urban planner, veterinarian, or social worker?

Crocker and colleagues (2010) discuss how researchers conducting qualitative research should acknowledge and embrace human imagination and creativity as a way to construct meaning. Thus, when doing qualitative research, it is important to remember that multiple interpretations of findings are okay. In fact, multiple interpretations are expected and valued. Although this might be a bit disconcerting to some, particularly those with a postpositivist worldview, it is key to highlight that the intent of all research is to learn as much as possible to inform a research question. In most cases, particularly if the intent is to understand experiences, meanings, and phenomena (i.e., qualitative research), multiple perspectives with diverse interpretations provide the greatest insight. For example, if we take an ankle injury that happens in a basketball game, that same injury can be experienced by different people in very different ways. The coach might see it as a threat to losing a big game; the athlete might see it as an excuse for poor performance; a fan might feel angry and upset at the opposing team; and the physical therapist might see it as an exciting challenge. All of these experiences of the injury are "true" from each different perspective. Thus, to say that there is only one meaning of injury is to discount the complexity of human experience.

Case Study

Excerpts of transcripts from four (fictional) one-on-one interviews about the meaning of sport for adolescent athletes are presented below. Read through all excerpts from the interviews and try to find two or three main themes that you think best represent the athletes' experiences. Use some of the general steps to qualitative data analysis described in this chapter to guide your process of theme development.

Transcript #1

Interviewer (I): Can you tell me about some of your experiences in sport?

Jean (J): They all suck. Sport sucks bad. I suck bad at sports.

I: What do you mean by "sports suck bad?"

J: I mean that they just aren't any fun. The kids who play sports are just real mean. They pretend they're all tough and better than you. Not cool. I just want to go outside and have some fun—run around a little. But then Riley always has to go bullying everyone, which makes sports no fun at all.

I: Can you tell me more about what makes you think you aren't very good at sports?

J: I don't know. I just suck. Seems like I'm always last no matter what we do.

I: Can you give me an example of what you mean?

J: Yesterday in phys ed class we went outside to play football. No one would pass me the ball. Ok, they passed me the ball once, but because I didn't catch it they didn't even throw me the ball again.

I: How did that make you feel?

J: It made me not want to even be there. Why should I run around for no reason with all these stupid kids laughing at me? I'd rather just be inside doing nothing.

I: If you could change sport to make it better, what would you do?

J: First, I'd get rid of all the goofs. They could go play their own games. The rest of us could go play by ourselves. Second, no one should care who wins. I mean, it's just a game—whether we win or lose in a football game during recess isn't a big deal. Except to Riley, who's just a big goof. I think bird watching should be a sport. Then we could all just go outside and have fun and no one would care what happens. That would be fun.

Transcript #2

Interviewer (I): Can you tell me about some of your experiences in sport?

Alexis (A): They're okay. It's not like I'm any great athlete or anything, but sometimes they're fun.

I: What makes them fun?

A: I guess winning is kinda fun. I hate losing, so winning makes things a lot more fun.

I: What happens if you don't win?

A: It's not *that* big of a deal, but I sure don't like it that's for sure. I especially don't like to lose to that little geek Blake. If you do, you're some kinda bad.

Continued

I: What do you like about winning?

A: It's just fun.

I: Can you tell me more about what makes winning fun?

A: I just like being better than everyone else. You know? It's like if you're not very good at something and somebody beats you at it you feel really bad about yourself for a while. That's why I like to win.

I: Why would somebody feel bad about themselves because they lost?

A: Because you find out how bad you really are. Before you lose you can think that you're all good and stuff. But when somebody beats you, you learn how bad you are.

I: What would happen if there was no winning and losing in sport?

A: There would be no point in it. What's the point in playing sport if you can't win?

I: What about being outside and running around to be healthy?

A: I think that is totally overrated. Maybe when you're old that stuff matters. But for me . . . no way. How many kids you heard of dying from being out of shape? None. If I need to do exercise when I'm older, that's what I'll do.

Transcript #3

Interviewer (I): Can you tell me about some of your experiences in sport?

Chen (C): Sure. Sports are good. They teach us all kinds of good values like sportsmanship.

I: Can you tell me more about what you mean?

C: Sure. I mean, if you're playing sports your coach makes you shake the other team's hands after to show you're a good sport.

I: Are teams always good sports?

C: Maybe not all of the time. But most of the time I'd say they are.

I: Can you tell me about a time when the other team wasn't a good sport?

C: Um . . . sure. On Saturday we were playing the Vipers and their star player Peyton was a total loser. After every score I'd hear Peyton yelling, "Who's yer daddy? Who's yer daddy?"

I: How did that make you feel?

C: Not too good. I wanted to scream in anger. But the funny part of the game was when our centre stuffed one of Peyton's shots and said, "Who's yer daddy? Who's yer daddy?"

I: How do you think other kids feel about playing sports?

C: Well, if you're good at them, you like them. If you're no good, you don't like them.

I: It's that simple?

C: Yeah, most of the time. But some kids don't really care how bad they are. They still keep on trying. Sometimes I wonder if they even know how bad they are.

I: What makes them bad at sports?

C: They're just all uncoordinated and stuff. I don't know. Me, I'm good at sports, so I don't know why everyone isn't good at them.

I: What are some of the reasons why you think they might not be good?

C: They probably don't care. Maybe their mom and dad never made them play sports when they were little. How am I supposed to know?

Transcript #4

Interviewer (I): Can you tell me about some of your experiences in sport?

Taylor (T): What do you mean?

I: What sports are you currently involved in?

T: Not too much. I play a little soccer. Mostly I just like to fight.

I: Is fighting a sport?

T: Yes.

I: What makes fighting a sport?

T: There is a winner and loser.

I: There is a winner and loser in chess. Is that a sport?

T: C'mon. That's way different. It's not like you have to move around to play chess. Fighting is a sport because you have to be strong to fight. If you're stronger, you win.

I: Is winning important?

T: Of course winning is important. You don't want to be some loser lying there on the ground with everyone laughing at you, do you? That's why I always win.

I: Can you tell me what would happen if you did lose?

T: I don't lose.

I: But if you did . . . ?

T: Well . . . I wouldn't like it. I probably wouldn't fight again that's for sure. Everyone would see you as a loser no matter what you did after that.

Continued

I: What happens when you lose when you play soccer then?

T: I don't like it, but it's different?

I: What makes it different?

T: Well, for one, it's not my fault when we lose. Our goalie is really, really crappy. If we had a good goalie we'd win all of our games. When I play goal we never lose. The coach wants me to play goal, but I score too many goals to be stuck in net.

Discussion Questions

1. What name would you give each theme that you developed?
2. How would you describe the essence of each theme in one or two sentences?
3. How were you able (or unable) to set aside your own assumptions of adolescent athletes' experiences in the data analysis process?
4. Did *your own* personal experiences in sport enhance your understanding of the adolescents' experiences and creation of themes, or did those personal experiences make it harder to identify the essence of *their* experiences? Or did your experience perhaps do both?
5. Would the outcome of your analysis be any different if we told you that the participants were all boys, all girls, or represented multiple genders?
6. If possible, find one or two other people to complete the same task (i.e., finding themes from the interview transcripts). Discuss similarities and differences in what was found across different people. In what ways is it both a strength and a weakness that different people (likely) identify different themes from the same set of transcripts?
7. What steps would you take next to increase confidence in your themes as accurate representations of the participants' experiences?
8. How would your results differ had we asked you to take a *deductive*, rather than *inductive*, approach to the data analysis by providing the themes in advance and asking you to code the transcripts using existing themes as a conceptual framework to organize the data?

Research Highlight

Ferguson and Philipenko (2016), at the University of Saskatchewan, studied the physical activity experiences of five First Nations students on a university campus. They used a qualitative narrative strategy of inquiry to generate data through talking circle and one-on-one interview methods. Of particular interest to the current chapter is their data analysis process, which included five key steps. First, they transcribed verbatim both the talking circle and the one-on-one interview data. Second, they read and re-read the transcripts multiple times to gain both a general and an intimate sense of the data. Third, they formally coded the data with a focus on the identification of broad categories or themes emerging from the data. Fourth, they then read and re-read the transcripts multiple times again to cross-check and verify that the themes they identified were the ones that best represented the experiences of the participants. Fifth, a narrative was constructed and presented, which integrated direct quotations from the participants and the researchers' interpretive and constructive processes (i.e., the themes they identified). Their research provides an effective example of how researchers might combine data generation via different methods (i.e., talking circle and one-on-one interviews) and use an integrated data analysis process to create a rich narrative of the students' experiences of physical activity. Using a systematic method of data analysis also gives us as readers increased confidence that narratives presented by the researchers are of sufficient quality to meaningfully inform their research question.

Further Reading

Ferguson, L., & Philipenko, N. (2016). "I would love to blast some pow music and just dance": First Nations students' experiences of physical activity on a university campus. *Qualitative Research in Sport, Exercise and Health, 8*, 180–93. doi:10.1080/2159676X.2015.1099563

Summary

Chapter 8 focused on common steps in qualitative data analysis, ranging from preparing transcriptions for analysis, to coding for content, to the creation of themes. There are many different approaches researchers can take to qualitative data analysis, but there tend to be six steps common across many types of research studies. These steps include (a) organizing and preparing the data, (b) reading or looking at all the data, (c) coding all the data, (d) generating descriptions or themes, (e) deciding how the findings will be represented, and (f) interpreting the findings. Ultimately, in qualitative research the goal is to understand experiences, meanings, and phenomena, and multiple perspectives with diverse interpretations provides the greatest insight.

Discussion Questions

1. What does it mean to say that qualitative data analysis is immediate, ongoing, and spiral?
2. Why is it important to not rush too quickly to coding (Step 3) of data in a qualitative research study?
3. In what cases would researchers lean towards using inductive, deductive, or combined inductive and deductive approaches to coding of qualitative data?
4. Why are multiple interpretations of qualitative data valuable?
5. What are some of the most likely challenges researchers face within each of the six steps in qualitative data analysis?

Recommended Readings

Elo, S., & Kyngäs, H. (2007). The qualitative content analysis process. *Journal of Advanced Nursing, 62*, 107–15. doi:10.1111/j.1365-2648.2007.04569.x

Humble, Á. M. (2012). Qualitative data analysis software: A call for understanding, detail, intentionality, and thoughtfulness. *Journal of Family Theory and Review, 4*, 122–37. doi: 10.1111/j.1756-2589.2012.00125.x

Sparkes, A. C., & Smith, B. (2014). *Qualitative research methods in sport, exercise and health: From process to product.* London: Routledge.

Woods, M., Paulus, T., Atkins, D. P., & Macklin, R. (2016). Advancing qualitative research using qualitative data analysis software (QDAS)? Reviewing potential versus practice in published studies using ATLAS.ti and NVivo, 1994–2013. *Social Science Computer Review, 34*, 597–617. doi:10.1177/0894439315596311

9 Evaluating the Merits of Qualitative Research Studies in Kinesiology

Learning Outcomes

By the end of this chapter, you should be able to:

- Identify strategies that can be used to contribute to the trustworthiness, rigour, and validation of a qualitative study.

- Explain the principle of methodological coherence.

- Apply criteria from a comprehensive checklist to judge qualitative research.

- Adopt a relativistic approach when considering the characterizing traits for evaluating qualitative research.

- Ethically assess qualitative research.

A Brief Primer on Evaluating Qualitative Research

As a result of reading the previous two chapters you should be more familiar with qualitative research, particularly in terms of the various study designs, methods of data generation, and data analysis approaches used in kinesiology. However, at this point you might be asking yourself, "That's all fine and dandy, but how do I know if a qualitative study is any good?" or "How do I distinguish the 'good' qualitative research from the 'bad'?", and maybe even "Qualitative and quantitative research are quite different from one another . . . so do I use the same or different criteria to evaluate the merits of each?" Well, you came to the right place for answers!

In Chapter 6 we discussed the concept of validity as a standard of evaluation for *quantitative* research studies. But most of the approaches to evaluate the merits of *qualitative* research are markedly different from those used to evaluate quantitative research. For instance, let's say you want to explore the meaning of sport for adolescent athletes and you deem that, based on taking a constructivist philosophical worldview and the purpose of your study, a qualitative study is the best approach (we will talk about the importance of ensuring your philosophical worldview and research design match a bit later in this chapter when we introduce methodological coherence). You decide that a phenomenological strategy of inquiry will provide insight into adolescent athletes' meanings of lived experiences of sport, and you proceed by purposefully recruiting a select group of adolescent athletes to participate in your study. The athletes are asked to keep personal diaries to document their experiences, and they participate in one-on-one interviews as well as a focus group discussion. After organizing your data (including transcribing the one-on-one interviews and focus group discussion), you conduct an inductive content analysis of your data and present the themes generated from the participants' meanings of sport as a *research poster* (stay tuned for Chapter 12 in which you will be introduced to a number of different ways that researchers can share the results of their research through various knowledge translation approaches). Clearly, in doing so you would want to have confidence in your study, and more specifically confidence that your conclusions were based on the research findings. In other words, you want to somehow consider the validity of your study. However, unlike in quantitative studies, there were no measures or physical instruments in your research; as a result, construct validity can't be used as a way to consider the merits of your research. Similarly, you did not introduce any sort of treatment or intervention to your study participants, so the quality of your study doesn't rest on internal validity or your ability to control for potential threats to internal validity.

Given that quantitative and qualitative research designs are inherently different from each other, qualitative research needs to be evaluated in ways other than the evaluation criteria presented in Chapter 6. The evaluation of qualitative research can include a number of considerations: (a) the trustworthiness of a study, (b) the degree of methodological coherence within a study, (c) whether certain criteria were included in a study, (d) how relevant those criteria are for different qualitative studies, and (e) the ethical soundness of a study. All are important to qualitative research and discussed throughout the sections that follow. An overview of the evaluation approaches covered in this chapter appears in Table 9.1.

Table 9.1 Qualitative evaluation approaches.

EVALUATION APPROACH	WHAT IS IT ALL ABOUT?	IMPORTANT NOTES	KEY REFERENCES
Trustworthiness	Convincing an audience that study findings are worth paying attention to	*Trustworthiness* is used synonymously with rigour and validation.	Guba, 1981 Morse et al., 2002 Creswell, 2014
Methodological coherence	Having all components of a research design align with one another	An armchair walkthrough can help researchers plan a coherent study.	Morse, 1999
Consolidated criteria for reporting qualitative research	Using a checklist to consider what is good research	Checklists include criteria about the research team, study design, analysis, and findings.	Tong, Sainsbury, and Craig, 2007
Relativistic approach to characterizing traits	Identifying study characteristics that may suggest high-quality research, depending on the context	Study quality is context-dependent (i.e., specific to the time, occasion, and purpose).	Sparkes and Smith, 2009 Sparkes and Smith, 2014 Schinke, Smith, and McGannon, 2013
Ethics	Being an ethically minded researcher	All research designs should have ethics as a foundation.	Davies and Dodd, 2002

Trustworthiness as a Starting Place for Evaluation

How do researchers conducting qualitative studies convince their audiences that the findings of a study are worth paying attention to and worth taking account of? The answer to this question, and corresponding strategies that may contribute to a study's merit, refers to the **trustworthiness** of a qualitative study (Guba, 1981). One place to start when considering the merits of a qualitative study is on four aspects of trustworthiness: the study's truth value, applicability, consistency, and neutrality.

1. The **truth value** of a qualitative study refers to its credibility. In other words, how true are the findings for the study participants? The extent to which the results and interpretations in a qualitative study are reflective of the participants' meanings and experiences is indicative of the study's truth value. Researchers conducting qualitative research should work to establish confidence in the truth of the findings for their participants.

2. **Applicability**, or transferability, refers to the extent to which the findings of a particular study may be applied to other contexts or with other participants. It is important to note that applicability in the qualitative sense is different than external validity, which was introduced when evaluating quantitative research in Chapter 6. Whereas researchers conducting quantitative studies may strive for study findings that are enduring in contexts other than the one under study, in qualitative research such generalizations are not possible (nor the goal) because phenomena are intimately connected to the context in which they are explored. As such, in qualitative studies, researchers should not attempt to generalize study findings to all contexts. Rather, the focus is on forming understandings that may be relevant from one context to the next depending on similarity between the contexts.

3. **Consistency** refers to the dependability of a study. In other words, would similar findings emerge if a study were replicated in similar circumstances? One of the defining features of the constructivist philosophical worldview (see Chapter 1) is that multiple realities exist. The assumption of multiple realities implies that participant insights, meanings, and perspectives are varied, and that even any one participant's meaning can evolve. As such, researchers conducting qualitative studies should seek to understand the variability of study findings or unique experiences that stem from the multiple realities assumption.

4. **Neutrality** essentially refers to the degree to which the findings of a study are based on the participants' meanings and experiences, and not merely a function of researchers' biases, motivations, interests, and perspectives. It is important for researchers to understand that their own meanings and experiences can play a role in the meaning-making process when conducting qualitative studies. As such, researchers should consider how their own experiences can impact the qualitative research process. This self-reflection process is known as researcher reflexivity and will be more fully outlined below.

You may have noticed some similarities between the four aspects of trustworthiness and key terms introduced in previous chapters that focus on quantitative research. For instance, attempting to have truth value in a qualitative study somewhat resembles the notion of controlling for potential threats to the internal validity of a quantitative study. However, striving for a single truth is somewhat incongruent with qualitative research, which is premised on multiple truths, meanings, and realities. The similarity between consistency as an aspect of trustworthiness in a qualitative study and reliability in quantitative research might be fairly obvious. However, while consistently finding the same or similar results among studies can be important in quantitative research, it is not an underlying goal of qualitative research. Neutrality is another example of an evaluation approach that is premised on quantitative standards in terms of the position of the researcher. However, unlike in quantitative research where the goal is to be objective, the subjective perspective that researchers adopt when conducting qualitative research can actually be a strength of qualitative research, assuming researchers are engaging in thoughtful elaboration on meanings as opposed to selectively interpreting and/or disregarding information (Haverkamp, 2005).

Although the four aspects of trustworthiness might include quantitative undertones, they can offer a starting place to evaluate qualitative research. There are even instances where qualitative research studies include elements of quantitative research, such as when researchers count the number of times certain words or phrases appear in qualitative interviews (a process known as quantitizing qualitative data, which we will talk about in Chapter 10). When describing the influence of families in the development of sport talent across three stages of sport involvement, Côté (1999) included "count data" by identifying the number of participants who contributed to the themes that emerged for each sport stage. For instance, in the specializing years (the second stage of sport involvement that is typically between the ages of 13 and 15 years), Côté counted the number of mothers, fathers, athletes, and siblings in his sample that discussed certain themes in their interviews. Three mothers, three fathers, four athletes, and four siblings contributed to discussion around the theme that parents make financial commitments to child-athletes, whereas one mother, one father, one athlete, and three siblings contributed to the theme about older siblings serving as role models of work ethic. Presenting this count data makes it possible for the reader of the Côté article to see who contributed to emergent study themes. Seeing count data in a qualitative study suggests that the distinction between qualitative and quantitative research can, at times, have grey areas.

Guba (1981) originally introduced trustworthiness as a way to evaluate the worth of naturalistic research (i.e., qualitative research). More recently, there has been a trend to move away from the use of the term trustworthiness. For instance, Morse and colleagues (2002) described the need to ensure *rigour* of qualitative research, and Creswell (2014) discussed a number of *validation strategies* that should be considered when evaluating qualitative research. Regardless of terminology, the various strategies used to support the trustworthiness, rigour, or validation of a qualitative study share many similarities. As such, the discussion in this section is grounded in the original trustworthiness work of Guba, which also provides a bit of a historical background on early approaches to evaluating qualitative research.

In thinking through the implications, it actually makes a lot of sense that researchers conducting qualitative studies would want their research to have trustworthiness, rigour, and validation. Let's say researchers explored the clinical expertise among occupational therapists by conducting a collective case study with eight occupational therapists. They conducted one-on-one interviews with the study participants and observed the clinicians during treatment sessions with their patients, and based on the data analysis, four themes of clinical expertise in occupational therapy were identified. These findings could have substantial implications for occupational therapy practice and education. As such, the researchers would want to ensure, as best as possible, that their results ring true to their participants, that the study has some applicability to other contexts or with other participants, that a level of consistency would emerge if the study were replicated in a similar context, and that the findings are not merely a result of the researchers' interests and perspectives. In other words evaluating the truth value, applicability, consistency, and neutrality of the research is important to evaluate the merits of the research.

Strategies to enhance trustworthiness, rigour, and validation

In an attempt to have a trustworthy, rigorous, and validated qualitative study, researchers can employ a variety of strategies that target different, or even multiple, phases of a research study, including the design of the study, data generation and fieldwork, or analysis and interpretation. Common strategies to enhance trustworthiness, rigour, and validation (some of which are easier to implement and are more common than others [Creswell, 2014]) are presented in Figure 9.1 and described below.

Audit trail

Establishing an **audit trail** makes it possible for someone external to the study to examine how the data were generated and analyzed, as well as how subsequent interpretations were made. An audit trail is a transparent description of the entire research process from the start of a research project to the reporting of findings. An external auditor assesses the degree to which the study processes are of high quality and measure up to acceptable practice by auditing events, influences, and the actions of the researcher. Agha et al. (2015), a research team from British Columbia, maintained an audit trail in their study of older adults' experiences using a DVD-delivered exercise program. As part of their audit trail, Agha et al. kept a detailed recollection of their analytical process, which included transcribing interviews, reading and coding the data, developing categories based on clusters of codes, and theme identification. Keeping this audit trail allowed an external reviewer to detect issues in the data analysis and assumptions made by the researchers.

Member check

Researchers can invite participants to **member check** data and study interpretations. Member checking consists of having study participants review the data they generated and/or emergent study findings, and providing study participants with the opportunity to add, alter, or delete information. For example, participants might be sent the transcript from their

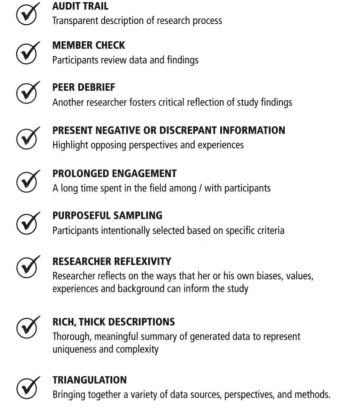

AUDIT TRAIL
Transparent description of research process

MEMBER CHECK
Participants review data and findings

PEER DEBRIEF
Another researcher fosters critical reflection of study findings

PRESENT NEGATIVE OR DISCREPANT INFORMATION
Highlight opposing perspectives and experiences

PROLONGED ENGAGEMENT
A long time spent in the field among / with participants

PURPOSEFUL SAMPLING
Participants intentionally selected based on specific criteria

RESEARCHER REFLEXIVITY
Researcher reflects on the ways that her or his own biases, values, experiences and background can inform the study

RICH, THICK DESCRIPTIONS
Thorough, meaningful summary of generated data to represent uniqueness and complexity

TRIANGULATION
Bringing together a variety of data sources, perspectives, and methods.

Figure 9.1 Common strategies to enhance trustworthiness, rigour, and validation.

individual interview or focus group, or invited to review themes that emerged from data analysis. The participants then have the opportunity to, for example, add further information to their transcript that clarifies a point they were trying to make in their interview, or make a suggestion on a theme that emerged from the data. Shannon (2016), a researcher from the University of New Brunswick, interviewed 17 adolescent female competitive dancers to better understand the factors that influence their continued participation in community-based competitive dance. Rather than providing participants with the full transcripts to review, participants were given the opportunity to provide feedback on the meanings that Shannon had drawn from the themes. More specifically, participants member checked the themes that were generated from the analysis of the interviews. Balish and Côté (2014), researchers at Queen's University, also included member checking in their research exploring community influences on athletic development. After the researchers interviewed 22 residents of an athletically successful community in Nova Scotia, participants were invited to check their interview transcripts for accuracy of their intended communications regarding community supports for developing athletic talent. The researchers also invited participants to review a summary of emergent study findings. Though Balish and Côté did not have disagreements from their participants regarding study findings, in general researchers need to consider how they might negotiate both (a) conflicts between their own interpretation of the data and potential differences with individual participants and (b) conflicting interpretations among multiple participants.

Peer debrief

Researchers can seek out other professionals who are able and willing to **peer debrief** with the researchers. The peer essentially pushes the researchers to critically reflect on the study findings in a way that perhaps the researchers have not yet considered. Peer debriefing also challenges researchers to ensure that their findings are grounded in the data that they collected, as opposed to being too heavily influenced by their own perspectives as researchers. Individuals serving the role of peer debriefer might include, but are not limited to, faculty colleagues or members of a thesis committee. Yi et al. (2015) included peer debriefing in their study of the health and wellness of urban Indigenous youth in Canada. They conducted semi-structured interviews and took field notes to understand the factors that influence, promote, and maintain the health and wellness of urban Indigenous youth in Canada. Yi and colleagues included peer debriefing at various phases of their study, particularly during data analysis in which they coded interview and field-note data, selected central concepts from those codes, and categorized emergent findings into themes and subthemes. In instances of disagreement between researchers and peer debriefers, the researchers thoroughly studied notes made during the coding process for further analysis, which allowed them to monitor their biases.

Present negative or discrepant information

Presenting **negative or discrepant information** that counters main study findings is a way to highlight opposing views or experiences and bring attention to individuals' unique perspectives. This technique reiterates the holistic nature of qualitative research by explicitly recognizing the complexity of a socially constructed world. Although primary themes may emerge from a given study, the larger picture is more nuanced than the study themes themselves. Presenting information that counters the main findings acknowledges this complexity. In their exploration of self-compassion in young women athletes' sport experiences, Ferguson et al. (2014) found that women athletes described self-compassion as advantageous in difficult sport situations by increasing positivity, perseverance, and responsibility. The researchers also discussed the apprehension expressed by some athletes in their research about fully embracing self-compassion because of concerns over settling for mediocrity in sport. Although this information appears to counter main study findings that self-compassion would be a useful resource in sport, presenting the contradicting information better acknowledges the complexity of the young women athletes' sport experiences.

Prolonged engagement

Prolonged engagement with participants in the field can serve many purposes and enhance the quality of the research. For instance, sustained time at a research site can help participants feel more natural in the presence of a researcher, while at the same time allowing researchers the opportunity to check their own perceptions. Persistent observation as a result of prolonged engagement can help researchers understand pervasive participant characteristics versus those that are irrelevant versus those that are atypical yet critical. Lisa Wozniak and her colleagues in Alberta spent six months in community recreational facilities qualitatively evaluating a lifestyle intervention for people with type II diabetes (Wozniak et al., 2015). They conducted interviews, engaged in research team observations, collected meeting minutes, and maintained systematic documentation of a Healthy Eating and Active Living for Diabetes intervention. As part of their sustained data generation, the researchers engaged at length with study participants, asking staff at the facilities to participate in three interviews throughout the duration of the intervention (i.e., baseline, midpoint, and post-intervention). The research team also had formal group meetings throughout the research process to debrief on their observations and check in on their own perspectives.

Purposeful sampling

Purposeful sampling of study participants who can best inform the researcher about the research question requires intentionally recruiting individuals that are information rich—those who are willing to share their experiences in great detail, shed light on specific phenomena being explored, or fully engage in the qualitative process. Purposeful sampling was introduced in Chapter 4 and discussed again in Chapter 7, and it is mentioned here to emphasize the importance of inviting not only participants who are appropriate for a study (i.e., the participants fit certain inclusion criteria for a study, such as being an older adult with chronic pain in a study that will explore older adults' lived experiences of chronic pain) but those who will meaningfully inform the topic being studied. In their grounded theory analysis of adolescents' lived experiences of type 2 diabetes, Protudjer, Dumontet, and McGavock (2014) from the University of Manitoba purposefully selected eight youth with diabetes and six primary caregivers to participate in their study. The youth and caregivers were intentionally selected to represent examples of successful self-management of diabetes.

Researcher reflexivity

Through **researcher reflexivity**, researchers position themselves by reflecting on their biases, values, experiences, and background to consider how these variables may shape or inform their research. Recall from Chapter 7 that researchers using a phenomenology strategy of inquiry will *bracket* their experiences with a phenomenon to acknowledge and set aside their own experiences so the focus can be on experiences of the study participants. Similar to this idea, reflexivity consists of two parts: (a) reflecting on one's experiences with the phenomenon/sample being explored, and (b) considering how one's experiences shape the research process. In their study of positive and negative body image experiences in middle age and older adult women, Bailey, Cline, and Gammage (2016) from Brock University included a reflexivity section in their published research article. The section on reflexivity overviews the entire research team, including research interests, training, and experience, as all three researchers were involved in the entire research process. The first author conducted interviews for data generation, so additional information was provided regarding her height, weight, and physical appearance to provide the reader with context about who was asking body image-related questions in the interviews.

Rich, thick descriptions

Rich, thick descriptions are created both when the data are generated and when study findings are presented. Collecting thorough descriptive data aligns with the meaning-making process that is inherent to qualitative research, and it allows researchers to gain greater understanding of the phenomenon of interest. Sharing or presenting research findings in a rich manner highlights the unique and complex experiences of the participants in a study. As noted in Chapter 8, providing a detailed description of the research setting is also important to provide context for the research. Kirby, Lévesque, and Wabano (2007) included a section on context in their study about adults' physical activity behaviours in a northern-rural Indigenous community. They situated the physical location of the Cree community they worked with, provided historical context of the Cree people, and further introduced the research setting by noting concerns over physical activity opportunities in the community.

Triangulation

Triangulation is a way to crosscheck, or triangulate, study findings and interpretations using a variety of data sources, perspectives, and methods. For instance, using multiple methods of data generation, such as one-on-one interviews and participant observation, in tandem with one another can help to overcome potential misinterpretations from any individual methods. If similar patterns of results emerge from different methods and contribute to the larger interpretation, the data are considered to be more trustworthy. The lifestyle intervention study by Wozniak et al. (2015) mentioned earlier when introducing prolonged engagement also provides an example of triangulation. The researchers used a variety of data sources and methods in an effort to provide a thorough assessment of the lifestyle intervention. Specifically, the researchers conducted multiple one-on-one interviews with study participants, engaged in research team observations and reflections, collected meeting minutes, and maintained systematic documentation of the intervention.

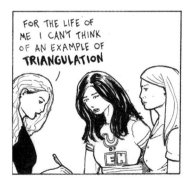
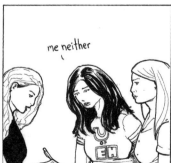
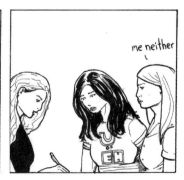

Case Study: Anaya's Story

Dr Ima Inquisitive's research team conducted a case study with the following purpose: to understand the personal, psychological, and social implications of a young girl's experiences with a spinal cord injury. They purposefully recruited a young girl who had experienced a spinal cord injury within the previous nine months to participate in their study. The researchers conducted semi-structured interviews and observations as their methods of data generation, coded the transcribed interviews and field notes, and engaged in a summative content analysis of the data. What appears below is the presentation of their case study.

Anaya was 10 years of age when she was in a life-threatening car accident and suffered a spinal cord injury. As a result, Anaya lost the use of her legs and now uses a wheelchair. Before her spinal cord injury, Anaya was a competitive figure skater and very committed to her sport. She trained three evenings a week, attended free skates two mornings a week, and competed nearly every weekend. In addition to figure skating, Anaya was very physically active. She spent a lot of her time outdoors, including cross-country skiing in the winter, playing tennis in the spring, knee boarding behind her parent's boat in the summer, and bicycling in the fall. In school, Anaya was always the first student dressed for physical education class, ready to participate in any activity the teacher had planned. Anaya and her friends spent most of their free time, including recess and noon hours, being active and setting up fun sport games after school.

Since the accident, Anaya has tried to remain active by adapting some of her activities to wheelchair activities. With the help of her parents, a local wheelchair ice skating club opened that she joined, and her school teacher introduced a few wheelchair-friendly activities during physical education class. Despite these efforts, Anaya is unable to be as active as she once was, and she explains that at times she struggles with feelings of disappointment. Whereas she used to be an outspoken role model in skating, Anaya visibly keeps to herself at the new skating club. Anaya has even started to avoid some physical activity environments, and her social status has changed; she stopped hanging out with some friends that she used to spend a lot of time with.

Interviews with Anaya suggest that she experienced some difficult emotions as a result of the physical changes in her life and at times is unsure how to cope with those changes. As she explains, "In the months that followed the accident . . . I was overwhelmed with what I was feeling, like emotions and stuff. I didn't know what my body could or couldn't do." Anaya had never experienced any significant emotional struggles before the accident, and she had not anticipated any dramatic changes. Though she is confused about how to manage her difficult emotions, she is not letting anyone help her: "This is my new life; no one else should have to deal with it." She further explained, "Some people act weird around me now, they think I am a different person on the inside. That makes me feel bad, so I don't spend much time with them anymore."

Discussion Questions

1. What specific techniques, if any, were used in an attempt to contribute to the trustworthiness, rigour, and validation of this case study?
2. Applying what you have learned about trustworthiness, rigour, and validation to this case study, consider whether Anaya's case study is an example of strong qualitative research.
3. How could the case study information be improved?

If researchers conducting qualitative studies employ a number of strategies that contribute to the trustworthiness of the study, does that ensure high-quality research? The answer is "no" ... or at least "not necessarily." There is no magic number or formula dictating that combining certain strategies or using a specific number of strategies will unequivocally result in a strong qualitative study. For instance, a sport psychology researcher working with Olympic athletes to understand the role of social support during the Olympics may spend prolonged time in the field, working with a select group of athletes for an extended period of time that began at the end of the previous Olympics; include multiple methods of data

Research Highlight

Given that many Canadian breast cancer survivors experience swelling in the upper body after cancer treatment (a condition called lymphedema), researchers at the University of Ottawa, University of Saskatchewan, and McGill University collaborated with healthcare practitioners across Canada to create a research program that explored arm disability after breast cancer. Led by Roanne Thomas-MacLean, Canada Research Chair in Qualitative Health Research with Marginalized Populations, the research team explored the impact and challenges of disabling factors following cancer treatment, including pain, range of motion restrictions, and lymphedema. Their program of research incorporated a variety of research designs and methods, including longitudinal surveys, clinical assessments, interviews, and ethnodrama. In one study, a grounded theory approach was adopted and the researchers conducted 40 semi-structured interviews across four research sites to explore the impact of arm disability (i.e., pain, range of motion restrictions, or lymphedema) on the everyday lives of breast cancer survivors. Of particular relevance to the topics discussed in this chapter, participants were purposefully selected for interviews, with inclusion criteria including (a) having been diagnosed with stage I, II, or III breast cancer, and (b) having arm morbidity (i.e., pain, range of motion restrictions, lymphedema, or self-reported swelling). The participants reported the importance of having family members' assistance while making adjustments to their lives, particularly their work lives, because of their arm disability. The emphasis on the social effects of arm disability highlights the complexity of disability and the need for rehabilitation that intersects various domains of survivors' lives. The experiences of these breast cancer survivors resulted in the development of an arm morbidity and disability model to inform healthcare professionals about the measurement of disability after breast cancer.

Further Readings

Thomas-MacLean, R., Spriggs, P., Quinlan, E., Towers, A., Hack, T., Tatemichi, S., . . . Tilley, A. (2010). Arm morbidity and disability: Reporting the current status from Canada. *Journal of Lymphoedema, 5*, 33–8.

Thomas-MacLean, R., Towers, A., Quinlan, E., Hack, T., Kwan, W., Miedema, B., . . . Graham, P. (2009). "This is a kind of betrayal": A qualitative study of disability after breast cancer. *Current Oncology, 16*, 26–32. doi:10.3747/co.v16i3.389

generation, such as interviews with athletes, coaches, and family members, observation, and collection of athletes' journals; maintain a personal journal to reflect on his own experiences; and publish his research in a peer-reviewed journal that describes five themes that emerged from his data analysis. Even though the sport psychology researcher did a number of things that contribute to the trustworthiness, rigour, and validation of his research, you now know that there are a number of things this researcher *didn't* do that may have added to the rigour of his study, such as inviting study participants to member check study themes, debriefing study findings with a colleague, and having an audit trail of his research. It is important to recognize that published research articles, such as the one described in this fictitious example, can still include flaws or areas for improvement. Evaluating the merits of a qualitative study can certainly start with identifying trustworthiness strategies, but there is much more to be considered when assessing qualitative research. It is time to move beyond the quantitative-infused language of trustworthiness and consider additional ways to evaluate qualitative research.

Additional Considerations for Evaluating Qualitative Research

In addition to considering the strategies used by researchers to work towards trustworthiness, rigour, and validation of a study, there are further ways to evaluate the merits of qualitative research. One approach is to examine the level of alignment among the various components of a research study—the coherence among the researchers' philosophical assumptions, research questions, study design, methods for data generation, data analysis, and interpretation. Crosschecking a study with a comprehensive "checklist" of criteria deemed to be reflective of strong research might also be useful when considering the merits of a qualitative study.

The principle of methodological coherence

It should come as no surprise that statements such as "Qualitative research is merely the reflection of a researcher's bias" and "Qualitative methods of data generation are sloppy" are outdated myths—if, of course, the qualitative study is done well. The role of researchers conducting qualitative studies is one that is very active, reflective, and engaged in the research process. Researchers are highly involved in an active meaning-making process, which includes taking the position of "research instrument" to generate data. Recall from Chapter 7 that researchers are key instruments in the qualitative research process. Given this critical role, it is essential that researchers be driven by a well-planned qualitative research design. This includes developing a strong purpose statement, asking important questions, generating the right data to inform those questions, and being a reflective and thoughtful researcher along the way.

Janice Morse (1999) proposed the principle of **methodological coherence** as an indicator of quality research. Methodological coherence requires alignment within a research design, including coherence among researchers' philosophical assumptions, research questions, study design, data generation, data analysis, and interpretation. Picture a thread that is woven through all of the parts of a qualitative research study. This thread should logically connect all the different aspects together and show how the various parts of the study correspond to one another. Imagine a situation where researchers are interested in the motivational climate of sport environments and propose the following research question: How is motivational climate created in elite sports? The researchers intend to explore the perceptions and behaviours of coaches, peers, and parents of elite athletes, and they plan to engage in one-on-one interviews with these individuals, as well as collect field observations during various sporting events (competitions, practices, team meetings, etc.). You might be thinking to yourself, "That is a great way to generate meaning from multiple perspectives on the motivational climate in elite sports!" But what if you found out that the researchers did not purposefully select participants from elite sport and instead recruited them from a novice soccer program? Indeed, participants could have knowledge of motivational climate in sport but likely not knowledge of *elite* sport. The study in this fictional example would have fairly low methodological coherence because the aspects of the study (i.e., research question and process of purposeful sampling) do not align with one another.

Methodological coherence should be evident in all aspects of the research. For instance, qualitative research designs are predominantly premised on a constructivist philosophical worldview. This means that the research question, strategy of inquiry, and methods of data generation should align with the constructivist approach. There should also be alignment between selected research methods and corresponding data analysis. For example, consider a group of researchers who are interested in better understanding the sedentary behaviours of kindergarten students. After engaging in focus group discussions with the students and collecting audiovisual data (e.g., video footage from observing kindergarten classrooms), the researchers' data analysis might be purely text-based; that is, the audiovisual data are not included in the analysis. In this example, there is misalignment within the study because the data analysis approach does not match the data that have been collected. Methodological coherence is essential for a strong qualitative study, and it should be considered at the design phase of a study to ensure the thread of coherence is woven throughout the study.

When planning a qualitative research study, Morse (1999) recommends engaging in an **armchair walkthrough** to develop a sense of one's research project, thereby enhancing methodological coherence. This walkthrough includes reflecting on all aspects of a qualitative study, from the types of questions that will be asked, to the kinds of data that are needed to inform that question, to how the specific data can be collected. Once those and other aspects have been envisioned, rigorous researchers will consider alternative approaches, including different questions that could be asked, the data-generation approach that best corresponds, the appropriate type of data analysis, and the best way to share the findings with the intended audience. An armchair walkthrough can be invaluable in providing researchers with a road map for what is to come. Keep in mind, however, that a key characteristic of qualitative research is that it is emergent and flexible; as such, the road map that results from a thorough armchair walkthrough is intended to be a source of confidence that researchers are being cognizant of the research processes moving forward with a well-conceived research plan.

Given the importance of methodological coherence as a way to evaluate qualitative research, the responsibility to be a reflexive researcher is perhaps even more important than previously considered. Researchers must not let assumptions, previous literature and knowledge, or personal agendas be the driving force behind their qualitative research. Rather, researchers need to consider their assumptions, how their beliefs inform the kinds of research questions being asked, preferences for certain forms of data, tendencies to analyze data in specific ways, and so on and so forth. By making existing knowledge and experiences explicit during the armchair walkthrough, or potentially bracketing one's assumptions, researchers can intentionally work towards conducting qualitative research that is methodologically coherent. Researchers dictate methodological coherence, and they need to be aware of this responsibility and walk through the research plan from the big picture aspects to the most intricate details.

Consolidated criteria for reporting qualitative research (COREQ)

Seeking a comprehensive protocol to adequately assess qualitative research, Tong, Sainsbury, and Craig (2007) reviewed the literature for criteria to evaluate qualitative research. At the time, several partial "checklists" were available that contained important criteria by which qualitative studies should be judged, but there existed no overarching framework for a comprehensive evaluation of qualitative research. They took it upon themselves to synthesize an initial pool of 22 pre-existing checklists to create one comprehensive list that researchers could use going forward to evaluate qualitative research. The result was the 32-item checklist containing **consolidated criteria for reporting qualitative research (COREQ)**. In the process of developing the COREQ, Tong, Sainsbury, and Craig were able to eliminate redundant items from original partial checklists, as well as items that were too broadly defined or impractical for researchers conducting qualitative studies to execute.

The COREQ is divided into three categories or domains with corresponding areas of focus: (a) research team and reflexivity (e.g., personal characteristics of the researchers, researchers' relationship with participants); (b) study design (e.g., theoretical framework, participant selection, research setting, data generation); and (c) analysis and findings (e.g., data analysis, reporting of research). The COREQ can be used as a guide to inform researchers of some important aspects to consider including in their qualitative research, as well as a way for the research audience to evaluate the merits of a qualitative study. Table 9.2 contains an adaptation of Tong, Sainsbury, and Craig's (2007) final 32-item COREQ checklist.

It is important to note (and probably apparent to you by now) that the COREQ was initially developed specifically for the evaluation of qualitative studies that included interviews and focus groups as the main method of data generation. As such, some of the items are particularly relevant to those qualitative approaches. The checklist is nonetheless a useful tool to review when considering the merits of a variety of qualitative studies. For instance, remember from Chapter 7 that *data saturation* refers to whether participants were recruited and data were collected until no new relevant knowledge was being obtained. Although data saturation is often discussed when considering qualitative research with interview and focus group data,

Table 9.2 Consolidated Criteria for Reporting Qualitative Research (COREQ) 32-Item Checklist (adapted from Tong, Sainsbury, and Craig, 2007).

DOMAIN AND CRITERIA	GUIDING QUESTION
Domain 1: Research term and reflexivity	
1. Researchers	Who conducted data generation?
2. Credentials	What were the researchers' credentials (e.g., Ph.D., M.D.)?
3. Occupation	What were the researchers' occupations at the time of the study?
4. Gender	Were the researchers men or women?
5. Experience and training	What experience or training did the researchers have?
6. Relationship established	Was a relationship established prior to study commencement?
7. Participant knowledge of the researchers	What did the participants know about the researchers (e.g., personal goals, reasons for doing the research)?
8. Researchers' characteristics	What characteristics were reported about the researchers?
Domain 2: Study design	
9. Methodological orientation and theory	What philosophical worldview was stated to underpin the study?
10. Sampling	How were participants selected (e..g., purposive, snowball)?
11. Methods of approach	How were participants approached (e.g., face to face, email)?
12. Sample size	How many participants were in the study?
13. Non-participation	How many people refused to participate or dropped out? Why?
14. Setting of data generation	Where was the data generated (e.g., home, clinic)?
15. Presence of non-participants	Was anyone other than the participants and researchers present?
16. Description of sample	What are the important characteristics of the sample?
17. Interview guide (if applicable)	Were questions, prompts, or guides provided by the researchers? Was this material pilot tested?
18. Repeat interviews (if applicable)	Were repeat interviews carried out? If yes, how many?
19. Audio/visual recording (if applicable)	Did the researchers use audio or visual recording to collect the data?
20. Field notes	Were field notes made during and/or after the data were generated?
21. Duration	What was the duration of the data generation?
22. Data saturation	Was data saturation achieved?
23. Transcripts returned (if applicable)	Were transcripts returned to participants for comment and/or correction?

Continued

Table 9.2 continued

Domain 3: Analysis and Findings	
24. Number of data coders	How many researchers coded the data?
25. Description of the coding system	Did the researchers provide a description of the coding system?
26. Derivation of themes	Were themes identified in advance or did themes emerge from the data?
27. Software (if applicable)	What software was used to manage the data?
28. Member checking	Did participants provide feedback on the findings?
29. Quotations presented	Were participant quotations presented to illustrate the themes/findings? Was each quotation identified (e.g., by participant pseudonym)?
30. Data and findings consistent	Was there consistency between the data presented and the findings?
31. Clarity of major themes	Were major themes clearly presented in the findings?
32. Clarity of minor themes	Is there a description of diverse cases or discussion of minor themes?

it is relevant to other qualitative approaches. Researchers who take an ethnographic approach to explore gender experiences of middle-year students in physical education classes might engage in participant observation, collect documentation on student records, and ask students to create drawings about their experiences. The researchers would want to cease data generation only when they believe that saturation has been achieved; that is, that no new knowledge would emerge if data generation were continued. The resultant data analysis and emergent themes from these forms of data generation would ideally stem from data saturation, just as if the researchers had been conducting interviews or focus groups.

Interestingly, the COREQ domains and corresponding criteria are somewhat a reflection of the principle of methodological coherence. That is, the specific items in the COREQ can be used as a checklist to evaluate pretty much the entire spectrum of a qualitative study, ranging from researchers' philosophical worldviews to the presentation or reporting of study findings, and everything in between. The COREQ checklist identifies a variety of specific details that qualitative research can be evaluated on, and the principle of methodological coherence reminds us of the thread that should be woven throughout a qualitative study to strengthen its quality.

Taking a Relativistic Approach to Evaluating Qualitative Research

In this chapter we have considered a number of approaches we can take when evaluating a qualitative study. A key take-home message is that there are no hard and fast rules that certain strategies will ultimately result in a quality research study. It is up to the researchers (and the readers and reviewers of that research) to evaluate and determine the merits of a study. Andrew Sparkes, Brett Smith, and their colleagues (e.g., Sparkes & Smith, 2009; 2014; Schinke, Smith, & McGannon, 2013) take a somewhat different approach for identifying the merits of a study. Rather than working within a pre-determined set of criteria, they take a relativistic approach to *characterizing traits* for evaluating qualitative research.

Characterizing traits are essentially criteria that *may* loosely allude to the quality of research, but are not necessarily indicative of strong research. That is, what researchers do in one study may contribute to its overall quality given the specific context (i.e., time, occasion, purpose) of that particular study, but implementing those same strategies to evaluate the quality of another study may not make it as rigorous given an entirely different context. Thus, characterizing traits are fluid and dynamic among research studies. Moreover, characterizing traits should be identified throughout the entire research process, as opposed to limiting evaluation to what was done during, say, data generation or data analysis.

In this type of approach, evaluating the merits of a qualitative study is not merely the result of adding together the number of pre-determined strategies or criteria that were used, with the more techniques used resulting in a better study. Consideration for certain strategies (e.g., trustworthiness, rigour, and validation strategies) and checklists (e.g., COREQ) might be good places to start when we are evaluating qualitative research, but these criteria need to be critically reflected upon within the context of any given study. Reflective researchers (and readers of research) evaluate *how* and *why* certain techniques were used within the context of the study. To strive for a high level of quality in any particular study, researchers need to challenge, change, modify, and interpret (and reinterpret!) evaluation criteria in an ongoing manner. In other words, the criteria to deem qualitative research as "good or "bad" is itself relative.

Every qualitative research study has a unique purpose with a unique context, and the criteria used to evaluate the merits of that study need to correspond to its distinctiveness. This does not imply that all research is accepted as good; research still needs to be held to high standards. The relativistic approach to evaluating qualitative research challenges readers to identify characterizing traits throughout the entire research process, to be reflective of changing contexts, and to be critical consumers of research. Furthermore, evaluators of qualitative research need to consider the merits of research in a fair and ethical way.

Critical Reflection Exercise

Return to Anaya's case study presented earlier in this chapter, and critically reflect upon the traits you had identified as indicators of "good" qualitative research, as well as the ways you indicated this research could be improved. Next, imagine that Anaya's doctor, Anaya's coach at the new figure skating club, and Anaya's best friend, Jordan, had also been interviewed for this case study. Anaya's doctor provides information about the

Continued

severity of Anaya's injury, describing the damage that occurred, but also indicating that Anaya will likely regain some, although minimal, movement in her lower body over time. Anaya's coach provides insight into Anaya's seemingly withdrawn demeanour at the new skating club, explaining that Anaya is able to master new choreography after she spends some time on her own to process and practise the basic movements. Finally, Jordan, Anaya's best friend, shares that she and Anaya have started a number of new hobbies since Anaya's accident. For instance, Jordan speaks at length about the book club the girls started in their class and brags about getting the chance to try out wheelchair figure skating with Anaya. Although some of the group of people that the girls used to spend the majority of their time with has changed, Jordan explains that she and Anaya have a lot of fun meeting new friends and trying new things.

Re-evaluate the merits of Anaya's case study with the new information that has been provided. Start by adopting a relativistic position in your evaluation and consider the new context of the modified case study. Next, reflect on your previously identified characterizing traits by challenging them in this new context. Do you need to modify the list of criteria that would indicate the merits (or weaknesses) of this case study? What traits are emerging that suggest this might be quality research? What is lacking? Take note of how your evaluation criteria, and the process to arrive at a conclusion, likely differed between the original and modified case studies.

Ethics: The Bottom Line for Evaluation

> . . . we need to accept that "quality" is a somewhat elusive phenomenon that cannot be pre-specified by methodological rules.
>
> Seale, 1999

The range of criteria to consider when evaluating qualitative research, from big picture philosophical questions to specific details about data generation, can be quite expansive (and perhaps a little overwhelming if qualitative research designs are new to you). Though we have made efforts to summarize and synthesize approaches for evaluating the merits of qualitative research, there is something almost intangible to the fluidity of qualitative research that makes it difficult to judge quality by a pre-determined list or by characterizing traits of strength. Furthermore, some of the differing approaches one can take to evaluate qualitative research can contradict one another; for instance, engaging in an armchair walkthrough and working towards methodological coherence are somewhat inconsistent with taking a relativistic approach and learning to live with uncertainty and flexibility. This is not to say that the criteria covered earlier in this chapter are not useful for evaluating qualitative research; the point we are trying to make is that there needs to be a base from which all evaluation should stem. That foundation is ethics.

Recall from Chapter 3 that engaging in ethical research is perhaps the most important responsibility of researchers. Ethics is an ongoing process in research, and researchers need to ensure they have respect for persons, demonstrate concern for the quality of their experiences, and treat people fairly and equitably throughout their research. Researchers need to continuously address tensions between the goals of their research and the rights of the participants. Being an ethically minded researcher can set the foundation for a strong study. Alternatively, engaging in ethically questionable ways is sure to result in weak research.

For example, in this chapter you learned that having participants member check their interview transcripts can be important to the trustworthiness, rigour, and validation of a study, and is also a criterion on the COREQ. Member checking can indeed be a great approach for researchers to check in with their study participants and to ensure the data they have shared is reflective of participants' experiences (or at least what they intended to share). But what happens if there is disagreement between the researchers and participants on the themes that emerged from qualitative data analysis? Or what if there is disagreement among the participants themselves? There is no lab manual that tells researchers what to do in these tricky instances. Having a strong ethical foundation can be critical in these types of situations so that researchers carefully consider how to move forward. Applying an ethical decision-making model, similar to the one outlined in Chapter 3, would be very useful in this scenario. After reflecting on the situation and working through an ethical decision-making process, the researchers might decide that they need to reanalyze the data. Or maybe a good way to negotiate this situation would be to have the participants involved in the data-analysis process. Perhaps allowing the findings to be presented in a manner such that multiple perspectives from different participants can be highlighted would be best. Clearly there is no one right way to move forward in this situation. What is important is that researchers return to a foundation of ethics to ensure the participants' rights are being considered and that the researchers are acting in an ethically defensible manner.

One way for researchers to be ethical is to infuse basic ethical principles into their research. For instance, respect for autonomy is demonstrated by obtaining informed consent from research participants. Researchers exercise justice when ensuring participants have a say in the themes that emerge from the data (return, for a moment, to the scenario presented in the previous paragraph). Nonmaleficence is at play when a researcher decides to end data generation because the topics in an interview are too painful and difficult for a participant to discuss. However, ethics are more than a set of principles or guidelines for research (Davies & Dodd, 2002). Researchers should strive to make sound ethical decisions throughout the entire research process, including when recruiting participants in a purposeful manner, gaining access to a group of participants or community (community-based research is discussed in Chapter 11), developing researcher-participant relationships, engaging in data generation with those participants, protecting participants' privacy, analyzing data, and sharing study findings.

Just as validity in quantitative studies is a matter of degree, so too are the merits of qualitative research. One thing that remains constant in both quantitative and qualitative approaches is that ethics are integral to the way researchers think about, approach, and do their research. Ethics can be, and should be, the foundation of *all* research in kinesiology.

Professional Highlight

Dr Stacy Irvine and Tim Irvine, Co-owners Totum Life Science, Toronto

....

Profile: The Irvines applied their university education in the field of kinesiology to the health and fitness industry through the development of their highly successful fitness and sports medicine facility, Totum Life Science, in Toronto, Ontario. Stacy and Tim completed their Bachelor's of Science and Master's of Science degrees at the University of Saskatchewan, all in the College of Kinesiology. Stacy went on to earn her Doctor of Chiropractic degree at the Canadian Memorial Chiropractic College. The Irvines take a multidisciplinary approach to their fitness and sports medicine facility, which includes individual and group training, sport performance, chiropractic and physiotherapy services, massage therapy, and naturopathy and nutrition services. Building on their kinesiology background, the Irvines believe in applying science to improve one's life, and this philosophy underlies the range of fitness and rehabilitation professional services offered at their facility. The Irvines place their trust in science to inform their daily practice and business approach; as such, a high level of rigour is needed in kinesiology-related research to inform these practitioners.

Further Resource

Totum Life Science website: http://totum.ca

Summary

Chapter 9 focused on evaluating the merits of a wide range of qualitative research designs used in kinesiology. The standards for qualitative research were applied to real-world examples of research in kinesiology. The specific focus of the chapter was on the application of trustworthiness, rigour, and validation, as well as additional criteria related specifically to the research team, study design, and data analysis when judging qualitative research in kinesiology. The principle of methodological coherence was introduced to emphasize the importance of congruency and alignment throughout an entire research design. The reader was cautioned against relying entirely on pre-determined checklists when assessing qualitative research, and instead taking a relativistic approach to characterizing traits of good research. The chapter concluded with a reminder about the importance of ethics, reinforcing that an ethically sound study is paramount when doing research.

Discussion Questions

1. Which strategies of trustworthiness, rigour, and validation most appropriately align with the truth value, applicability, consistency, and neutrality of a qualitative study? Table 9.3 might be useful for categorization. There may be some strategies that fall in more than one category.

Table 9.3 Template to describe the strategies of trustworthiness, rigour, and validation aligning with each aspect of trustworthiness.

ASPECT OF TRUSTWORTHINESS	SPECIFIC STRATEGIES
Truth value	
Applicability	
Consistency	
Neutrality	

2. What is the principle of methodological coherence? In your answer, be sure to explain why it is important that the various aspects of a qualitative research design align with one another.
3. Find and read a qualitative research article within your kinesiology-related area of interest. After reading the article, return to the COREQ items in Table 9.2 and identify the criteria the researchers' report/include in their study and those that are omitted. If you could go back to the researchers and ask for clarification or more information, what would you ask?
4. How might you take a relativistic position when evaluating qualitative research in kinesiology?
5. Imagine that you are conducting an ethnography on the culture of personal training. You just spent eight months interacting with personal trainers and their clients, including extensive fieldwork where you observed a number of personal trainers working with their clients. You generated a lot of data in your observations of initial consults, endurance training, and high intensity workouts. You also developed close working relationships with a number of the personal trainers, and you recently found out that one of the trainers is keeping portions of the money she receives from a few clients rather than giving it all back to the business (the business runs such that all personal trainers are paid out of one pooled fund). What implications does this situation have, if any, for your research? Walk through an ethical decision-making process as to how you, the researcher, might proceed (see Chapter 3 if you need a refresher on an example of an ethical decision-making model).
6. What are five key questions you might ask a researcher at a scientific conference to adequately evaluate the merits of her or his qualitative research study?

Recommended Readings

Davies, D., & Dodd, J. (2002). Qualitative research and the question of rigor. *Qualitative Health Research, 12,* 279–89. doi:10.1177/104973230201200211

Morse, J. M., Barrett, M., Mayan, M., Olson, K., & Spiers, J. (2002). Verification strategies for establishing reliability and validity in qualitative research. *International Journal of Qualitative Methods, 1,* 13–22. doi:10.1177/160940690200100202

Tong, A., Sainsbury, P., & Craig, J. (2007). Consolidated criteria for reporting qualitative research (COREQ): A 32-item checklist for interviews and focus groups. *International Journal for Quality in Health Care, 19,* 349–57. doi:10.1093/intqhc/mzm042

10 Mixed Methods Research

Learning Outcomes

By the end of this chapter, you should be able to:

- Describe mixed methods research.

- Explain when researchers should use mixed methods research.

- Identify various ways to combine quantitative and qualitative research into a mixed methods design.

- Consider how to integrate quantitative and qualitative data analysis approaches for analyzing data in mixed methods research.

- List the strengths and challenges of mixed methods research.

- Appreciate that mixed methods research is more than simply adding quantitative research and qualitative research together.

Introduction to Mixed Methods Research

A lot of information about research designs has been presented in the previous nine chapters of this textbook. For instance, *quantitative research designs* are often used to test theory, examine the status of variables, investigate differences among groups, and explore relationships among variables. Measurement validity and reliability were introduced, as well as a variety of statistical techniques to analyze numerical data. Various threats to the validity of a quantitative study and potential strategies to control for threats to internal and external validity were also overviewed. *Qualitative research designs* were introduced for gaining in-depth understanding of complex phenomena and meanings of experiences. A range of methods for qualitative data generation were presented including interviews, observations, written documents, and arts-based approaches. Central to qualitative research are the inclusion of the researcher as an integral part of the meaning-making process, an emergent and flexible study design, the generation (collection) of non-numerical data, and the inclusion of (typically) a smaller number of participants. These are only a few highlights of the substantial amount of information we have covered on quantitative and qualitative designs in kinesiology-related research. Table 10.1 outlines key characteristics of quantitative and qualitative research designs.

Table 10.1 The defining characteristics of quantitative research designs and qualitative research designs.

KEY CHARACTERISTICS OF QUANTITATIVE RESEARCH	KEY CHARACTERISTICS OF QUALITATIVE RESEARCH
• Objectivity, or protection against bias • Theory testing • Typically large sample sizes • Random selection • Measurement of variables • Numerical data • Validity and reliability • Statistics • Internal and external validity	• Multiple meanings and complexity of experiences • Emergent and flexible design • Natural setting • Purposeful sampling • Typically small sample sizes • Non-numerical data • Inductive and deductive data analysis

As you become more knowledgeable about research in kinesiology-related fields, you might be asking yourself, "What if researchers want to use both quantitative and qualitative approaches within one study?" Well, quantitative and qualitative research approaches *can* be integrated into one study, and that is what mixed methods research is all about. **Mixed methods research** is an approach to inquiry that combines quantitative and qualitative forms of research. In a sense, mixed methods research is simply a systematic and purposeful mixing of both approaches in a study (or across a series of studies).

Refer back to Table 10.1, this time through the lens of a mixed methods researcher. Rather than completely separating the quantitative characteristics from the qualitative characteristics, imagine that the columns separating the quantitative and qualitative elements become blurred and come together into one study. A number of questions might immediately come to mind, such as, "How do researchers recruit participants for a mixed methods study?" "What data analysis approach can be used to analyze numerical and non-numerical data?" and perhaps the most difficult question of all "How do researchers reconcile differing philosophical worldviews that typically underlie quantitative and qualitative studies?" Keeping in mind that many of these questions do not have simple answers, by the end of this chapter you should have a solid foundation of mixed methods research knowledge. More than anything, this foundation should include an appreciation that mixed methods research is more than simply collecting and analyzing quantitative and qualitative kinds of data (Creswell & Plano Clark, 2011). Authentic mixed methods research involves using quantitative and qualitative approaches in tandem so that the overall strength of a study is greater than either quantitative or qualitative research on its own.

When should researchers do a mixed methods study?

Mixed methods research is becoming increasingly common within kinesiology as a way to answer all kinds of research questions including, but not limited to, evaluation of exercise programs, measurement of physical activity, development of sport programs for young women and youth, and the informing of physical education strategies. For example, a research team at the University of Waterloo conducted a mixed methods study to examine the perceived acceptability of wearable activity trackers for older adults living with chronic illness (Mercer et al., 2016). A sample of 32 older adults living with a chronic illness were asked to wear five different activity trackers (i.e., a standard pedometer and four novel activity trackers) for at least three days per device. After testing each device, participants completed a technology acceptance questionnaire that assessed perceived usefulness, perceived ease of use, attitude towards using, behavioural intention to use, and actual use. After testing all five devices, participants engaged in focus groups to discuss user acceptance of the activity trackers. All four of the novel activity trackers were rated similarly in the technology survey and were rated higher than the standard pedometer. The standard pedometer was constantly rated as the least preferred option. A thematic analysis of the qualitative data resulted in findings suggesting that older adults may benefit from devices that are compatible with their personal computers and the inclusion of comprehensive manuals for interpreting the data generated by activity tracking devices. The researchers concluded that there may be meaningful potential in using activity trackers to help older adults increase awareness of their level of physical activity and to become more active; however, barriers to using activity trackers need to be considered prior to their adoption.

Another example of a mixed methods study comes from a group of researchers in Atlantic Canada. Robinson and Randall (2016) focused on the current state and possible future of physical education in Canada's four Atlantic provinces using large-scale surveys and focus groups. An online survey was completed by physical educators that inquired about who is responsible for teaching physical education in Atlantic Canadian schools, qualifications and experiences of Atlantic Canadian physical educators, and the nature of physical education programs in Atlantic Canada. Eight online focus groups were conducted after quantitative data were analyzed. The focus-group discussions were structured to learn more about the future of physical education in Atlantic Canada. More specifically, the focus groups supported the exploration of participants' suggestions for changes to core content to make physical education an important and positive feature of schools in Atlantic Canada. Findings suggested that physical educators in Atlantic Canada are largely satisfied with the state of physical education, with little to no perceived need for internal reform within the discipline. Results from the focus groups suggested that any changes to physical education in Atlantic Canada should be physical educator–informed.

How did the researchers in the above examples decide to use a mixed methods design for their study? Put another way, why did the researchers decide to include both quantitative and qualitative phases? After all, ". . . mixing methods for no good reason other than the sake of it can produce disjointed and unfocussed research" (Mason, 2006a, p. 3). In any research study, the research question is what drives the direction of the research. Once researchers pose a question to be answered, the research design should match or correspond in a way that will best answer that question. Some research questions will lead to quantitative research designs. For instance, asking which metabolic and reproductive biomarkers are associated with breast density is likely to be best answered by implementing a quantitative research design, perhaps by collecting numerical data obtained from mammograms and blood samples. Other research questions lead to qualitative research designs. Inquiring about parents' perceptions of the Canadian Sedentary Behaviour Guidelines for the Early Years (Tremblay et al., 2012) corresponds to a qualitative research design, perhaps through focus group discussions with a group of parents. As highlighted throughout this book, research questions dictate the appropriate research design.

Sometimes the research question lends itself to being informed with both quantitative and qualitative components, and mixed methods research is most appropriate. For example, a mixed methods research design would likely be appropriate if researchers wanted to explore age-related patterns and experiences of chronic cancer-related pain in younger and older patients. The researchers could collect quantitative data on variables such as pain intensity, pain management, and functional ability to generate age-related trajectories of pain in younger and older adults. They could also qualitatively focus on understanding patients' pain as part of the cancer experience through separate focus groups for the two age categories. One unique thing about mixed methods research designs is that the quantitative component and qualitative component will each inform the research question in distinct ways. In the chronic cancer pain example, the quantitative findings provide insight into potential differences in pain intensity and functionality between younger and older cancer patients, while the qualitative findings offer rich insight into the complexity of the chronic pain experience for different age groups. Implementing a quantitative research design or a qualitative research design would have only partially informed the research question.

Researchers' personal characteristics also play a role in determining the specific research design. Their philosophical worldviews, education, training, and past research experience will influence the research design choice. In fact, researchers' philosophical worldviews will dictate the types of research questions that are even asked. Researchers who adopt a postpositivist worldview, for example, are likely to ask research questions that are best answered through quantitative research designs. Recall from Chapter 1 that postpositivism is premised on the belief of objectivity and finding one single truth in research. Researchers who operate from this lens will ask research questions that tend to align with the characteristics of quantitative research, such as collecting numerical data, measuring variables, and doing statistical analyses to find the answer to the question. Researchers with a postpositivist worldview are also less likely to ask research questions that correspond with qualitative research designs, because their philosophy is not premised on understanding multiple meanings and experiences. On the other hand, mixed methods research designs are largely undertaken by researchers with a pragmatist philosophical worldview, where the focus is on doing what works to find solutions to problems. Pragmatism is premised on the idea that the best approach to research is to do what works at the time for the particular research question, and therefore incorporate any designs that are appropriate to address the research question. A mixed methods research design works well for researchers with a pragmatist worldview because quantitative *and* qualitative methods provide the best understanding of their research and solution to their research questions.

The skills, training, and experiences that researchers have can also influence the type of research design that is used. A researcher who has a research lab focused on the narratives of online bullying, has developed a qualitative research graduate program, and teaches an undergraduate course on qualitative research methods is probably unlikely to have the requisite abilities and knowledge to independently conduct a pre- and post-test experimental study on the differences in cortisol levels (stress) following an episode of cyberbullying (recall experimental designs from Chapter 4). The point of this fictitious example is to highlight that researchers likely have certain skill sets and experiences that align with certain research designs over others. As such, the creation of research teams is an excellent strategy to bring together a diverse group of researchers who may have various training and experience (and philosophical worldviews) that, when combined, can generate diverse research designs. One example of a mixed methods research team is the Monitoring Activities of Teenagers to Comprehend their Habits (MATCH) study, led by Mathieu Bélanger in New Brunswick. The MATCH study includes both quantitative (e.g., surveys) and qualitative (e.g., individual interviews) data collection tools to understand physical activity experiences in youth over time (Bélanger et al., 2013). The purpose of the multidisciplinary team is to develop new ways of keeping more youth active with a focus on studying children starting in grade 5 and following them throughout primary and secondary school during times when physical activity levels decrease significantly.

Research Highlight

A team of researchers at the University of Manitoba conducted a mixed methods study to assess the feasibility and lived experiences of a peer-supported community-based life-style intervention for youth with type II diabetes (Huynh et al., 2015). Twelve Indigenous youth participated in a 16-week after-school intervention that was premised on peer support. Four university students and four adolescents served as peer mentors and delivered the physical activity and healthy eating intervention. Following the intervention, five youth and two mothers participated in semi-structured interviews to discuss challenges living with type II diabetes and the perceived benefits of participating in the intervention. Anthropometrics (e.g., waist circumference) and cardiometabolic risks (e.g., blood pressure) did not change from pre- to post-intervention. However, the perceived psychological and social (psycho-social) outcomes of intervention participation suggest an emphasis on relationship-building when designing behaviour modification for Indigenous youth living with type II diabetes. This mixed methods research study provides an excellent example of drawing upon both quantitative and qualitative research approaches in one study because, although there were no statistically significant findings from the quantitative measures, the qualitative data that were generated provides support for important psycho-social outcomes of the intervention.

Further Reading

Huynh, E., Rand, D., McNeill, C., Brown, S., Senechal, M., Wicklow, B., . . . McGavock, J. (2015). Beating diabetes together: A mixed-methods analysis of a feasibility study of intensive life-style intervention for youth with type 2 diabetes. *Canadian Journal of Diabetes, 39*, 484–90. doi:10.1016/j.jcjd.2015.09.093

Writing Exercise

For the following three research descriptions, explain how you might conduct the research study utilizing a mixed methods research design. Specifically, consider the following questions for each description:

- In what order would you conduct the quantitative and qualitative components of the study? What is your rationale for that order?
- Which research component would you give more priority, the quantitative component or the qualitative component (or, alternatively, would both components have equal weighting?). Again, explain your rationale for your choice.

1. Professional sport is an attractive and billion-dollar industry that employs many people in Canada. Among those employed in professional sport organizations are coaches, who are important members in the management of a sport organization. Professional coaches perform multiple roles that ensure that the sport organization is able to achieve its goals and objectives. The purpose of this study is to examine the management of professional sport from a coach perspective.
2. Low back pain is among the most commonly reported reasons that manual labour workers are referred to physical therapists and chiropractors. However, many individuals suffering from severe or repeated low back pain episodes continue to work, even if their jobs require a substantial amount of manual labour. This is troubling as frequent episodes of low back pain often result in long-term sick leave or permanent disability from work. The purpose of this study is to find out why manual labour workers continue to work with low back pain episodes.
3. Obesity and type II diabetes rates are on the rise in Canada. Children and youth are an important demographic to focus on, as developing healthy habits at an early age can result in healthy lifestyles later in life. Developing programs that emphasize creative physical activity options and fun ways to eat healthily may help develop healthy behaviours in children and youth. The purpose of this study is to explore the impact of a physical activity and healthy eating intervention on children and youth across Canada.

Planning Mixed Methods Research

Combining quantitative and qualitative research approaches in a mixed methods research design requires a lot of planning. The combination of quantitative and qualitative research methods can take many forms, and researchers conducting mixed methods studies have to decide if the quantitative and qualitative methods will be conducted simultaneously or sequentially (one following the other). Researchers also need to decide if one of the components will have greater emphasis in their mixed methods research or if there will be equal weighting between the quantitative and qualitative components. It is also critical that researchers consider how they plan to merge or connect the quantitative and qualitative data and results. When planning mixed methods research, researchers need to consider many things including the implementation timing, priority, and integration of the quantitative and qualitative components.

Implementation sequence

There are two general ways to plan the timing of the quantitative and qualitative components within mixed methods research: concurrently and sequentially. Conducting the quantitative and qualitative components at the same time is known as a **concurrent mixed methods research design**. In concurrent designs, researchers collect their quantitative and qualitative data at essentially the same time. Other mixed methods research designs call for a two-phase, sequential approach to data collection, whereby the quantitative and qualitative components are done one after the other. In a **sequential mixed methods research design**, data collected during the first phase informs data collection in the second phase. After collecting and fully analyzing data from the first phase, findings are incorporated into and inform subsequent plans for data collection. We will go into further detail and provide specific examples of concurrent and sequential mixed methods research designs a bit later in this chapter.

To add some complexity to these two general implementation approaches, another way that mixed methods research can be implemented is having separate quantitative and qualitative studies conducted over a longer period of time, all aimed at answering a broader research question (Creswell & Plano Clark, 2011). A larger mixed methods program of research is evident when researchers conduct a number of individual quantitative studies and qualitative studies all focused on one research topic. When the individual studies are looked at as pieces of a larger whole, the larger program of research represents a mixed methods approach. Jennifer Brunet at the University of Ottawa conducts research aimed at identifying and understanding processes that influence breast cancer patient/survivors' physical activity motivation and behaviour, and her study designs include both quantitative approaches (e.g., examining physical activity motivations and behaviour; Brunet & Sabiston, 2011) and qualitative approaches (e.g., exploring barriers to physical activity participation; Brunet et al., 2013). Taking a step back from each individual study, her research reflects a mixed methods program of research intended to increase physical activity levels among individuals reporting low levels of physical activity, such as cancer patients/survivors.

Priority

Another important aspect for researchers to consider when planning mixed methods research is whether one of the research components (quantitative or qualitative) will have greater priority than the other. Priority refers to the weight or emphasis assigned to the quantitative and qualitative research components. For instance, a mixed methods study can prioritize the qualitative component of the research and give less attention to the quantitative component. Woodgate and Sigurdson (2015) conducted a mixed methods study to determine the impact of a school-based, youth-led cardiovascular health promotion intervention on youth's capacity for health promotion. The intervention included a variety of activities, such as a healthy food workshop and a web-based health promotion project, intended to educate, empower, and support youth's knowledge and skills for cardiovascular health promotion. For the quantitative component, participants completed a positive youth development questionnaire before and after the program to determine if there were changes in character, competence, caring, connection, and confidence after the intervention. For the qualitative component, the participants took part in three focus groups to ascertain their perspectives on the processes involved in the intervention activities and to consider lessons learned and improvements for the future. The participants also completed written journals after each intervention activity to explore ongoing experiences in the intervention. The researchers directly stated that the qualitative component was given greater emphasis in their study. Even if the researchers had not indicated that the quantitative component was embedded within the larger qualitative focus, there were certain indicators that suggest the qualitative component was allotted greater weight. The study spanned two school years (a total of 22 months), which reflects the characteristic of spending prolonged time in the field (you were introduced to prolonged time in the field as a strategy to potentially enhance the rigour of qualitative research in Chapter 9). The amount of qualitative data that was collected exceeded the amount of quantitative data. Numerical data were generated from two questionnaires, whereas multiple focus groups and journals generated qualitative data. Not all researchers doing mixed methods studies specify which component of their research is given greater weight. However, looking for clues such as the number of participants, time spent in the field, amount of numerical versus non-numerical data, and greater reporting of quantitative or qualitative findings can indicate which component of a mixed methods study was given greater priority.

Integration

Mixed methods research designs require the mixing, or purposeful integration, of the quantitative and qualitative components. Integration can occur at various stages of the mixed methods research process, including data collection, data analysis, and data interpretation phases. As previously noted, sometimes mixed methods research occurs over the course of multiple and separate quantitative studies and qualitative studies that together provide a larger mixed methods research program. In this instance, the integration of the quantitative and qualitative studies might occur at the knowledge translation stage, whereby the knowledge gained from the various studies is synthesized, disseminated, exchanged, and applied to certain audiences (stay tuned for more on knowledge translation in Chapter 12).

Decisions about when and how to integrate quantitative and qualitative components in mixed methods studies relates back to the research question and initial research planning (Andrew & Halcomb, 2009). Having congruence between the study purpose and integration approach is critical in mixed methods research. It is important that researchers plan their mixed methods research with a clear idea of how the different components will inform one another and how the quantitative and qualitative components provide distinct answers to the research question. Failing to plan how the research components will be mixed leads to researchers blindly collecting data and then trying to make sense of the process. Integration should never be an afterthought! The *armchair walkthrough* discussed in Chapter 9, in which researchers reflect on all aspects of a research study before its implementation, might be relevant when planning how to integrate a coherent mixed methods study.

Integrating quantitative and qualitative components often—though not always—includes converging or merging the data at the analysis phase. It is important that researchers consider how they will analyze the various data they are planning to collect. Depending largely on the timing of the research components (i.e., concurrent or sequential), the quantitative and qualitative data might be analyzed separately in its original form and then brought together after independent data analysis. A **side-by-side comparison** is done when quantitative and qualitative data are analyzed separately; one set of findings is presented followed by the other. For example, researchers might first present qualitative research findings and then compare them with quantitative statistical results. Alternatively, researchers might report the quantitative statistical results and then discuss the qualitative findings that support or refute the statistical results. Kathryn Bills, a graduate student researcher at the University of Victoria at the time, employed a mixed methods study to examine senior community parks in British Columbia, particularly park visitation levels, types of utilization, park accessibility, and infrastructure (Bills, 2012). Data collection consisted of questionnaires, park observations, and one-on-one interviews with seniors and park recreation staff. The questionnaire included questions about overall health, senior community park awareness, and physical activity patterns. Observations of community parks were taken for seven days to produce visitation and usage patterns. The interviews were intended to elaborate on initial quantitative results, including older adults' individual experiences with community parks and recreation staff's opinions of park programming and planning. Quantitative results revealed under-utilization of the community parks and a discrepancy between individuals aware of the parks and those who visit more than once a month. Qualitative results uncovered why the park may be underutilized, including identifying aspects of the park that require improvement as well as infrastructure shortcomings.

Quantitative and qualitative data might also be analyzed independently for each phase in cases in which researchers need the findings from one phase of the research to plan or inform the next phase of the research. For instance, if the quantitative phase is done before the qualitative phase, the quantitative results might be used to inform the types of questions that are asked in the qualitative phase. On the other hand, if the qualitative phase is done before the quantitative phase, the qualitative results might facilitate the development or identification of measures or instruments to be used in the quantitative phase. In their investigation of how the general population responds to learning about living with a chronic condition, McTaggart-Cowan et al. (2012) conducted semi-structured interviews with members of the general population that included listening to and reflecting on recordings of patients with rheumatoid arthritis discussing adaptations to living with their condition. Following thematic analysis of the qualitative data, participants' responses during the interviews were used to generate items for a questionnaire to be used in a subsequent quantitative phase. The questionnaire was developed to evaluate the general population's rationales for changing health values after being informed about adaptations to chronic disease, and items were derived using the language of the participants in the qualitative component.

Another option for mixed methods data integration is known as **data transformation**, whereby one form of data is converted into the other form of data (Andrew & Halcomb, 2009). Researchers can either *qualitize* numerical data or *quantitize* qualitative data. Qualitizing data might consist of taking numerical data to provide a description of a sample. For example, longitudinal numerical data on the mental health status of Canadians could be used to provide detailed descriptions of mental health patterns. Coupled with qualitative data on the mental health experiences of individuals, the larger data integration might weave between details of individual lives and the patterns of groups of lives. To transform qualitative data into quantitative data (i.e., quantitize qualitative data), qualitative codes or themes are often changed into quantitative variables, counted, and then included as numerical data. Counting reflects the numbered nature of phenomena, with frequency suggesting the importance of various emergent themes (though frequency and importance are not necessarily synonymous). For example, data generated from one-on-one interviews with university teachers about their students' behaviour in class could be transformed into quantitative data through frequency counting, and then used to develop a descriptive list of student behaviour. Researchers could count the number of times that teachers use certain language in their interviews, such as smartphones and Instagram, to develop a hierarchical list of students' off-task behaviour during university courses.

Case Study: Naomi's Story

Naomi is 19 years old and in her second year of university. She is very energetic and enthusiastic, and has always been very physically active. One of Naomi's passions is cheerleading, and she has been engaged competitively for a number of years. When Naomi started university she continued to travel back and forth between cities in order to stay connected with her original cheer club. Realizing the burden this was taking (financially, travel time, extra time away from her studies, etc.), Naomi decided to try out for one of the local competitive cheer clubs. Naomi talked one of her friends, Martina, who is also a competitive cheerleader, into trying out with her so that they could both take a risk together—one that they hoped would pay off in terms of making the local cheer club to continue their passion. The tryouts are at 7:00 p.m. on Tuesday night.

Naomi and Martina are full of nervous energy as they drive to the tryout, and they express to each other that they both want to make an excellent first impression and are incredibly excited for what is to come. Naomi and Martina park their car and walk towards the gymnasium where the tryouts are being held. The girls open the door and walk into a gymnasium full of noise, excitement, and energy from a room full of other young women. The girls step inside and Naomi begins to take off her jacket, change her shoes, and get prepared. She notices Martina has stopped in her tracks and is staring at the room full of young women who are busily preparing themselves and practising their routines for the tryouts. Naomi asks Martina, "Hey, what's wrong?" Martina slowly replies, "Look around . . . what do you see?" Naomi, getting somewhat impatient with Martina's sudden change of energy, decides to engage with Martina, stops what she is doing, and stands next to her friend to see what she is looking at. Martina goes on, "We are the only Indigenous girls here. *Everyone* else is white." Naomi didn't know what to say, nor had she perceived the environment in the manner that Martina had. But Martina was right. All Naomi could see was white. Sure there were the usual high pony-tails, performance make-up, and bright-coloured attire that all cheer girls tended to wear, but there were no other visibly First Nations girls in the entire gym.

Naomi picked up her bag, and the girls turned around and walked out of the gym to go home.

Continued

Discussion Questions

1. Using Naomi's case study as a starting point, develop a research question that you could explore using a mixed methods research design.
2. Identify the quantitative elements of your research study. Who will be your participants? How many participants will you select? What will your participants do? What measures or instruments will be included?
3. Consider the qualitative elements of your research study. In particular, who will be your participants? What strategy of inquiry (e.g., narrative, grounded theory, qualitative description) will you use? What forms of data will you generate?
4. Consider how you will combine the quantitative and qualitative components of your study. For instance, which component will be given more weighting—quantitative or qualitative—and why? Will you conduct the quantitative and qualitative components one after the other or at the same time? Why? How will you combine the quantitative and qualitative data together; in other words, how will you analyze your numerical and non-numerical data?

Mixed Methods Research Designs

As previously introduced, the combination of quantitative and qualitative research approaches can take many forms, including mixed methods research designs in which quantitative and qualitative methods are conducted either simultaneously or one following the other (Creswell, 2014).

In concurrent mixed methods research designs (also called *convergent* designs), quantitative and qualitative data are collected at about the same time. A key assumption within this approach is that both quantitative and qualitative data provide different types of information, and together they provide insights into the research question that are greater than either approach on its own. The quantitative data can take a variety of numerical forms, including observational checklists, instrument data, or survey data (as discussed in Chapter 4). Similarly, the qualitative data can be generated using any of the forms presented in Chapter 7, including interviews, observation, written documents, and visual data. Concurrent designs can be a means for establishing triangulation as is the case when more than one method is employed to see if results converge (recall triangulation as a strategy to enhance the rigour of qualitative research presented in Chapter 9). Although quantitative and qualitative data are collected at the same time in concurrent designs, the data might be given equal or unequal *priority* as previously discussed. In **concurrent nested designs** one of the methods dominates while the other one is nested or embedded within it. The nested method may be of secondary interest or intended to answer a specific subtopic of interest that is connected with the primary research question. Concurrent mixed methods research designs are depicted in Figure 10.1.

An example of a concurrent mixed methods research design is a study by William Harvey and his colleagues at McGill University (Harvey et al., 2009). They conducted interviews with six boys who were diagnosed with attention deficit hyperactivity disorder (ADHD) and six age-matched boys without ADHD. The interview data were converged with assessments on the

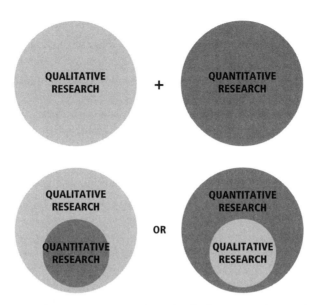

Figure 10.1 Depiction of concurrent mixed methods designs with equal priority (top panel) and concurrent nested designs (bottom panel).

Test of Gross Motor Development-2 that was used to examine skill and movement in loco-motor (e.g., running, leaping) and object (e.g., catching, kicking) control. Based on the findings, boys with ADHD were not as proficient at locomotor or object control when compared to age-matched boys without ADHD. The boys with ADHD also described their physical activity experiences with less detail and knowledge about movement, and expressed unfavourable experiences in physical activity generally. Using a concurrent mixed methods design allowed the researchers to get an in-depth description of the physical activity experiences of boys with ADHD, as well as make comparisons to boys who were not diagnosed with ADHD and collect information that can be used to inform tailored programs.

Important decisions need to be made when conducting any research study regarding the choice of a study sample, including *who* and *how many* people will participate. These issues become particularly complex when doing mixed methods research. Will individuals participating in one component of the research also participate in the other component? For instance, should participants who provide quantitative data also generate qualitative data? As for sample size, in Chapters 4 and 7 you learned that quantitative studies typically include larger sample sizes in order to conduct meaningful statistical analyses, whereas qualitative studies tend to include fewer study participants to gather rich information on a smaller sample. You might be asking yourself, "What sample size do researchers use in a concurrent mixed methods research design?" Sometimes researchers doing a concurrent mixed methods research study will collect data from the same number of participants, representing either the same participants or two different groups of participants, for both the quantitative and the qualitative components. This unquestionably means that either the traditionally larger quantitative sample size will be reduced, potentially impacting the statistical analyses that are available, or the typically smaller qualitative sample size will be increased, thereby likely limiting the amount of data generated from any one individual. Another approach that some researchers take is to honour the traditional approaches of having a larger sample size in quantitative research and smaller sample size in qualitative research by including only a subset of the participants from the quantitative component in the qualitative component.

Sequential mixed methods research designs involve two distinct phases in which researchers collect one form of data in the first phase, analyze the data, and then use the results from that first phase to inform the second phase. Sequential mixed methods designs allow researchers to clarify the results of one method through the use of a second method. How do researchers doing a sequential mixed methods study decide whether the quantitative phase or qualitative phase will be implemented first? The research purpose and research questions should guide the particular sequence of data collection.

A team of researchers in Toronto, Ontario, conducted a mixed methods study to evaluate a new clinical reasoning instrument to examine Canadian orthopaedic manual physical therapists (Yeung et al., 2015). They recruited 11 Canadian orthopaedic manual physical therapy examiners to complete an electronic questionnaire that reviewed the instrument. In a subsequent qualitative phase, the examiners participated in semi-structured telephone interviews to elaborate on questionnaire responses regarding the feasibility and acceptability of the instrument. This is an example of an **explanatory sequential mixed methods design**, in which the quantitative data are collected in the first phase and the qualitative data are collected in the second phase. An explanatory sequential mixed methods design is depicted in Figure 10.2.

The intent of explanatory sequential mixed methods designs is to have the qualitative data help explain in more detail the initial quantitative results. Perhaps not surprising, this specific type of sequential design is tailored more to researchers with strong quantitative backgrounds. As shown in our example, a typical procedure consists of collecting quantitative numerical data (e.g., survey data) in the first phase, analyzing the data, then following up with qualitative data generation (e.g., one-on-one interviews) to help explain and better understand the quantitative findings. The quantitative results often inform the types of participants to be purposefully selected for the qualitative phase, as well as the types of questions that will be asked of the participants during qualitative data generation. Typical quantitative sampling procedures take place for the quantitative phase, such as random selection, stratified random sampling, or

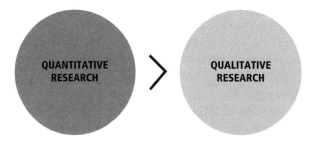

Figure 10.2 Illustration of an explanatory sequential mixed methods design.

systematic sampling (recall these types of sampling procedures from Chapter 4). As discussed with concurrent mixed methods designs, a similar decision has to be made with sequential mixed methods designs as to whether the qualitative sample should consist of individuals who were in the initial quantitative phase. There is no one right answer to this question, and researchers need to reflect on their study purpose to consider the most appropriate strategy to best inform their research questions. Yeung et al. (2015) had the same orthopaedic manual physical therapy examiners participate in the quantitative and qualitative phases of their explanatory sequential mixed methods study. The researchers positioned their study as a pilot test of the clinical reasoning instrument, so although the size of the sample was smaller than is typical for quantitative studies, the number of participants was deemed sufficient for a pilot study. Having the same participants in both phases of their study allowed the researchers to get an understanding of the participants' rationale for their quantitative ratings of the instrument. In other words, it made sense to have follow-up interviews with the same study participants to hear their explanations and insight. Moreover, the interview guide used in the qualitative phase was developed partially based on questionnaire responses from the quantitative phase.

There are also **exploratory sequential mixed methods designs**, which is the reverse of explanatory sequential mixed methods designs (see Figure 10.3). Once again there are two distinct phases, but exploratory sequential designs start with a qualitative phase followed by a quantitative phase. Researchers begin by exploring a research question with qualitative data and analysis, and then use the second quantitative phase to build on the results of the initial phase.

Professional Highlight

Dianna Moulden, Registered Sport Physiotherapist, Manual Therapist, and Nutritionist

....

Profile: To become a leader in the healthcare industry, Dianna began her journey at McMaster University with an undergraduate Honours degree in Kinesiology. Following her work as a kinesiologist with underprivileged individuals in Hamilton, Ontario, Dianna went on to obtain a diploma in Holistic Nutrition. Wanting to create a niche within the healthcare industry and having the desire to treat the "whole" individual, she received a Master's of Science degree in Physiotherapy and a Master's of Clinical Science degree in Manipulative Therapy. Working with educated practitioners within her community, Dianna serves the Hamilton sports community on a holistic level by identifying the links between nutrition, injuries, health, and performance. Similar to how mixed methods research designs incorporate multiple forms of research for a greater result than if only one research design were chosen, Dianna integrates multiple treatment approaches when working with her clients to achieve their strength, mobility, function, nutrition, and life goals. Her clientele ranges from professional athletes to active community members, and she strives to keep her skill set current in order to provide the most effective client-centred rehabilitation care possible.

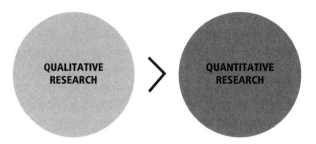

Figure 10.3 Illustration of an exploratory sequential mixed methods design.

Quite often, the intent of exploratory sequential designs is measurement development in which the goal is to develop strong measures or instruments with specific samples of populations (informed through the initial qualitative phase). After the instrument is developed, researchers then use the measure with a larger sample (in the quantitative phase). The qualitative data can inform writing of scale items through participant quotes, grouping of items on the measure by codes, and suggesting themes to categorize codes into subscales. For example, Andrée Castonguay from Concordia University collected narratives from older adolescents and young adults who provided descriptions of situations and events that led to feelings of body-related pride. These narratives were used to inform the development of questions that have become part of the Body and Appearance Self-Conscious Emotions scale (Castonguay et al., 2014) and the Body-Related Self-Conscious Emotions Fitness Instrument (Castonguay et al., 2016). Specifically, the narratives and actual quotes from participants were transformed into a pool of items to measure body-related pride, guilt, and shame. These items were then evaluated by experts in emotion and body image, tested in samples of older adolescents and young adults, and informed the final instruments that can be used to measure body-related self-conscious emotions.

The study participants in exploratory designs will most often consist of different participants for the qualitative and quantitative phases. A good procedure is to draw both the qualitative and quantitative samples from the same population, but make sure the individuals for each specific sample are not the same. For example, Castonguay et al. (2014, 2016) sampled from Quebec post-secondary education colleges and university programs to generate initial narrative data and then tested the instruments with *different* samples from the same general population. The time lapse between studies helped ensure non-overlap in sampling. This was important to ensure that participants who contributed to initial instrument development in the qualitative phase were not surveyed with the tool in the subsequent quantitative phase, which would have introduced confounding factors into the study.

Benefits of mixed methods research

The examples of mixed methods studies that you have read in this chapter highlight the advantages of mixed methods research. Some of the benefits include (a) neutralizing weaknesses and maximizing strengths of quantitative and qualitative designs, (b) triangulating, (c) improving comprehensiveness, (d) developing and testing instruments, (e) assisting sampling, and (f) enhancing generalization (Sparkes, 2015). Capitalizing on the strengths of quantitative and qualitative methods by bringing them together can help to overcome or neutralize the limitations of each method in isolation. Including both quantitative and qualitative data allows for greater validity or rigour of a study through triangulation of data collection methods. Further, using multiple methods provides a more comprehensive or complete picture of the study variables. As already discussed in this chapter, mixed methods studies can assist in the development, testing, and refinement of measures or instruments for use in future studies. When quantitative methods are employed first they can assist with purposeful sampling for subsequent qualitative methods. On the other hand, quantitative methods can enhance the transferability of qualitative findings from the first phase in a subsequent quantitative phase.

Kinesiology programs across Canada tend to be very multidisciplinary in nature; biomechanics, bone health, cardiovascular physiology, growth and development, Indigenous health, motor control, musculoskeletal health, neuromuscular adaptations, nutrition, sport psychology, and women's health are only a few of the areas that are investigated by kinesiology researchers and their colleagues. Having the option of conducting mixed methods research can expand the types of questions that are explored in a broad-ranging field of study. From using population-level health data to develop physical activity and diet programs, informing the representation of athletes in the media, developing new measures for movement and skills, and testing disease diagnostic protocols, researchers who conduct mixed methods research are not limited to using any specific types of designs. Having both quantitative and qualitative design options allows kinesiology researchers to think outside the box and find ways to best answer their research questions. Also, and very importantly, having a background in mixed methods research helps researchers interpret, critique, and understand a wide range of research studies conducted in the field, including the very challenges discussed in the following section that are inherent to combining quantitative and qualitative research approaches.

Challenges of mixed methods research

As critical consumers of information, it is important to weigh the benefits of mixed methods research against the challenges it poses. This is for good reason, because there can be a lot of challenges with doing mixed methods research. Some potential barriers to mixed methods research include (a) blending philosophical worldviews that traditionally underlie quantitative and qualitative research; (b) bringing together researchers with differing philosophical worldviews, education, and experience; (c) navigating timelines and access to resources; (d) making sampling and analysis decisions; and (e) resolving publication and evaluation challenges.

The pragmatist philosophical worldview was introduced in Chapter 1, and we returned to it during this chapter as the underlying philosophical worldview that typically guides researchers conducting mixed methods studies. However, there is still some concern, particularly from researchers who might eschew pragmatism, about blending knowledge that is gained from both quantitative approaches and qualitative approaches. Rather than struggle with reconciling different forms of knowledge by forcing one research approach to fit the other,

Mason (2006b) suggests that researchers think more in terms of meshing or linking data from different approaches to allow their distinctiveness to be held in creative tension. Researchers can gain a more comprehensive understanding of human experience by bringing together measurable and generalizable aspects with unique experiences.

The amount of time, effort, and work required to enable a collaborative mixed methods research team and execute a successful mixed methods research study should not be taken lightly. We hope that you have gained an appreciation for the amount of time it takes to do any research study. Generating a research question, carefully planning the most appropriate research design, obtaining institutional ethical approval and any other required approvals (e.g., school board, health region), recruiting participants, collecting data, analyzing data, and reporting the findings all require a great deal of time and effort. Now consider doing all of those components (and the many details that go into each component) in a mixed methods study. In some ways it means doing *double* the amount of work! Resources such as study personnel, finances to pay research assistants and purchase study materials and supplies, and access to instruments and equipment can easily be spread thin in a mixed methods study. Perhaps one of the most important resources that researchers never seem to have enough of is time. The amount of time it takes to conduct a mixed methods study can be substantial, and researchers need to consider this important element when planning their research.

Sampling has already been discussed a few times in this book, and sampling decisions in mixed methods research can be challenging. As with all studies, sampling strategies in mixed methods research should both stem logically from the research questions and be ethical (Andrew & Halcomb, 2009). Part of a researcher's ethical commitment includes not placing study participants under unnecessary burden. The question of burden becomes complex when deciding whether participants in one phase should also participate in the other phase of a mixed methods study. Perhaps having participants involved in both the quantitative and the qualitative phases is the best choice based on the research question. However, if the procedures of the study seem excessive in terms of time commitment or another form of burden, researchers need to default to ethical principles and ethical decision-making to drive their sampling strategy (refer to Chapter 3 for an overview of an ethical decision-making process). Moreover, mixed methods research designs often combine more than one sampling strategy to satisfy the quantitative and qualitative phases, so the sampling strategies utilized need to be appropriate, meaningful, and ethical. Unnecessary data collection or overuse of participants' time should be avoided because it places burden on participants.

You have already been introduced to a few options that researchers have when analyzing data in a mixed methods study. Deciding when and how to integrate quantitative and qualitative data is no easy task. But what about the challenge that might arise when contradictory findings are produced between the quantitative and qualitative components? Integrating findings in mixed methods research can be challenging, particularly if the findings suggest divergent conclusions. Ferguson et al. (2012) had a seemingly inconsistent finding between their quantitative and qualitative phases when exploring the relationship between women's physical activity and psychological well-being. Their initial quantitative phase resulted in no relationship between women's physical activity and psychological well-being; however, their subsequent qualitative phase found that being physically active was described as contributing to women's well-being. When the results from one form of data contradict results from the other form of data, what are researchers to do? Well, one thing that researchers should *not* do is fall victim to forms of reporting bias; for instance, **positive reporting bias** is the selective reveal or suppression of information. Analyzing one form of data in a direct effort to support or match the other form of data is simply not good research. Dismissing conflicting findings does similar injustice to the research. Indeed, contradictory findings in kinesiology might actually be quite telling about the holistic and complex nature of human movement (assuming the contradictory findings are based on rigorous research, of course). Ferguson et al. found that level of physical activity was not related to psychological well-being, as indicated by the lack of a statistically significant correlation in their quantitative phase. What emerged in subsequent one-on-one interviews was that physical activity level is less important to the women's well-being than what they experience while they are active. It is when the women are goal setting, relationship building, self-reflecting, and working on self-development during physical activity that it contributes to their well-being. This is an example of a mixed methods study in which the quantitative and qualitative phases each inform the research question in distinct ways, and the combination of the two phases provides greater insight than each phase alone. In other words, without the other phase included, only part of the story on women's physical activity and well-being would have been told.

The mixed methods study by Ferguson and colleagues (2012) was published in an academic journal, which is a common way that researchers present their study findings. However, one challenge when publishing a mixed methods study pertains to the amount of space that is allocated to a single journal article. Journals often have policies in place that limit the number of pages for each article, such as the recommended 20 pages in the *Medicine & Science in Sports & Exercise* journal. Having limited space might not be conducive to a mixed methods research study that will often include multiple or lengthier sections in the article allocated to sampling strategies, data collection, and data analysis. As such, researchers need to make decisions about how to condense their mixed methods research for the purpose of publication, or consider if publishing their findings in a journal is the best approach for presenting their research. There are a variety of ways that researchers are able to share their findings (e.g., short film, online tools), and you will be introduced to a number of options in Chapter 12.

Another challenge with mixed methods research designs is evaluation; what criteria are appropriate for judging a mixed methods study? Criteria for evaluating quantitative and qualitative research designs were covered in Chapters 6 and 9, respectively. Some researchers favour the separation of evaluation criteria for the quantitative and qualitative components of a mixed methods design (Sparkes, 2015). In this case, things like the validity and reliability of instruments in the quantitative component would be evaluated, and identifying characterizing traits that might suggest rigour of the qualitative component might be considered. It is inappropriate to judge a quantitative study using qualitative criteria and vice versa; choosing to consider separately the quality of the quantitative and qualitative components might make sense if each component is discrete in a mixed methods study. At other times, simply assessing the individual components when evaluating mixed methods studies might be too limiting because mixed

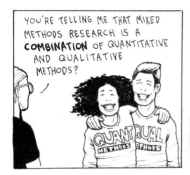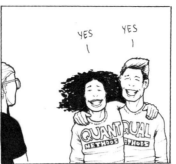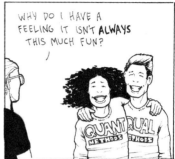

methods research is more than just the sum of its quantitative and qualitative components. It is important that standards of quantitative and qualitative research are not compromised in a mixed methods study, which can be a challenge for researchers. Expanding the range of criteria used to judge mixed methods research, and creating novel combinations of judgment criteria, requires thoughtful consideration.

Mixed methods research designs clearly have the potential to further the development of knowledge in kinesiology research. The topics studied in kinesiology are varied and complex; rather than isolate our research strategies, we may be able to improve and extend our knowledge by drawing on different approaches. The field of kinesiology will continue to mature in terms of novel research designs and combination of research methods. Care should be taken to facilitate the development of rigorous mixed methods frameworks to support the creativity and challenges faced by researchers doing mixed methods research.

Summary

Chapter 10 introduced mixed methods research designs. Characteristics of mixed methods research were described, and the reader was presented with the different ways to implement quantitative and qualitative research through concurrent and sequential designs. Options for the timing and priority of quantitative and qualitative components in mixed methods studies were introduced. Strategies for integrating mixed methods data were also discussed, including side-by-side comparison of quantitative and qualitative results as well as data transformation for analyzing mixed methods data. The chapter concluded with an overview of the benefits and challenges of mixed methods research.

Discussion Questions

1. In your own words, what is mixed methods research?
2. What might a mixed methods research study look like in your area of interest? Use Table 10.2 to help organize your research plan.

Table 10.2 Research planning table.

RESEARCH ASPECT	YOUR RESEARCH PLAN
Research question	
Rationale for using mixed methods	
Mixed methods research design	
Rationale for mixed methods design	
Quantitative data collection	
Qualitative data collection	
Weighting	
Rationale for weighting	
Sampling strategy	
Integration approach	
Anticipated challenges	

3. A journalist for the university paper wants to highlight your recent mixed methods research study in the next online edition of the paper. For part of her article she wants to know why you did a mixed methods study instead of a quantitative or qualitative study. How do you respond?
4. What are the differences between a concurrent mixed methods research design and a sequential mixed methods research design? In your answer be sure to include the distinguishing features of each design.
5. What are the similarities and differences between side-by-side comparison and data transformation as ways to integrate data in a mixed methods study?

Recommended Readings

Andrew, S., & Halcomb, E. J. (Eds.). (2009). *Mixed methods research for nursing and the health sciences.* Chichester: Wiley-Blackwell.

Creswell, J. W., & Plano Clark, V. L. (2011). *Designing and conducting mixed methods research* (2nd ed.). Thousand Oaks, CA: Sage.

Sparkes, A. C. (2015). Developing mixed methods research in sport and exercise psychology: Critical reflections on five points of controversy. *Psychology of Sport and Exercise, 16,* 49–59. doi:10.1016/j.psychsport.2014.08.014

11 Participatory Action Research

Learning Outcomes

By the end of this chapter, you should be able to:

- Summarize the defining features of participatory action research.
- Apply a participatory action research design.
- Justify participatory action research as a respectful approach for engaging in research with underrepresented research populations.
- Assess the inherent challenges of engaging in participatory action research.

Introduction to Participatory Action Research

Participatory action research (PAR) has a rich history in various academic disciplines, yet PAR is only starting to gain momentum within the field of kinesiology. PAR emerged, in part, in response to a distrust of traditional postpositivist research that typically does not include participants as active agents in the production of knowledge (remember from Chapter 1, postpositivism is premised on the notion that there is an objective truth to be discovered through research). Research driven by a postpositivist philosophical worldview was critiqued for being inadequate in providing insight into the social and cultural issues that are deeply embedded in human experiences, whereas those committed to PAR have a clear commitment to social justice. Participatory research approaches are relevant to research in kinesiology, particularly to those researchers who seek to understand experiences of those affected by or excluded from sport and physical activity opportunities (Frisby et al., 2005). The unique transformative power of PAR, which can and should be applied in kinesiology settings, has been aptly summarized by Brydon-Miller and colleagues who stated:

> We believe passionately in the power of participatory action research to push us to challenge and unsettle existing structures of power and privilege, to provide opportunities for those least often heard to share their knowledge and wisdom, and for people to work together to bring about positive social change and to create more just and equitable political and social systems. (Brydon-Miller et al., 2011, p. 396)

PAR has been described as a particularly unique and emerging research approach that not only co-generates knowledge with participants, but also results in practical outcomes for participants. Within PAR, research is conducted alongside or *with* participants, rather than *on* participants. Unlike most other research designs, PAR is typically approached by researchers with political and social agendas who seek to engage community members as active participants in identifying and addressing community issues. Recall from Chapter 1 that it is likely a transformative philosophical worldview that guides those who engage in PAR. Researchers who approach their studies from a transformative worldview, which may also be referred to as participatory or advocacy worldviews, have identified the need for research to be closely connected with politics and to have some sort of an action agenda that advocates for groups that have been underrepresented in research.

A concise overview of the history of PAR has been provided by Kemmis and McTaggart (2008), who attributed social psychologist Kurt Lewin and his work related to community action programs in the 1940s for providing the stimulus to action research movements within various academic disciplines (see Lewin, 1946). In your reading of the vast array of kinesiology research that has been published in peer-reviewed journals, you may have come across not only the term PAR but also other similar approaches such as participatory research, action research, and community-based participatory research (CBPR). **Action research** is typically conceptualized as the broader framework that encompasses PAR and the various other approaches. These terms are sometimes used interchangeably, yet some scholars (e.g., Kemmis & McTaggart) have written about the differences among each approach. Despite differences among the various action research approaches, there are some common threads that weave through them. Importantly, the various approaches are collaborative and they result in direct benefits to participants. Within this chapter we will refer primarily to PAR, but we will also draw upon examples of CBPR that have recently been employed by kinesiology researchers in Canada.

Defining Features of PAR

Recall from Chapter 7 that many qualitative strategies of inquiry are quite collaborative (e.g., narrative) and some qualitative strategies of inquiry result in direct benefits to participants through advocacy for underrepresented groups (e.g., critical ethnography). With this in mind, how does a novice researcher distinguish PAR from other forms of inquiry? How exactly *is* PAR defined? Participatory action research has been described by Brydon-Miller and colleagues as "the sum of its individual terms" (Brydon-Miller et al., 2011, p. 388). They described how PAR is *participatory* in that all people (researchers and participants) are involved in all phases of the research process. They also explained how *action* is central to the PAR process in that the primary goal of research is to create positive change to address participant-identified injustices. Lastly, they described how *research* is a social process of gathering and asserting knowledge, which belongs to all people.

The study design by which researchers engage in PAR is often considered a defining feature of this research approach. Such study designs (e.g., action research spiral) will be described in the following section. However, given that PAR can be approached or designed in a number of ways, it is important to identify some of the other defining or key features of this research approach. In addition to the study design, Kemmis and McTaggart (2008) described PAR as having seven key features:

1. *Social process:* Researchers and participants who engage in PAR are committed to examining relationships and particularly how those relationships exist in our social world. Individually and collectively, those involved in PAR seek to understand how they are shaped or formed in relation to one another.
2. *Participatory:* Unlike most other research approaches, those involved in PAR are engaged throughout the various phases of the research process, from the identification of research questions, to the generation of knowledge, interpretation of findings, and the resulting action.
3. *Practical and collaborative:* Participants and researchers work together to examine the various social practices that connect them with others and to understand how to enhance such interactions. Interactions are enhanced through real-world action strategies that address real-life issues.
4. *Emancipatory:* With a commitment to addressing social injustices, PAR supports participants in recovering or freeing themselves from the constraints of social structures. It is not the researchers themselves but the collaborative and participatory nature of PAR that supports this emancipation.
5. *Critical:* PAR provides the foundation for addressing irrational and unjust constraints that are inherent in the social context within which people interact.
6. *Reflexive:* Practices are transformed within PAR in an effort to address social injustices, and this process of transformation occurs through cycles of action and reflection among and between all those involved (e.g., participants, researchers).
7. *Process to transform both theory and practice*: Theory and practice hold equal standing within PAR. Recall from Chapter 2 that a theory is an explanation of observed patterns or supposition about a relationship among phenomena. Those engaged in PAR are committed both to enhancing such theory and to addressing real-life issues through critical reasoning.

Writing Exercise

Using a kinesiology-related library database (e.g., SPORT Discus), retrieve a peer-reviewed journal article that is relevant to kinesiology and has specifically stated that the study was PAR. After reading the study, write down your answers to the following questions:

1. Which of the seven defining features of PAR are specifically identified in the paper?
2. Which of the defining features of PAR were likely included in the research process, but were *not* specifically described in the paper?
3. What doubts, if any, do you have that this study is indeed a PAR study?

You will remember from Chapter 7 that there are various qualitative strategies of inquiry that incorporate some of the above-mentioned defining features (e.g., reflexive, critical). When a research study is reflective of all seven defining features, it is likely PAR. However, is it necessary to include *all* defining features in order to be PAR? The simple answer is "no." Given that PAR is employed across various disciplines and settings, and given that there is no one "right way" to do PAR, there is great variability regarding what does and does not constitute PAR. For instance, Amy Carpenter and her colleagues (i.e., Carpenter et al., 2008) from the University of Manitoba described their community-based PAR study that involved the initiation of an Indigenous youth mentorship program focused on providing an after-school physical activity, education, and nutrition program. The authors described how the research issue (i.e., need for more physical activity opportunities in the school community) was defined by Indigenous youth. Relationships were established among researchers, youth, and school officials, and a flexible data collection protocol for gaining insights into how to address the issue were employed (e.g., conversations of planning sessions were recorded). The PAR resulted in the development of a mentorship program, which consisted of 10 to 12 Indigenous high school students who developed and designed weekly physical activity programs and snacks that could accommodate up to 25 children.

Carpenter et al.'s (2008) PAR study is reflective of a number of the defining features of PAR, with the most obvious being that it was a participatory and collaborative process that resulted in very practical outcomes for youth. Other PAR studies you come across might not be so clear with respect to how they incorporate the defining features of PAR. The authors might not articulate who defined the research issue (i.e., researchers or participants), and the practical outcomes or action strategies might not be clear. Given that you will come across various studies that are defined as PAR, when making judgments about PAR we encourage you to draw upon the works of various scholars including Kemmis and McTaggart (2008), who have spent a great deal of their academic careers identifying defining features of this approach so that researchers have common ground from which to evaluate PAR.

When trying to evaluate the merits of PAR we also encourage you to go back to Chapter 9 in this book and consider the overview we provided of Schinke, Smith, and McGannon's (2013) work, which supports a relativistic approach for evaluating research. In their work they identified a number of characterizing traits that support researchers in making judgments about the quality of research. For instance, characterizing traits include the extent to which the research is *community driven* and community partners are involved in the identification of research questions and methods. Researchers might also want to consider the extent to which there was *prolonged engagement and consultation*. Such engagement likely plays a critical role in the establishment and nurturing of relationships, which can support ongoing collaboration. As well, it might be important to identify *project deliverables* and the extent to which community members receive mutual benefits and practical outcomes from their engagement in the research process. Such characterizing traits are simply considerations to support researchers in evaluating participatory and community-driven forms of research and should not be applied as strict criteria. The following research highlight from Schinke et al. (2013) provides a practical example of how various characterizing traits (e.g., prolonged engagement and consultation, project deliverables) contributed to the quality of their research with an Indigenous community.

Research Highlight

Robert Schinke, who holds a Canada Research Chair in Multicultural Sport and Physical Activity at Laurentian University, and his colleagues described the necessary transformation of a sport research project that was "steeped in post-positivism" to a CBPR approach (Schinke et al., 2013). They discussed how the project was initiated in 2003 with an Indigenous community in northeastern Ontario, but the research topic and questions were conceptualized by the mainstream researcher and there was no input or consultation with the community. As such, the data collection processes applied in the project resulted in descriptive numerical data that did not include or represent the perspectives of their Indigenous participants, and the results were deemed culturally unsuitable. Since 2006, as Schinke et al. describe, the project has been much more collaborative in nature and adheres to the tenets of CBPR. Specifically, the mainstream researchers have worked with the community to co-develop relevant research questions. As well, the community is involved in all aspects of the research process including the generation of meaningful research through talking circles, the interpretation of research, and the sharing of the research with other local communities and research communities. Importantly, the research has resulted in practical outcomes for the community. At the time of the research publication, the CBPR had supported a youth leadership adventure program that was in its sixth year of existence and the research resulted in the creation of a leadership manual that was developed by the community for their sport staff and youth. The research described by Schinke et al. demonstrates that a participatory approach was essential to developing a meaningful and enduring sport development project.

Further Reading

Schinke, R. J., McGannon, K. R., Watson, J., & Busanich, R. (2013). Moving toward trust and partnership: An example of sport-related community-based participatory action research with Aboriginal people and mainstream academics. *Journal of Aggression, Conflict and Peace Research, 5,* 201–10. doi:10.1108/jacpr-11-2012-0012

Research Process

Given that PAR is employed in various academic disciplines (e.g., kinesiology, education, sociology) and settings (e.g., schools, neighbourhoods, hospitals), the manner in which PAR is designed and carried out will also vary. Unlike many other qualitative or quantitative research designs, there is no distinct set of guidelines to follow for designing a PAR project. As well, and importantly, PAR is not a linear process. Unlike other research designs that typically occur in a consecutive format from development of the research question to data generation, data analysis, and data interpretation, PAR is typically thought of as a cyclical and iterative process (this cyclical and iterative process will become clearer in the following section when we describe the action research spiral). There is no one way to do PAR, and within this chapter we describe two research processes or study designs for carrying out PAR, including the **action research spiral** and a **five-phase participatory action research approach**.

Action research spiral

The early writings of Kurt Lewin serve as a foundation for understanding the PAR process as one that is cyclical and requires ongoing planning, executing, and reconnaissance (Lewin, 1946). He described how the action research process starts with *planning,* whereby the plan for addressing the overall research objective and first action step is identified. The next step in the research process involves *executing* the initial plan through action. Following the execution is the *reconnaissance* or fact-finding step, whereby the action is evaluated and new insights and basis for re-planning is established. From here, a new spiral or cycle of re-planning, executing, and reconnaissance takes place. This spiral continues until the overall objectives and actions are achieved.

Lewin (1946) described the spiral research process within the context of the broader action research framework. More recently, Kemmis and McTaggart (2008) situated their description of the action research spiral specifically within the context of PAR, explaining how the process occurs through a spiral of self-reflective cycles that include planning, acting and observing, and reflecting (see Figure 11.1).

The various stages or steps of the spiral are relatively self-explanatory. Researchers, working closely with participants and communities, begin with a *plan* for a change, they *act* and *observe* with respect to the change process and anticipated consequences, and then they *reflect* on such processes and consequences. Based on this first cycle, the researchers and participants then re-plan, act and observe again, and then reflect again. It is critical to note that although this PAR process is depicted as a neat spiral, the design should be conceptualized as more of a fluid and responsive process in which the various stages may overlap. As well, the collaborative nature of each phase of the spiral within the PAR process should be emphasized. Participants and researchers work together to plan, to act and observe, and to reflect during each cycle.

A recent PAR project led by Sarah Oosman, within the School of Physical Therapy at the University of Saskatchewan, employed the action research spiral in a PAR project that engaged Métis community members in informing the design of a comprehensive school health intervention (Oosman et al., 2016). Oosman and her colleagues described how a Métis community research coordinator and community advisory board supported the planning, acting and observing, and reflecting that represent the PAR action cycles. The community advisory board was particularly important in terms of the *planning* as their combined input insured that multiple Métis perspectives (e.g., two Elders, a teacher, the mayor) informed the project. These multiple perspectives were very apparent in the *acting and observing* phase of the research, whereby

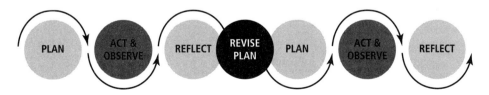

Figure 11.1 The action research spiral.

Source: Informed by Kemmis, S., & McTaggart, R. (2008). Participatory action research: Communicative action and the public sphere. In N.K. Denzin & Y.S. Lincoln (Eds.), *Strategies of qualitative inquiry* (3rd ed., pp. 271–330). Thousand Oaks, CA: Sage Publications. Reprinted by permission of the publisher (Taylor & Francis Ltd, http://www.tandfonline.com).

Métis-specific activities such as jigging and fiddling were integrated into programming. Reflecting occurred through regular communication between and among the community research team via face-to-face meetings and teleconference calls. Through such communication it was possible to identify new action items that would subsequently serve as the foundation for a new cycle of planning, acting and observing, and reflection.

You may have noticed that many of the examples shared in this chapter thus far have focused on working with Indigenous populations. However, it is critical to acknowledge that PAR is not restricted to research with Indigenous peoples. As you will read a little later in this chapter, participatory approaches can serve as a respectful process for engaging underrepresented populations (including Indigenous peoples) in research. There are a growing number of exemplary kinesiology-related PAR studies that have focused on engaging with Indigenous populations and, as such, we felt compelled to share such studies to help enhance your understanding of PAR processes.

Five-phase participatory action research approach

The spiral process described above might not have the detail that some researchers prefer when conceptualizing, engaging in, or writing about PAR. As such, Stringer and Genat (2004) described a five-phase action research model that outlines more detail in terms of the activities that researchers and participants engage in when trying to systematically identify and address the issue or problem. The five phases in Stringer and Genat's framework include (a) the research design, (b) data gathering, (c) data analysis, (d) communication, and (e) action. They explained how the *research design* is focused on initiating the study by developing a picture of the study in terms of key issues and the people that are affected. *Data gathering* is a process whereby participants' perspectives are explored, and key features of such experiences are then identified in the *data analysis*. *Communication* takes place through a number of avenues including the writing of reports, and *action* is the process whereby solutions are created for the issues identified. Similar to the action research spiral, this five-phase action research approach should be envisioned as a cyclical process that is iterative and often can involve overlap among the phases.

A similar five-phase research approach was also outlined by a team of researchers led by kinesiology scholar Wendy Frisby from the University of British Columbia (Frisby et al., 2005). Within their own PAR research, they described how the five-phase research process includes:

- Setting the research question
- Building trust
- Data collection
- Data analysis
- Communicating results for action

By simply observing the descriptive headings for each phase that have been given to the five-phase approaches described by Frisby et al. (2005) and Stringer and Genat (2004), we see that the two processes are clearly very similar. Notably, Stringer and Genat did not include *building trust* as a specific phase, yet they do describe how the development of relationships (and ultimately trust) is a working principle of PAR. As well, similar to Stringer and Genat, the five-phase approach presented by Frisby et al. does not necessarily occur in a linear fashion and the five components must constantly be negotiated among researchers and participants.

Frisby et al. (2005) provided a detailed example of how a five-phase research approach was applied to their research with a community-based organization called Women Organizing Activities for Women (WOAW). Members of WOAW included various women on low income as well as community partners. As presented earlier in this chapter, a defining feature of PAR is that it is emancipatory; that is, the research is focused on addressing social injustices. Within Frisby et al.'s PAR, members of WOAW sought to address the social injustices of various practices and policies that restrict access to community-based recreation programs for women on low income. Table 11.1 outlines the five-phase research process reported by Frisby et al.

Table 11.1 An example of the five-phase PAR research process.

PHASES OF THE PAR APPROACH	EXAMPLE FROM FRISBY ET AL., (2005)
Setting the research questions	The PAR team hosted a workshop whereby members of WOAW were provided with the opportunity to: <ul><li>Identify some of the barriers and benefits of participation in recreation programs</li><li>Identify strategies that would support their inclusion in community-based recreation programs</li><li>Initiate ongoing conversations among researchers and WOAW members</li><li>Identify research questions (e.g., "What are the lay meanings of physical inactivity, stress, and social isolation for this diverse group of women on low income?"; p. 373).</li></ul>
Building trust	Building and maintaining trust among members of WOAW and the research team took place over a three-year period. Trust was established through many processes including open discussions regarding the research process, the creation of an environment that values women's diverse perspectives, and biannual meetings to discuss issues related to the research funds and budget.
Data collection	Interviews and group discussion (i.e., "researcher parties") were the primary sources of data generation.
Data analysis	Data were analyzed by research team members, and preliminary findings were presented to members of WOAW for feedback and evaluation.
Communicating results for action	Usually this is the final phase of the PAR process, yet in this study the communication of results unfolded throughout the entire research process. Action occurred on many levels including the individual level (e.g., personal action whereby women on low income reduced their social isolation by coming together to talk about injustices they face), and at an organizational level (e.g., community organizations made changes to policies in response to findings from the research).

Source: Frisby et al., 2005

Professional Highlight

Dr Wendy Frisby, Professor (retired), School of Kinesiology, Faculty of Education, University of British Columbia

....

Profile: Dr Frisby is well-known for her engagement in community-based sport and recreation research focused on the inclusion of marginalized groups. Her program of research has played a significant role in demonstrating the applicability of PAR within the field of kinesiology. She has written about her commitment to, and the inherent challenges of, engaging in PAR from within university settings (e.g., Frisby et al., 2005). Within her research she has also documented the integral role of feminist theories in informing action research (e.g., Frisby, Maguire, & Reid, 2009). Consistent with the emancipatory feature of PAR, Dr Frisby has worked to address social injustices by ensuring that her research findings were translated not only to academic audiences, but to the general public, government agencies, and non-profit organizations. As a result of her research excellence, Dr Frisby received numerous accolades including her recognition in 2011 as one of the Most Influential Women in Sport and Physical Activity by the Canadian Association for Women in Sport. Participatory action research is relatively rare when considered among the range of study designs employed in kinesiology, and Dr Frisby is a leader in this approach to research.

Further Readings

Frisby, W., Maguire, P., & Reid, C (2009). The "f" word has everything to do with it: How feminist theories inform action research. *Action Research, 7*, 13–29. doi:10.1177/1476750308099595

Frisby, W., Reid, C. J., Millar, S., & Hoeber, L. (2005). Putting "participatory" into participatory forms of action research. *Journal of Sport Management, 19*, 367–86.

The brief description of the five-phase PAR approach in Table 11.1 provides a kinesiology-specific example of the transformative nature of this approach to research. Researchers who engage in PAR may apply research designs that are more flexible (e.g., action research spiral) or that have slightly more structure (e.g., five-phase participatory action research design). Regardless of the chosen approach, researchers should embrace the notion that PAR is emergent and flexible and that it may need to be modified over time to fit the needs of the entire research team.

Data generation and data analysis

In the above section we provided brief descriptions of the five-phase participatory action research approaches outlined by Stringer and Genat (2004) and Frisby et al. (2005). However, you might still have questions about *how* to engage in data generation and data analysis within PAR. Throughout this book we have provided detailed descriptions of measures (Chapter 4) and data analysis (Chapter 5) that are typically used in quantitative research. We also provided an overview of various qualitative processes of data generation (Chapter 7) and data analysis (Chapter 8). With this knowledge of the various options for data generation and analysis, we encourage researchers and participants involved in PAR to work collaboratively to identify the most relevant measures or processes of data generation for addressing the research questions. There are no specific measures or processes that must be used in PAR. Instead, the intent is to identity processes of data generation that will extend understandings of the issues being explored. Of course, given that methodological coherence (remember this term from Chapter 9) is paramount to all research, your processes of data analysis should align with your chosen processes of data generation, which naturally stem from the collaboratively developed research questions.

Although PAR does not have required processes for data generation, there are measures or processes that are common within PAR. For instance, given that PAR is founded on the belief that people of all ages hold a deep understanding of their own lives and can be active participants in identifying and addressing community issues, *one-on-one interviews* and *group interviews* are often used within PAR. *Observation* is also used within PAR; this process of data generation supports researchers in seeing, hearing, and experiencing the social situation or injustice that is experienced by participants. Participants may also share *personal diaries* and *photographs*, or create various types of *visual artwork*, to shed light on their experiences with the social issues that are being explored within the research. Qualitative processes of data generation are typically more common within PAR that is conducted by kinesiology researchers, but it is possible to include quantitative measures. For instance, *surveys* or *questionnaires*

Case Study

Isabella recently graduated with a kinesiology degree and her provincial government has hired her as a Physical Activity Coordinator. Isabella is expected to work with a small (300 people) community to identify strategies for addressing the high rates of physical inactivity experienced by their community; it is important to keep in mind that these inactivity rates are similar to those of all Canadians. Recognizing that she can not address this issue alone, she makes meaningful connections with leaders within the community. To address the issue, Isabella's new team initiates a PAR study using the five-phase participatory action research approach as described by Frisby et al. (2005). The team's goal is to identify and take action to address the physical inactivity within the community. Keeping in mind the defining features of PAR, including the collaborative nature of this research approach, answer the following questions:

Discussion Questions

1. What strategies will Isabella's team employ in *setting the research questions*?
    a. Assuming she successfully engaged participants in setting the research questions, what is a possible research question?
2. How will Isabella's team work to *develop (and maintain) trust* among all team members?
3. What processes of *data generation* and *data analysis* could be used to address the research questions?
4. The last phase of Isabella's research involves *communicating results for action*.
    a. To which audiences should Isabella communicate her findings?
    b. How should Isabella communicate her findings?
    c. Describe some of the action strategies that could occur as a result of Isabella's PAR.

might be used as a relatively inexpensive process for acquiring information from large groups of people. Through surveys or questionnaires, information might be sought about experiences of social injustices, or such measures might be used to gain insight into proposed forms of action to address social injustices.

In terms of data analysis, we encourage you to refer back to the previous chapters in this book that describe relevant quantitative (Chapter 5) and qualitative (Chapter 8) data analysis approaches for the data that are generated through PAR. As well, Chapter 10 provides a concise overview of how to analyze data in mixed methods studies that include both quantitative and qualitative forms of data. There is flexibility within PAR with respect to how to engage in data generation and data analysis and, given the iterative and responsive nature of PAR, processes of data generation and data analysis may also change slightly (or even entirely) over the duration of the research project.

Role of Theory in PAR

Remember from Chapter 7 that we described the role of theory in qualitative research, and that theory can be used as a theoretical lens to guide a study or as an interpretive framework for helping to make sense of findings. Theory can be used in similar ways within PAR. Theories,

Writing Exercise

Go back to the *case study* that was just presented in this chapter. Imagine now that you are working specifically with an Indigenous community and your research team was guided by a theory, namely the Integrated Indigenous-Ecological Model (we briefly alluded to this model when describing a qualitative study in Chapter 7). This theory or model as described by Lavallée and Lévesque (2013) is a contextually relevant model that has been defined specifically for sport, recreation, and physical activity promotion in Indigenous communities. This model draws upon the strengths of Western and Indigenous perspectives by acknowledging that sport, recreation, and physical activity opportunities should be delivered at each of the six ecological leverage points (i.e., intrapersonal, interpersonal, organizational, community, policy, mother earth) in order to strengthen or enhance overall health (i.e., physical, mental, spiritual, emotional).

A concise overview of the Integrated Indigenous-Ecological Model is provided on page 26 of the *Everybody gets to play™ First Nations, Inuit & Métis Supplement* (Canadian Parks and Recreation Association, 2009). Access this document, review the model, and write down your answers to the following questions:

1. What action strategy, at *each of the six ecological leverage points* (e.g., intrapersonal, organizational), could be implemented to address physical inactivity?
2. How did the use of this theory inform, enhance, or change the action strategies that you initially identified in the original case study?
3. Using a library database with which you are familiar (e.g., PsycINFO), identify a different theory that is often used in kinesiology, which could be used to inform your team's action strategies. How could this theory guide your PAR or help you to make sense of the findings?

such as feminist theories or various other critical theories, naturally *guide* or inform PAR by calling into question the power imbalances that often serve as the foundation of social injustices. Theories may also play a critical role by helping to *make sense* of findings and to identify action strategies to include in a study. Discipline-specific theories, such as theories commonly used by those in kinesiology, combined with the knowledge that is shared by participants can also inform actions or practices within PAR.

Theory can play a central role in informing our PAR practices and, at the same time, theory can be generated through practice. As such, theory will likely play a role in PAR whether it is explicitly acknowledged or not.

Process for Engaging Underrepresented Populations in Research

The participatory or advocacy worldviews that typically guide PAR have supported the necessary inclusion of underrepresented populations in kinesiology research. Underrepresented populations have distinct and important experiential knowledge that can be respectfully explored through PAR approaches. Arguably, it is necessary to include participants from diverse and underrepresented populations if we are to deepen understandings of phenomena and experiences that are studied within kinesiology. As was presented in Chapter 6, we need to be critical of research that simply draws upon WEIRD (Western, educated, industrialized, rich, and democratic) samples as they do not adequately represent, nor do they optimize on, the experiences of diverse populations (Henrich, Heine, & Norenzayan, 2010). Researchers (e.g., Messner & Musto, 2014) have also described how issues of culture and race, for example, provide a "fascinating blank slate" for sport researchers. Issues around culture, ethnicity, and gender, to name a few, can be explored when underrepresented populations are included in research.

Research approaches such as PAR provide an opportunity to respectfully engage underrepresented populations in mutually beneficial, relevant, and respectful research. The defining features of PAR, such as its participatory, collaborative, and transformative nature, support the inclusion of populations that may otherwise be apprehensive or even opposed to participating in research approaches that are guided by postpositivist philosophical worldviews. For instance, the voices of Indigenous youth have generally been overlooked in kinesiology research, and our team has worked with Indigenous youth on various PAR projects focused on body image, sport, and physical activity (e.g., McHugh, Kingsley, & Coppola, 2013; McHugh & Kowalski, 2011). In the above section you also read about the PAR projects led by Frisby et al. (2005) that involved low-income women, and Frisby (2011) has also engaged in participatory research alongside Chinese immigrant women in Vancouver. A PAR approach was used by Giesbrecht and colleagues from the University of British Columbia to develop a wheelchair skills home program for older adults with restricted mobility (Giesbrecht et al., 2014). A team from Dalhousie University also used a PAR approach in their research that was focused on improving Black women's health in rural and remote communities in Nova Scotia (Etowa et al., 2007). These Canadian-specific and kinesiology-related

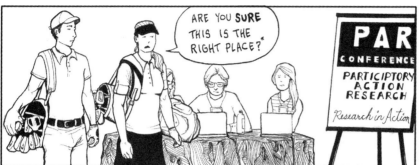
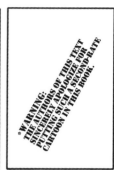

PAR projects are a few examples that represent the necessary emergence of PAR within kinesiology. Populations that have traditionally been overlooked in kinesiology research are emerging at the *forefront* of participatory approaches.

Inherent Challenges of PAR

We have provided numerous examples to describe how PAR can advance knowledge, as well as how PAR results in mutually beneficial outcomes or action for participants and researchers. Despite the many benefits, PAR is also accompanied by a number of inherent challenges. Within our own experiences of PAR, we certainly have encountered these challenges. Given that PAR is flexible and emergent, and there is no one "right way" to engage in PAR, we are unable to provide specifics as to how researchers should work to address such challenges. Instead, we have shared some examples of how we (and other kinesiology researchers) have navigated such challenges in the hopes that such knowledge may be transferable to other contexts. In the following sections we identify the challenges associated with (a) establishing and nurturing relationships, (b) ensuring ongoing participant collaboration, and (c) identifying various levels of action.

Establishing and nurturing relationships

The establishment and maintenance of trust and relationships are central to the success of PAR. Various researchers have written about the need for developing and nurturing relationships, yet much less has been written about the actual *process* by which relationships are developed and nurtured. It is relatively well understood that the establishment of meaningful relationships takes time, and Heather Castleden and her colleagues from Dalhousie University described the challenges experienced as a result of this time commitment. Castleden, Morgan, and Lamb (2012) interviewed Canadian university researchers who engage in participatory research approaches, and it was emphasized that spending time in the communities within which they want to engage in research is an essential component in establishing relationships. One participant in their study stated:

> My Dean asked me two years into my project why I hadn't published yet out of it and he had no idea what I was talking about when I told him I spent the first year drinking tea, you know? [laughter] Because it took several visits to the community, a lot of patience and sitting down and talking to people and deciding how would be the best way of going about doing this, getting them to a point where they trusted me to be a partner in doing [research] with them and to do it the right way, before we ever really even embarked on collecting any kind of data. (Castleden et al., 2012, p. 168)

The experiences shared by this Canadian researcher who engages in participatory research provides a small glimpse into the challenges experienced by those engaged in PAR. Researchers doing PAR have a strong understanding of the importance of developing relationships and they are committed to the process. However, researchers typically have numerous other university-related obligations, such as teaching and various service commitments, and therefore feel challenged with the time commitment that is often necessary to establish and maintain the relationships that are necessary for PAR. These challenges, combined with pressures from universities and research funding agencies to regularly publish research findings in a timely manner, contribute to the complexities associated with establishing and nurturing relationships for PAR.

It is well established that relationships are central to the success of PAR, and some Canadian universities are becoming more aware and supportive of researchers who experience challenges when engaging in PAR. In Chapter 3, the TCPS 2 was highlighted as a joint policy of the three federal funding agencies in Canada, that provide funding for Canadian researchers. In the ninth chapter of the TCPS 2, which is focused on research that involves Indigenous peoples in Canada, there is a clear statement about the importance of engaging in participatory approaches that are founded on respectful relationships. Article 9.12 of the TCPS 2 states:

> As part of the community engagement process, researchers and communities should consider applying a collaborative and participatory approach as appropriate to the nature of the research, and the level of ongoing engagement desired by the community.

In describing the application of this article, the TCPS 2 outlines respectful relationships as a key component in participatory research. Given that researchers must adhere to such ethics guidelines when engaging in research, it is necessary for universities to acknowledge and support researchers who work hard to engage in ethical research practices. Indeed, many would argue that universities still have a long way to go in terms of supporting those who engage in PAR, but we are confident that we are on the cusp of a positive shift within Canadian universities to support such participatory research approaches.

Ensuring ongoing participant collaboration

Researchers and community partners (i.e., participants) in PAR work together to engage in all phases of the research process, from identifying research questions to developing action initiatives and sharing research findings. Researchers who engage in PAR work to alleviate the power imbalances that have been common in more traditional or postpositivist approaches. Within traditional or postpositivist approaches, researchers will typically work alone or as part of a team of researchers to develop research questions, conduct the study, and analyze findings. Researchers who engage in PAR, however, typically try to foster a sense of shared ownership, whereby researchers and participants have shared control of the research processes and outcomes.

Although researchers might approach their work with honest and clear intentions of full collaboration, the contributions of researchers and participants may vary depending on the specific phase of the research. For instance, PAR researchers typically share the commonly held belief that a participant "is an expert in the matters of his or her everyday life" (Boog, 2003, p. 435), and these matters are typically the very social issues that are addressed in PAR. As such, when considering the *five-phase participatory action research approach,* participants will likely play a very active role in setting research questions, building trust, data collection, and communicating findings for action phases. There may also be strong efforts on behalf of the researchers and participants to have equal participation in the data analysis phase. However, our own previous research with Indigenous youth has highlighted a number of challenges, including lack of time and even interest on the part of the youth to be involved in data analysis. It is critical to acknowledge that the involvement of participants and researchers can take many forms throughout the research process as a result of differing expertise and interests. As well, the extent of participant involvement in certain phases may need to be negotiated. It is important for researchers to respect the level of involvement that is preferred by participants. For instance, participants may not be interested in being involved in the line-by-line analysis of interview transcripts but want to provide critical feedback on preliminary findings within the data analysis phase. Collaboration on the data analysis therefore may occur, but it may not be in the way imagined. The trust that has been established within PAR relationships is paramount, as it will serve as a foundation for navigating the extent and level of involvement by all team members (researchers and participants) throughout the various phases of the research process.

Identifying action

Earlier in this chapter you were asked to engage in an exercise whereby you were to retrieve a peer-reviewed journal that describes a PAR study that is relevant to kinesiology. Did that study clearly describe action initiatives that were derived from the study? Did you find yourself asking "Where is the action in this PAR study?" Researchers do not always clearly articulate the various levels of action that have occurred in their research, nor do they always clearly describe the impact that the action has had on the issue at hand. This lack of description could be the result of various factors including page restrictions in peer-reviewed journals (i.e., lack of space does not support a detailed description), the researchers not being aware of the various action initiatives or the related impacts, or the possibility that very little (or no) action resulted from the study. In other instances, the action might take place only *after* the study has already been published!

Our experiences with PAR suggest that researchers should be aware that action can occur on various levels, from individual-level action to broader societal- or policy-level action. In reading PAR studies, it is possible to get caught up in the belief that action must occur at a societal level to address the injustices or the issues experienced by participants. However, a team of researchers led by Colleen Reid from the British Columbia Centre of Excellence for Women's Health argued that action can take many forms and be implemented at various levels (Reid, Tom, & Frisby, 2006). They described how action can occur on individual or collective levels and that some actions may be implemented while other actions simply remain a hope for the future. Given that PAR is often carried out in collaboration with populations that have traditionally been overlooked in research, the engagement in the research process itself may constitute individual-level action. Action can also be more collective and make a broader impact on communities. For instance, in our PAR work with Indigenous youth we made active changes to the school community as a result of our research (see McHugh & Kowalski, 2011). Recognizing the impact that physical activity and food have on the body image experiences of youth, we made concrete changes to physical activity opportunities that were available in the school (e.g., created lunch-time physical activity programming including yoga and badminton) and to food that was available within the school (e.g., introduced a weekly salad bar at a minimal cost). Communication of research findings to broad audiences (e.g., academic and public audiences) through various outlets including media and peer-reviewed publications can also be a form of action in that awareness is created. Such awareness is likely paramount to the development of policies (i.e., societal-level action) that are necessary to begin addressing the issues and injustices that are foundational to PAR.

Writing Exercise

Given the inherent challenges of engaging in PAR, various researchers have documented their experiences of how they navigated such challenges. Using a kinesiology-related library database, access a study that has used a participatory approach (e.g., PAR, CBPR) and has documented at least one PAR-related challenge that was encountered. Write down your answers to the following questions:

1. What challenge(s) did the researchers experience?
2. How did the researchers address the challenge(s)? If the researchers did not provide such information, how do you think the researchers *should* have addressed the challenge(s)?
3. In what ways do the benefits or outcomes of the research outweigh the challenges experienced?

Summary

Within this chapter you have been presented with a general overview of the history of PAR as a research approach and the contemporary role of PAR within the field of kinesiology. Recognizing that PAR approaches can vary across disciplines, you were provided with an overview of the seven defining features of PAR. As well, we described two processes or designs for carrying out PAR, which included the *action research spiral* and a *five-phase participatory action research approach*. Drawing upon the knowledge gained from earlier chapters, we shared an overview of common approaches for engaging in processes of data collection and data analysis within PAR. We also described the role of theory in PAR. Given the defining features of PAR, we described how this approach to research is an ideal and often necessary approach for engaging underrepresented populations in kinesiology research. Finally, we ended this chapter by describing the inherent challenges of engaging in PAR and we shared our own PAR experiences of working to address these challenges.

Discussion Questions

1. In what ways is PAR transformative?
2. What are four of the seven defining features of PAR?
3. Consider the two PAR approaches described in detail in this chapter (i.e., action research spiral and five-phase participatory action research approach), and identify a social issue that you think could be explored in a kinesiology research study. Given your knowledge of each approach, what approach would you likely use to engage in PAR? Why did you choose this approach?
4. How can theory be used in PAR?
5. How is PAR an ideal approach for engaging underrepresented populations in kinesiology research?

Recommended Readings

Brydon-Miller, M., Kral, M., Maguire, P., Noffke, S., & Sabhlok, A. (2011). Jazz and the banyan tree: Roots and riffs on participatory action research. In N. K. Denzin & Y. S. Lincoln (Eds.), *The SAGE handbook of qualitative research* (4th ed., pp. 387–400). Thousand Oaks, Sage Publications.

Frisby, W., Reid, C. J., Millar, S., & Hoeber, L. (2005). Putting "participatory" into participatory forms of action research. *Journal of Sport Management, 19*, 367–86.

Kemmis, S., & McTaggart, R. (2008). Participatory action research: Communicative action and the public sphere. In N. K. Denzin & Y. S. Lincoln (Eds.), *Strategies of qualitative inquiry* (3rd ed., pp. 271–330). Thousand Oaks, CA: Sage Publications.

12 Knowledge Translation

Learning Outcomes

By the end of this chapter, you should be able to:

- Define knowledge translation.
- Illustrate the anatomy of a journal article.
- Identify a variety of traditional and innovative knowledge translation strategies.
- Discuss how researchers choose knowledge translation strategies for their research.

What Is Knowledge Translation?

Although not explicitly, you have already been introduced to knowledge translation throughout this book. For instance, Chapters 8, 9, and 10 included sections on how researchers might choose to present the findings of their studies. In Chapter 9 we identified research posters as a way that researchers might choose to present their study findings to an audience. Publishing research findings in journal articles was discussed in Chapters 8 and 10 as another way that researchers often share their research. To get a sense for the popularity of journal articles, just consider the countless examples of published journal articles we have included throughout this book! As discussed in Chapter 8, journal articles represent only *one* option for researchers to share their study findings. In fact, this book is actually a form of knowledge translation about the research process in kinesiology. Sharing research findings, insights, and experiences is what knowledge translation is all about.

Although there are differing ways to *label* the method of presenting or reporting of research-related information (e.g., knowledge mobilization, knowledge sharing, knowledge translation), the Canadian Institutes of Health Research (CIHR, 2015), one of the three federal funding agencies in Canada, defines **knowledge translation** as a process that includes the *synthesis*, *dissemination*, *exchange*, and *application* of knowledge. Knowledge translation, often referred to as "KT," is a dynamic process and one that needs to be ethically sound. The knowledge translation process takes place within a complex system of interactions between researchers and *knowledge users*.

A **knowledge user** is any individual who is likely to be able to use the knowledge gained through research to make informed decisions about policies, programs, and practices. A knowledge user can be, but is not limited to, practitioners, policymakers, educators, decision-makers, healthcare administrators, community members, or individuals in a health charity, patient group, private sector organization, or media outlet. The interactions between researchers and knowledge users can vary in intensity, complexity, and level of engagement depending on the nature of the research and the findings, as well as the needs of the particular knowledge user.

Writing Exercise

Read the following research summary, adapted from Robinovitch et al. (2013), and respond to the questions that follow.

Imagine that you conduct a quantitative study to examine the causes and circumstances of falls in elderly people. You partner with long-term care facilities, and digital cameras are installed in common areas at the facilities so you can collect and review video footage when falls occur. You review each fall video with a validated survey that includes questions about the fall initiation, in particular the cause of the fall and activity occurring at the time of the fall. You find that the primary cause of falls was shifting of bodyweight (e.g., an improperly placed step during walking) and trips or stumbles. The most common activity at the time of the fall was walking forward, followed by standing quietly. You conclude that your objective evidence shows new avenues for prevention of fall injury in long-term care facilities.

1. Identify at least three ways that you might present your research findings.
2. How might you report your research findings to individuals in the healthcare profession?
3. How might you share your research findings with elderly people and their care providers?
4. How might you report your research findings to peers in your research methods course?
5. Looking at your responses to questions 1 to 4, explain why you might present your research in different ways to different people.

Core elements of knowledge translation

According to CIHR, there are four fundamental elements of knowledge translation:

- Synthesis
- Dissemination
- Exchange
- Ethically sound application of knowledge

The **synthesis** of knowledge requires contextualizing and integrating findings from individual research studies within the larger body of knowledge on a topic. Examples of synthesizing knowledge include systematic reviews, narrative reviews, meta-analyses, and practical guidelines. Bérubé et al. (2016) conducted a narrative review on adult chronic pain risk factors and protective factors. Their review included studies that met the following criteria: (a) descriptive or retrospective studies, (b) cross-sectional or longitudinal studies, and (c) previous narrative or systematic reviews. Through their review, the researchers found that patients who scored high in psychological risk factors (such as anxiety, pain catastrophizing, and pain-related fear) were more likely to develop chronic pain and accompanying impairments. Pain self-efficacy and pain acceptance were both identified as protective factors that could improve daily functioning and quality of life for the individual. As a result of their narrative review, and subsequent synthesis of knowledge, the researchers concluded that cognitive-behavioural interventions applied at the acute phase of chronic pain could limit chronic pain.

Knowledge **dissemination** entails identifying a particular audience and tailoring the knowledge exchange to that audience, including both the message and the medium. Dissemination examples include providing summaries for knowledge users, delivering educational sessions with patients, and media engagement. Debora Matthews from Dalhousie University was recognized for her ability to communicate her Canadian oral health research to the public, dental professionals, and policymakers. Dr Matthews received the 2013 CIHR Institute of Musculoskeletal Health and Arthritis Research Ambassadors Knowledge Translation Award for disseminating her scientific research into improved health for Canadians, more effective health services and products, and a strengthened healthcare system. As the director of the Network for Canadian Oral Health Research, Dr Matthews translates clinical research knowledge into clear and useful formats for clinicians and their patients. In addition to a bilingual website designed to promote knowledge sharing among Canadian oral health researchers and the broader community, knowledge dissemination within the network includes a blog that provides critical summaries of evidence-based research related to oral health, a search engine for clinicians, team-building workshops on engaging Indigenous voices to address oral health disparities, and a national registry of oral health research-related resources.

Knowledge **exchange** includes engagement between researchers and knowledge users that results in mutual learning through planning, producing, disseminating, and applying existing or new research. Noreen Willows from the University of Alberta is a population health researcher who investigates cultural meanings of food and health. As part of her research that examines obesity in First Nations communities, Dr Willows works closely with community members to find solutions to health problems. Her team of researchers and community members work together to develop tailored and community-based interventions, as well as to build capacity to alleviate food insecurity. For example, a workshop between researchers and 15 community members resulted in action plans to improve community food security, such as developing hunting, fishing, and gardening programs to provide food for school meals. The workshop, which was premised on collaborative decision-making, is one example of how Dr Willows exchanges knowledge by engaging in reciprocal learning through her community-driven research.

The **application** of knowledge translation strategies, which refers specifically to putting knowledge into practice, should be consistent with ethical principles (recall from Chapter 3 the ethical principles of autonomy, nonmaleficence, beneficence, justice, fidelity, and veracity), social values, and legal regulatory frameworks. The Kahnawake Schools Diabetes Prevention Project (KSDPP) is a community-based participatory research project aimed at diabetes prevention in the Mohawk community of Kahnawake in Quebec. The KSDPP is a partnership between the community and researchers affiliated with McGill University, University of Montreal, and Queen's University. The partnership involves working cooperatively and collaboratively throughout the research process, including developing research questions; determining methodology; generating, analyzing, and interpreting data; and the dissemination of research experiences and results. An important part of the KSDPP was the evolution of a Code of Research Ethics that was written by the researchers in conjunction with the community in the first year of the project. The Code of Research Ethics includes the obligations and procedures that guide the partners to achieve the goals of the project, reflects the principles of participatory research, and ensures that the Kahnawake community is a full partner for the entire research process, including the application of knowledge gained through the project. The KSDPP Code of Research Ethics, including a section dedicated to how knowledge is put into practice, is available online.

It might appear that there is overlap between some of the elements of knowledge translation, making it difficult to separate them from one another. However, synthesizing, disseminating, exchanging, and applying knowledge are all integral parts of the knowledge translation process.

Knowledge translation process

There are generally two ways to plan the timing of knowledge translation activities: (a) activities that occur at the end of a research study or project, and (b) activities that are integrated or ongoing throughout the duration of a research study or project.

End-of-project knowledge translation consists of sharing knowledge that was gained during a project, and this knowledge is presented after a project has been completed. Typical end-of project knowledge translation approaches include disseminating and communicating

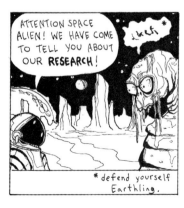
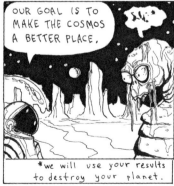
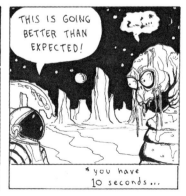

research to peers through published journal articles and conference presentations. However, these are not the only options for end-of-project knowledge translation. Researchers need to tailor the information or message they disseminate, as well as the medium through which they communicate that information, to be appropriate for a specific audience. For example, researchers who conducted a study on the benefits of dynamic stretching and wanted to share their findings with a group of athletic therapists would want to tailor their knowledge translation approach so it is appropriate for that audience. One option might be to offer interactive educational sessions on dynamic stretching for athletic therapists. The message that is shared (i.e., the benefits of dynamic stretching) is presented in a way that resonates with the audience (i.e., through practical workshops with athletic therapists).

Integrated knowledge translation involves the active engagement between researchers and knowledge users throughout the entire research process. Researchers and knowledge users work together to collaboratively shape the research process; therefore, the synthesis, dissemination, exchange, and application of knowledge is ongoing throughout the research project. The partnership between researchers and knowledge users in integrated knowledge translation can include collaboratively determining research questions

Professional Highlight

Dr Kerry McGannon, Associate Professor, Faculty of Health, Laurentian University

Profile: Dr McGannon's research focuses on the social and cultural influences of sport and physical activity participation. More specifically, Dr McGannon explores the construction of self-identity, interpretations of sport and physical activity, and psychological experiences of health behaviours. Her research stems from a Cultural Sport Psychology theoretical perspective, whereby athletes' cultural heritage is considered for meaningful understandings of marginalized and minority sport populations. The overall goal of her research, which consists of primarily qualitative research methodologies, is to produce knowledge to support and create space and opportunities for individuals as cultural beings in physical activity contexts to improve well-being. Some of Dr McGannon's knowledge translation strategies include publishing in journal articles, academic books, and chapters; presenting at national and international conference presentations; and using social media to share her research.

Further Readings

McGannon, K. R., Busanich, R., Witcher, C. S. G., & Schinke, R. J. (2014). A social ecological exploration of physical activity influences among rural men and women across life stages. *Qualitative Research in Sport, Exercise and Health, 6,* 517–36. doi:10.1080/2159676X.2013.819374

McGannon, K. R., & Smith, B. (2015). Centralizing culture in cultural sport psychology research: The potential of narrative inquiry and discursive psychology. *Psychology of Sport and Exercise, 17,* 79–87. doi:10.1016/j.psychsport.2014.07.010

and methodology, collecting data, developing instruments, analyzing data, interpreting findings, and disseminating knowledge. The integrated knowledge translation approach is sometimes referred to as collaborative research, action-oriented research, co-production of knowledge, or participatory action research, all of which were introduced in Chapter 11. The philosophy behind integrated knowledge translation is that effective knowledge translation rests on engagement with knowledge users even before the research begins, and many funding agencies request that integrated research teams are developed early in the research process. Salsberg et al. (2015) conducted a critical review of participatory research to identify key strategies for fostering a researcher–community partnership that can be essential for integrated knowledge translation. The five most frequently used strategies are (a) forming an advisory committee consisting of researchers and knowledge users, (b) developing a research agreement, (c) using group facilitation techniques, (d) hiring co-researchers or partners from the community, and (e) ensuring frequent communication. These practical strategies can foster successful participatory action research and, in turn, integrate knowledge translation throughout the research process.

Knowledge Translation Strategies

Now that you have been introduced to knowledge translation, it is time to consider tangible strategies that researchers use to synthesize, disseminate, exchange, and apply the knowledge gained from their research, either at the end of their projects or integrated throughout their research. The knowledge translation strategies presented in this chapter are organized into two broad domains: (a) traditional and (b) innovative. Traditional knowledge translation strategies include, but are not limited to, published journal articles and various forms of conference presentations. The traditional strategies have a strong reputation and long history in academics. Researchers continue to become more and more innovative with knowledge translation, which is at least partially a reflection of their engagement with knowledge users. As a result,

Table 12.1 Summary of knowledge translation approaches.

TRADITIONAL KNOWLEDGE TRANSLATION APPROACHES	INNOVATIVE KNOWLEDGE TRANSLATION APPROACHES
Publications Examples include journal articles, guidelines, manuals, reports	**Text-based** Examples include stories, narratives, fictional narratives, poetic representation
Conference presentations Examples include verbal presentations, poster presentations, symposia	**Media-based** Examples include social media, websites, online tools, TED talks, three-minute thesis competition
	Arts-based Examples include short film, interpretive dance, ethnodrama, visual art, musical performances
	Relationship-oriented Examples include community engagement, gatherings

the innovative domain includes dramatic, artistic, electronic, and relationship-based ways to exchange knowledge. The traditional and innovative domains are not necessarily mutually exclusive, and there are some specific knowledge translation strategies that cross over between the domains. We chose to categorize specific knowledge translation strategies into these two broad domains for sake of organization and to emphasize the innovation that continues to occur as researchers push the boundaries of synthesizing, disseminating, exchanging, and applying knowledge. An overview of the knowledge translation domains, corresponding categories, and specific examples of knowledge translation strategies appear in Table 12.1.

Traditional Knowledge Translation Approaches

Publications

Published journal articles are probably the most familiar form of knowledge translation. After completing a research study, researchers develop a manuscript (a written report of their research), and submit it to the editor of a journal in hopes of having it accepted for publication and shared with the academic community. Quite often the editor of a journal will send the manuscript to a few select experts in the research area to have it undergo peer-review. This process, known as the **peer-review process**, dates back to the 1700s when materials for publication in royal societies were subject to inspection by a select group of individuals who were knowledgeable in the area and whose recommendation was influential in the fate of the materials and documents (Spier, 2002). Today, peer-reviewed research articles are ones that have undergone critical review from experts in the respective field, and as a result may have been returned to the authors for modification and revision prior to the manuscript being published. The revise and resubmit aspect of the peer-review process ensures (or strives to ensure) high-calibre research appears in journals. The peer-review process plays a significant role in determining which manuscripts are accepted for publication, and therefore which research studies get disseminated to the academic community through this form of knowledge translation. Since the early 2000s, more and more journals have provided open-access publication options for researchers to consider in order for the general population to have greater access to research articles. For instance, some journals are fully open access, meaning that all of the articles included in the journal are freely available to the wider public. Other journals are more of a hybrid and include articles that are open access and others that are not, with researchers having the option to choose whether their article will be open access. Open-access journal articles often require researchers to cover publication costs to provide access to online articles free to the general public. Journals that do not have open access options often require subscriptions, site licences, or pay-per-view for the general public to access articles. Although there is typically a fee to publish an open-access journal article, a big advantage of open-access publications is often the potential to reach a larger audience.

Anatomy of a journal article

Published journal articles tend to follow a fairly standard format. If you performed a literature search in an area of interest you would likely find that most of the articles are structured in a similar way to include specific information for the academic community. Research publications include a comprehensive title on the first page of the article, as well as an abbreviated title that appears on subsequent pages. A typical research article is often organized around the following headings: *Abstract, Introduction, Method, Results,* and *Discussion,* and these elements are depicted in Table 12.2. Within these headings some research articles might include subheadings for further organization, such as a literature review subsection in the Introduction, a measures subsection in the Method, a subsection on specific hypothesis testing in the Results, or a subsection on study strengths and limitations in the Discussion.

The **Abstract** is essentially a scientific summary of the research study. The Abstract should be brief yet comprehensive and allow readers to survey the contents of an article quickly. One approach to writing an abstract is to consider how to concisely summarize the content of the study for the benefit of someone who knows nothing about what was done in the study. Every journal will have specific guidelines on what should be included in the Abstract, but typically it will briefly outline the research question/problem, present why the problem is worth studying,

Table 12.2 The anatomy of a standard research publication.

COMMON STRUCTURE OF A RESEARCH PUBLICATION	
Title	• Comprehensive title • Short running title
Abstract	Summary of background, purpose, methods, results, conclusion
Key terms	3–5 important words or descriptors
Introduction	Review of literature • What is known • Deficiencies in existing research Purpose or study aims
Method	• Participant information and sampling procedures • Measures (quantitative study) or strategy of inquiry (qualitative study) • Study procedure • Data analysis
Results	Preliminary or descriptive results • Main results • Tables, charts, diagrams, maps, and figures
Discussion	Summary of findings • Compare and contrast findings with other work • Strengths and limitations of the study • Potential directions for future research The importance of the study
References	Using appropriate citation style

and describe study participants, data collection methods, analysis approach, main findings, and study implications or conclusions. Most journals request that researchers list a handful of **key terms** (e.g., three to five) at the end of the Abstract that reflect the focus of the study and are used for indexing articles in search engines. Researchers should therefore carefully select key terms that not only best represent their research, but also words their audience might use in electronic searches to access their research. Journals will also specify a word limit for the length of an abstract. For instance, the *Journal of Applied Physiology* outlines that abstracts for their journal should be one paragraph consisting of no more than 250 words. Although brief, the importance of the Abstract should not be underestimated. Most people have their first, or even only, contact with an article by reviewing the Abstract. First impressions are sometimes everything!

The **Introduction** should answer the question "What is this paper about?" More specifically, the Introduction should ease the reader into the study topic and lead them logically toward the research question and purpose statement (recall research questions and purpose statements from Chapter 2). A literature review is included in the Introduction, overviewing previous studies that are relevant to the research topic. The literature review provides context for the reader by outlining and critiquing what is already known about the topic, as well as identifying gaps in previous research that the study will address. In other words, readers should get a firm sense of what has already been done in the research area and what the current study will offer after reading the literature review. The Introduction should conclude with a formal statement of the purpose of the research.

Details about how the study was conducted are presented in the **Method**. A complete description of the methods allows the reader to evaluate the appropriateness of the methods used, and permits researchers to replicate the study. Several subsections might appear in the Method, such as participant information (i.e., identifying characteristics of study participants), sampling procedures (i.e., explaining how participants were recruited or selected), measures (i.e., information about the measurement instruments or tools used to collect data, including evidence of validity and reliability), procedure (i.e., describing what the participants were required to do), and data analysis (i.e., overviewing how the data were analyzed). We have tried to introduce you to most, if not all, of the different aspects often found in the Method. For instance, Chapter 4 included a discussion of sampling methods and various instruments, tools, and measures used for data collection in quantitative research. Similarly, Chapter 7 included an overview of sampling methods and processes of data generation in qualitative research. Entire chapters were dedicated to data analysis in quantitative and qualitative research in Chapters 5 and 8, respectively. Another important element to include in the Method is that ethical approval was obtained to conduct the study. It is common to see a phrase in published journal articles stating (or similar to) "ethical approval was obtained from the Research Ethics Board prior to participant recruitment" (recall our discussion of Research Ethics Boards in Chapter 3). Though this statement is brief, it is essential to include as evidence that the research adhered to ethical guidelines.

For a lot of readers the **Results** is the most interesting section because it tells the reader what was found in the study in relation to the study purpose. It is important to report all results, including those that run counter to expectation. Hiding uncomfortable or unexpected findings by omission is not acceptable (or ethically responsible). The American Psychological Association (2010), which prepared the stylistic and formatting manual used by many social science researchers in kinesiology, specifies that "accurate, unbiased, complete and insightful reporting of the analytic treatment of data (be it quantitative or qualitative) must be a component of all research reports" (pp. 32–3). The ways to present research findings are varied, and can differ substantially between and within quantitative and qualitative research studies.

Almost all Results sections will include written text. Additional ways to present study findings include tables, charts, diagrams, maps, and figures. For example, in their investigation of knee joint kinematics, kinetics, and muscle activity patterns during a stepping-down task, Sanchez-Ramirez and colleagues (2016) presented their results with written text, tables, and figures. The written text includes a description of the results from hypothesis testing and presentation of corresponding *p*-values to indicate statistically significant findings (recall our discussion of *p*-values in Chapter 5). The tables consist of results reported in numerical form, including the means and standard deviations of muscle activity for the experimental and control groups in their study. The figures depict graphical illustrations of different muscle contractions during the stepping-down task. In a different study of pediatric nurses' perceptions of work-related stressors in medical and surgical units, De Almeida Vicente et al. (2016) from the Montreal Children's Hospital and McGill University presented their findings as written text and in table form. The written text is lengthier than in our previous example and is organized around three emergent themes. Within each theme the researchers present quotations from participants to support and address the study themes. The table reports information about the study participants, including age, gender, and education and work experience as a nurse.

The key point we are trying to make in presenting the above examples is that both sets of researchers utilize multiple ways of presenting their study findings in the Results. Sometimes the same approach is used in both studies (i.e., written text and tables), but there are also unique elements to each study (i.e., amount of written text, what is reported in the tables). How the Results are presented will vary according to the research approach and specific research design, the research question or purpose, and for whom the research is being published. The bottom line is that it is crucial that relevant and sufficient information be presented in the Results to support any claims that are made and to justify study conclusions.

After presenting the Results, it is time to evaluate and interpret the findings in reference to the original research question. The **Discussion** will incorporate any conclusions that might be drawn from the research findings. In doing so, it is important to return to the original research questions and study purpose to consider how the study findings are situated within the larger body of literature. Identifying similarities and differences between the results and the work of others is one way to contextualize, confirm, or clarify conclusions. The Discussion should also include consideration for the strengths and limitations of the study. Addressing potential directions for future research is another element that is often included in the Discussion. Ending the Discussion with commentary on the importance of the study or the primary contribution made to the literature is one approach to justify why readers should attend to the findings.

A study out of the University of Winnipeg by Gregg, O, and Hall (2016) provides an example of a published journal article that follows the structure outlined above. Gregg, O, and Hall examined the relationship between athletes' goals and their use of imagery, and their research was published in the *Psychology of Sport and Exercise* journal. The article starts with the title of the study and information about the researchers (including institutional affiliations), and presents an abstract to provide a brief summary of the entire research project (including study objective, method, results, and conclusion). The Introduction includes an overview of the pertinent literature to their research area, including a focus on elite athletes, consideration of different types of goals, and athletes' use of imagery as a psychological skill in sport. The Introduction also outlines previous research that has examined goals and imagery, and identifies gaps or omissions that have yet to be considered. Close to the end of the Introduction the researchers identify the aim (objective or purpose) of their study, which was to investigate the relationship between goal orientations and imagery ability. Their Method follows a common approach often seen in a published journal article and includes subsections for participants (indicating that 112 female and 160 male athletes representing four sports participated in the study), measures (including a subheading for each measure of imagery and goal orientation, with corresponding validity and reliability information), procedure (including a note that ethical approval and informed consent were obtained), and data analysis (containing a clear description of the statistical analyses that were used). Organizing the Method with these subheadings allows the reader to easily locate certain sections of the study to identify the corresponding information. The Results presents the findings of their data analysis, and the researchers included additional subheadings to further organize and highlight their results. For instance, the subheading "Differences in Cognitive Imagery Ability" outlines that female athletes reported having significantly more clear and vivid internal imagery perspective than male athletes. An interpretation of study findings, including those that were and were not expected, appears in the Discussion section. The researchers once again chose to organize this section with subheadings to direct the reader's attention accordingly to topics on "Motivational Imagery Ability" and "Cognitive Imagery Ability." After the Discussion, the reference section appears and includes all of the resources the researchers cited within the body of their article.

The journal article presenting the study by Gregg, O, and Hall (2016) follows a fairly typical format and is organized into certain sections and subsections that are labelled with headings and subheadings. It is important to note that although journal articles tend to follow the structure outlined in this chapter, not *all* articles have this particular organization or use these specific headings. For instance, a qualitative article might include an additional "strategy of inquiry" subheading in the Method section but not a "measures" subheading. A mixed methods article might include double the number of headings that are typically found in an article in order to organize both the quantitative and qualitative components. Although you may come across variations among journal articles, the anatomy of research articles tends to include many of the pieces presented in this chapter.

Other forms of publications

Researchers can publish their research in ways other than the typical peer-reviewed journal article. Mark Tremblay (University of Ottawa) is the director of the Healthy Active Living and Obesity research group (HALO) at the Children's Hospital of Eastern Ontario

Research Institute and is a renowned researcher for his work on childhood obesity, physical activity and health measurement, and knowledge translation. In addition to publishing over 275 peer-reviewed journal articles and book chapters, Dr Tremblay has published his research in many different forms. For instance, he is the Chief Scientific Officer of the ParticipACTION Report Card, which is an annual comprehensive assessment of child and youth physical activity in Canada (ParticipACTION, 2016). In addition to grading daily physical activity behaviours (e.g., organized sport, active transportation), the Report Card includes movement guidelines, sedentary behaviour guidelines, and sleep guidelines, and discusses a number of settings and sources of influence on health behaviours (e.g., school, family, and peers). The Report Card is published online as both a highlight summary report and a full report that includes background information on the methodology, analysis, findings, and references.

As another example, Health Canada published "Eating Well with Canada's Food Guide— First Nations, Inuit and Métis," which is a tailored food guide that was created to reflect the values, traditions, and food choices of Indigenous peoples in Canada (http://www.hc-sc.gc.ca/fn-an/food-guide-aliment/fnim-pnim/index-eng.php). The guide includes both traditional foods (e.g., moose stew, blueberries) and store-bought foods (e.g., pasta, peanut butter), and explains how traditional foods can be used in combination with store-bought foods for healthy eating. Unique images and content are included in the guide, such as pictures of foods that are generally available in rural and remote locations. The guide has healthy eating recommendations that can be used by individuals, families, and communities, and includes dietary information that is based on science.

Conference proceedings

Another traditional knowledge translation approach centres on conferences at which researchers present and discuss their research in person to an audience. Depending on the conference, the audience might consist of fellow researchers, community members, knowledge users, or even the general public. One benefit of conference presentations for knowledge translation is that they usually include some level of interaction between the presenter(s) and the audience. Like publications, conferences also provide an important channel for exchanging information between researchers.

The number of municipal, provincial, national, and international conferences at which Canadian researchers doing kinesiology-related research present their work is a list that is too long (and continuously growing) to generate here. Researchers normally have three formats for conference presentations: (a) verbal, (b) poster, and (c) symposium. For an oral or **verbal presentation**, a researcher speaks in front of an audience at a conference to deliver an overview of her or his research in a limited amount of time (often 10 to 20 minutes, depending on the conference). Given the short amount of time, researchers often limit their presentation to the essential features of a study, omitting many of the details that might appear in a published journal article. Visual aids are typically included in the form of slides through computer presentation software. Audience interaction tends to occur at the end of the verbal presentation, with a small amount of time allotted for questions and answers between members of the audience and the presenting researcher(s). As an example, researchers from the University of Ottawa gave a verbal presentation on their attention demand research in the motor control and learning domain at the *North American Society for the Psychology of Sport and Physical Activity* conference in Portland, Oregon (Saunders et al., 2015). Following a traditional journal article structure, the presentation began by verbally overviewing important background information on attention demand and vision. The study objectives were introduced, which were to determine if an anterior load, the occlusion of vision, or both increase attention demand when navigating an obstacle. Next, details were provided on the 16 study participants as well as what the participants did for the study (i.e., procedure), which was perform an obstacle task while carrying no load, a clear five-kilogram load, and an opaque load. Key results were then presented, highlighting that carrying an anterior load during an obstacle task does not negatively impact attention demand. The presenting researcher (usually the first author listed on the conference abstract) had a total of 15 minutes to deliver the presentation, which included 3 minutes for questions from the audience at the end of the presentation.

A **poster presentation** consists of researchers creating posters that depict summaries of their research. Poster presentations often take place in a large room with posters placed on the walls or on poster stands. Poster presentations are scheduled for specific periods during a conference, and researchers stand by their poster while interested (or pretending to be interested) individuals walk around, read the material, and discuss items of their choosing with the researchers. Conference organizers instruct researchers on the format of poster presentations, including size and orientation. The *Canadian Society for Exercise Physiology,* for example, instructs researchers to create posters that are landscape orientation and are no bigger than 6 feet wide and 4 feet high. One advantage of poster presentations is that the audience can have detailed discussions with the researchers, as opposed to being restricted to the short time limit for questions in a typical verbal presentation. Longer and more in-depth conversations can take place during poster presentations, benefitting both the researcher and the audience. A team of researchers affiliated with the Sport Injury Prevention Research Centre in Calgary, Alberta, presented a poster on injury rates and risk factors in youth rock climbers at the *International Olympic Committee World Conference on Prevention of Injury and Illness in Sport* in Monaco (Woollings et al., 2014). Their poster included brief, bullet-point background information; presented a clear research objective; outlined their research methods (including the study design); presented results in table, text, and figure formats; and highlighted key study findings situated within the larger body of literature. The poster also included all of the researchers' information, including institutional or organizational affiliations, as well as logos from each institution, organization, and funding agency. As evident in this example, many poster presentations follow a traditional journal structure—only in an abbreviated and eye-catching manner. Some researchers are creative with their poster presentations and integrate the use of technology, such as adding small shelves for electronic tablets to display photographs or animated results, to add extra dynamism to a traditionally static medium. For example, a graduate student researcher from the University of Saskatchewan included an electronic tablet as part of her poster presentation at the *Canadian Society for Psychomotor Learning and Sport Psychology* conference when sharing her research on women athletes' body and eating attitudes (Killham, Kowalski, & Duckham, 2015). The tablet was included as an interactive medium to continuously stream quotes from the qualitative component of her mixed methods study that highlighted athletes' experiences of body image and self-attitudes.

Researchers can also present their study findings as a **symposium** at a conference. A symposium is a formal gathering of experts in a specific area of research who each present their research on a particular topic. The defining characteristic of a symposium is that it covers a single topic, with multiple verbal presentations all focused on that topic. At the 2015 *Canadian Society for Psychomotor Learning and Sport Psychology* conference, a group of Canadian and international motor control researchers led by Matthew Heath (University of Western Ontario) delivered a symposium on Fitts' (1954) law. Presentations included introducing Fitts' law (i.e., a logarithmic formula for predicting the time required to move to a target), exploring ramifications of the law, discussing explanations for the law, and overviewing studies that tested the law. The group of researchers indicated that the aim of their symposium was to generate debate regarding Fitts' work as a law-based phenomenon in the movement sciences. Unlike the typical verbal presentation format at a conference, a symposium often includes lengthier discussion and engagement with the audience at the end of the session after all researchers have delivered their presentations.

Many, though not all, conferences publish the abstracts of the studies that are presented at a conference, which is why we were able to provide corresponding citation information for each conference presentation in this chapter.

Case Study: Team KINect's Story

The KINect research team received a large research grant to develop, validate, and implement the use of a new tool for measuring physical activity levels. After a few years of research, the researchers developed a 15-minute tool, collected evidence of validity and reliability, published several validation studies in peer-reviewed journals, and presented their research at academic conferences across the country. KINect researchers envisioned that family physicians would administer this 15-minute tool to their patients during annual checkups, at which point personal recommendations could be made to patients who do not meet the recommended amount of physical activity outlined in the Canadian Physical Activity Guidelines. Now at the end of their grant funding, Team KINect is wondering why their tool is not being widely used, and they are at a loss as to why they cannot move their findings into practice.

Discussion Questions

1. How might Team KINect's research approach have allowed them to anticipate barriers to their tool being used?
2. Could they have identified and approached potential knowledge users before they began their research? If so, who?
3. What recommendations might you offer Team KINect for end-of-project knowledge translation?
4. What recommendations might you offer Team KINect for integrated knowledge translation?

Innovative Knowledge Translation Approaches

Developing knowledge translation approaches that actively engage researchers, community members, health professionals, practitioners, policymakers, and the general public are imperative to raising awareness of research findings and facilitate the use of those findings. Innovative knowledge translation through arts-based, text-based, media-based, and relationship-oriented approaches expand the possibilities of synthesizing, disseminating, exchanging, and applying knowledge.

Arts-based

Arts-based research was briefly introduced in Chapter 7 as a form of visual data that can be generated in qualitative research. Integrating art into research is becoming more common, and Canada's federal funding agencies have recognized the impact of arts-based research and the use of art as a knowledge translation approach. Kate Tilleczek at the University of Prince Edward Island was funded by CIHR to increase understanding of the theory and practice of arts-based knowledge translation by exploring the contribution of arts-based research specifically within health research. Premised on the belief that arts-based research methods highlight human aspects of medicine and healthcare in ways that lower barriers and improve understanding of health, Dr Tilleczek explored both arts-based knowledge creation and knowledge dissemination.

The move towards a performance medium for knowledge translation requires researchers to extend themselves beyond their traditional training and typical experiences. Arts-based knowledge translation can take many forms, and performing data can be a powerful way of presenting research (Sparkes & Smith, 2014). Some examples of arts-based knowledge translation include short film, interpretive dance, ethnodrama and theatrical performances, visual art, and musical performances.

Software programs, cutting-edge technology, and instantaneous access to an ever-available audience through social media make short filmmaking a popular option for innovative knowledge translation. Nick Holt (who was also the focus of our Research Highlight in Chapter 1) examined why people participate in ultramarathons and created a **short film** of the Canadian Death Race, which is a 125-kilometre marathon course that begins and ends with a 1280-metre plateau, includes three mountain summits, and has 2100 metres of elevation change. The short film provides the audience with an engaging and emotionally charged look at the highs and lows of the gruelling event. Race participants provide dialogue and video documentation of their own journeys before, during, and after the race. The short film, entitled *Canadian Death Race 2012—Research Study*, is available online.

Interpretive dance is an arts-based knowledge translation approach that has the potential to educate audiences by taking an unconventional and provocative approach to disseminating research. As a knowledge translation approach, interpretive dance consists of developing a dance performance to communicate research. Dance can be an effective way to share research findings, enhance awareness and understanding of a research topic, and highlight the importance of the aesthetical and visceral impact of the performance. International "Dance Your Ph.D." contests have existed for over half a decade. One kinesiology-related interpretive dance consisted of a mixture of ballet, modern, and Chinese classical dance to present research on brain blood vessel dynamics during exercise. The dance, appropriately titled "Brain Blood Vessel Dynamics during Exercise," is also available online. Another example of the use of dance as a creative and affective form of knowledge translation comes from Danielle Peers at the University of Alberta who studies disability in relation to sport, art, and social justice and uses performance art as knowledge translation at festivals, workshops, and conferences.

Ethnodrama is the act of dramatizing data through script writing that then becomes the basis for a film or theatrical performance. Specifically, ethnodrama combines ethnography (recall from Chapter 7) and drama into a written play script consisting of dramatized selections of data (Sparkes & Smith, 2014). Production companies collaborate with researchers to create original and interpretive scripts that engage audiences both cognitively and emotionally through a theatrical performance. Ethnodramas attempt to remain true to the participants whose stories contributed to the research, since the script is based on the data they shared. A group of researchers at Western University created an ethnodrama based on their ethnographic study that followed people living with dementia over an 18-month period to examine relationships in home-based dementia care (Speechley et al., 2015). Data generation for this study consisted of interviews and observations (field notes), and data analysis resulted in four emergent themes that represented integral care processes that shape and influence home-based dementia care. The researchers wanted to present their research as an ethnodrama to make the results of their research more engaging and interesting, and thus spark critical dialogue that could revise and improve home-based dementia care decisions. The researchers collaborated with a playwright who used the data and themes to create the structure and story line of a play called *Advocating for Hilda*. A theatre director was hired to cast and direct the play, and both video and theatre versions of the play were created. The video version of the play can be viewed online.

Another arts-based knowledge translation strategy that relies on engagement of the senses is the various forms of **visual art**. Paintings, images, and photographs, for example, can be powerful tools for sharing knowledge as they convey information that is difficult to describe in words. Moola et al. (2015) investigated how children in Hamilton experience their environment, specifically their access to walking routes and physical spaces. The researchers collected and worked with children's visual productions, including drawings, photographs, PowerPoint presentations, videos, and maps, which together were complex expressions of their spatial experiences and perceptions of environmental change. The use of visual images allowed the children to convey their literal and symbolic experiences, and the researchers were subsequently able to identify a number of environmental barriers (e.g., pollution, graffiti) and community strengths (e.g., community gardens, cultural diversity).

Music is another way that research findings can be communicated to an audience. **Musical performances** engage audiences on a bodily level in ways that are fundamentally different than visual art (Sparkes & Smith, 2014). Musical composition is a meaning-making process in which new knowledge and understandings can emerge, and can be an empowering experience. A benefit of musical performances as an arts-based knowledge translation approach is that music can be particularly effective for audiences with literacy challenges. Colleen Dell (2011) from the University of Saskatchewan translated the findings from her research on drug addiction into a song and music video, "From Stilettos to Moccasins." The research project examined the role of identity and stigma in Indigenous women's healing from drug abuse in Canada. Indigenous women healing from drug abuse and individuals helping them on their journeys wrote the song. The singer is a Cree singer/songwriter, and a professional production company directed the video. The music video can be seen online.

Something you might be noticing as we provide examples of innovative knowledge translation approaches is that sometimes the line between data generation and data presentation (i.e., knowledge translation) is blurred. For instance, video footage and documents such as photographs were introduced in Chapter 7 as examples of qualitative data, and now we have discussed short films and visual art as ways to synthesize, disseminate, exchange, and apply knowledge. Although at first this may seem confusing, remember that integrated knowledge translation consists of ongoing interaction between knowledge users and researchers throughout the duration of a research project. Given this constant engagement between researchers and their audience, there can certainly be overlap when collecting data and sharing research knowledge. It may not always be possible to separate data generation from knowledge translation.

Research Highlight

A team of researchers led by Carla Rice at the University of Guelph established the Re-Visioning Differences Media Arts Laboratory (REDLAB), a mobile media laboratory and expressive arts institute dedicated to exploring ways that arts-informed research can create opportunities for marginalized individuals and communities. Through her research, Dr Rice challenges stereotypes and aims to understand how technology and art can transform the views that the public and policymakers have about people who embody differences such as physical impairments and altered appearances. Through Project Re-Vision, Rice et al. (2015) investigated the power of image and story by exploring representations and meanings of disability through digital stories, which are short videos of visual images (e.g., photographs, artwork) paired with audio recordings of personal narratives. The researchers asked people with physical impairments and healthcare providers to each make a digital story that illustrates meanings of disability, and the published research article includes access information for readers to view the digital stories online. The videos explore themes of vulnerability, centralizing bodies that have previously been marginalized, resistance to dominant ways of thinking about disability, as well as reflection upon the social and biological processes that produce our bodies. This line of inquiry has the potential to shift stereotypical images and attitudes, and ultimately improve teaching, learning, and care practices within Canada. Overall, Dr Rice and her colleagues conduct research that includes innovative mediums such as photography, digital storytelling, autobiographical films, and research-based drama to create alternative and empowering representations of differences. The REDLAB and Project Re-Vision are effective examples of knowledge translation strategies intended to engage diverse audiences.

Further Reading

Rice, C., Chandler, E., Harrison, E., Liddiard, K., & Ferrari, M. (2015). Project Re-Vision: Disability at the edges of representation. *Disability & Society, 30,* 513–27. doi:10.1080/09687599.2015.1037950

Text-based

Storytelling is probably one of the oldest forms of knowledge sharing known to humanity. Indigenous knowledge, for instance, rests on oral tradition derived from practical experience and storytelling, which helps to develop wisdom that can be passed on to younger generations (Baskin, 2005). **Stories** are a medium through which meanings can be communicated in order to make sense of life experiences and convey knowledge. Furthermore, stories are a mode of communication that is familiar to policymakers, as well as the general public, so information can be more easily communicated. Stamatakis, McBride, and Brownson (2010) explored the use of stories to translate the health benefits of physical activity to policymakers, as data alone may be unlikely to make a compelling argument. The researchers expressed that a well-executed, evidence-based story can improve translation of research into policy by enhancing understanding of the problem of physical inactivity, improving the content of the messages included, and framing evidence in a way that emphasizes the most salient points for policymakers.

Although it was presented as a qualitative strategy of inquiry in Chapter 7, **narratives** allow researchers to share their research through storytelling. As a form of knowledge translation, narratives communicate realities of individuals through the power of language. Narratives have a plot that sequentially connects events over time to provide an explanation (Sparkes & Smith, 2014). The development of narratives often requires collaboration between researchers and participants, with the resulting narratives being a co-constructed retelling of experiences and interpretations (Clandinin & Connelly, 2000). A well-written narrative can draw readers into the research problem and connect them to the complexities of the research. Researchers from Vancouver, British Columbia explored young adults' experiences of smoking, quitting, and healthy lifestyles, and presented their findings in narrative form (Haines-Saah et al., 2013). Qualitative data generation included photographs, one-on-one interviews, and focus groups with 12 participants. The researchers developed two narratives based on the participants' data and incorporated their photographs in a unique photo-narrative approach to present study findings. One narrative considered the influence of Vancouver's health culture on smoking cessation, and another narrative presented discourse on the struggle between outdoor spaces as enabling or preventing smoking behaviour.

Fiction can be a valuable tool for exchanging information, especially when researchers seek to advocate for diverse groups. Through fiction, research findings may have a greater likelihood of reaching the general public, who may not normally access or read traditional research findings (Block & Weatherford, 2013). **Fictional narratives** can engage a reader in the emotional aspects of a research experience by imagining being a part of another world. An example of a fictional narrative was presented in Chapter 8 in which a graduate student researcher created a fictional story, using a detailed description of the woman's house as an initial metaphor, to represent women's experiences of a mindfulness-based yoga program. The story was created from the patterns and themes that emerged in her data collection, which included journal entries and field notes.

Poetry can also be a way to retell lived experiences and translate knowledge from research. **Poetic representation** takes place when researchers transform their data into a poem-like presentation (Glesne, 1997). Essentially, research data are compressed into a consistent pattern of verse in poem form. Poetic representation often includes the exact words from research participants by arranging them to create a meaningful representation of the data. Creating the poem requires significant word reduction while also illuminating wholeness and interconnection among ideas. Research findings are filtered through the researcher, who takes the position as a poet, and the medium (i.e., the poem) is part of the message. The following is a poetic representation provided by West and Bloomquist (2015), who investigated the concept of trust by university educators:

Trusting Others

I don't think it happens automatically with a snap of the fingers.
I think you have to work to create an atmosphere
where students learn to trust their peers
and faculty learn to trust each other.

You can't just wiggle your nose and it's done.

You have to earn it
and work for it,
especially in a first year class room.

With my first-years
    I did think-pair-shares and lots of group assignments.
These groupings were intended to foster critical thinking,
    make my students think outside their comfort zones,
    consider alternative point of views,
    and play devil's advocate.

But there isn't always trust between students.
Sometimes they have more trust in the system
or in their prof or textbook or whatever the content may be.

Students need to know they can trust themselves and the teacher and each other.

Reprinted with permission from the authors.

West and Bloomquist (2015) interviewed six university-level teachers about trust within the university and developed poems by coding the data, condensing words, shaping poems, and cross-checking the data. As is evident in the example provided, writing up research as poems allows participant's natural pauses, repetitions, and rhythms to be honoured, making a more accurate representation of the data.

Media-based

Social media was already mentioned in this chapter when highlighting short films as an option for innovative arts-based knowledge translation. Social media is increasingly popular for researchers to disseminate their research findings because the findings can be made immediately available to the general public. Social media also offers powerful approaches for researchers to reach large numbers of individuals to connect, support, and learn from each other. From developing Facebook pages to highlight research findings, sharing images of up-to-date research occurrences over Instagram, and tweeting out brief research updates on Twitter accounts, social media is an immediate, free, and readily available way to share research with the general public. A multidisciplinary research group at the University of British Columbia, including medicine and nursing researchers, examined the various dynamics at play in the use of social media when promoting health and wellness research (Ho & Peter Wall Workshop Participants, 2014). They concluded that social media has the power to engage the general public, health professionals, researchers, and innovators to work together to promote health and wellness. However, key questions need to be considered, including how to improve different segments of the general public's access to information and knowledge contained in social media (e.g., individuals living in remote locations with limited Internet access), how to incentivize health professionals to embrace social media and work with the public to maximize on the power of this medium to support health and wellness, and how to build credibility of research-based information that is exchanged over social media.

In addition to social media there are other media-based options that researchers can use to synthesize, disseminate, exchange, and apply knowledge from their research. Many kinesiology researchers develop **websites** about their research labs, which often include updated information about previous and current research projects. For example, Catherine Sabiston has a website for her Health Behaviour and Emotion Lab out of the Faculty of Kinesiology and Physical Education at the University of Toronto. The website is an up-to-date information hub that overviews members of her research team; provides details of current research (including status updates on progress); lists publications, abstracts, conference presentations, and community outreach activities; and links to relevant websites related to her research area (e.g., Canadian Breast Cancer Foundation).

Another example of the use of the Internet for knowledge translation is through the development of **online tools**. Salim Yusuf, the founder and executive director of the Population Health Research Institute at McMaster University, worked with his network of global health researchers to develop the *Canadian Hypertension Education Program*, which is a large-scale program intended to improve the quality of cardiovascular disease care and patient outcomes. The online tools include updated standardized clinical practice guidelines to detract, treat, and control hypertension; educational materials for professionals and the public (e.g., blood pressure log and blood pressure monitoring postcard); and even a downloadable app that is intended to serve as a rapid resource for clinicians who diagnose or treat patients with hypertension.

TED talks are short online talks (usually 18 minutes or less in duration) that originally intended to bring together great thinkers in technology, entertainment, and design, and today cover a vast range of topics in more than 100 languages. The mission of the TED organization is to spread ideas, which is reflective of the heart of knowledge translation. Kathleen Martin Ginis (University of British Columbia–Okanagan) delivered a TED talk that focused on Canada's physical inactivity crisis, and the importance of self-control as a personal resource to maintain an exercise program.

Canada's **National 3-Minute Thesis Competition**, operated through the Canadian Association for Graduate Studies (http://www.cags.ca/index.php) is another example of using electronic media to translate knowledge from research. The National 3-Minute Thesis Competition is a virtual academic research communication competition that is held annually, and is only open to master's or doctoral students. The competition is premised on the importance of researchers needing to present their ideas and results to the public as efficiently and in as engaging a way as possible. As such, the thesis competition is designed to make research accessible by improving the communication skills of graduate student researchers. Competitors from around the country are invited to present the complexities of their research in an engaging and accessible way before a live audience. The presentations are taped and disseminated over the Internet. The competitors have three minutes to present their research, they are allowed one take of their presentation, they can include only one slide, and no props are allowed.

Relationship-oriented

Going beyond written, visual, or virtual forms of knowledge translation, other innovative approaches for synthesizing, disseminating, exchanging, and applying knowledge include gatherings of people involved and interested in research. Research **gatherings** to exchange knowledge are often premised on relationship building and interactions between researchers and various knowledge users. Gatherings provide another forum for researchers to share information, and to engage researchers with knowledge users. Participatory action research, which was covered in Chapter 11, often includes gatherings (whether formally or informally acknowledged), where community engagement is emphasized and reciprocal knowledge exchange between researchers and community members is put into practice. An annual gathering hosted by CIHR, known as the Pathways Annual Gathering, brings together researchers and Indigenous community partners to discuss progress of research in areas related to health promotion and health equity for Indigenous peoples. Part of the intent of the gathering is to facilitate cross-learning, knowledge exchange, and relationship building among researchers, community members, partners, and other stakeholders.

Selecting Knowledge Translation Strategies

There are clearly a variety of ways that researchers can synthesize, disseminate, exchange, and apply the knowledge gained from their research and during their research. So, how do researchers choose their knowledge translation strategies? As we have discussed numerous times in this text when making decisions about other aspects of the research process, the choice of which knowledge translation strategy to use should be driven primarily by the research question or purpose. Two other important factors to consider are the intended audience and ethically sound strategies. For instance, researchers engaged in a healthy eating participatory action research project with a First Nations community will likely want to include community engagement and gatherings as part of their integrated knowledge translation approach, as these strategies align with many of ethical principles underlying chapter nine of the *Tri-Council Policy Statement: Ethical Conduct for Researchers Involving Humans* (which we discussed in Chapter 3 and is one of the most recently developed ethics policies for engaging in research with Indigenous peoples in Canada). As another example, researchers who examine the rate of concussions in Canadian Interuniversity Sport will want to consider an appropriate knowledge translation approach that targets the audience they are trying to reach. Perhaps the researchers could deliver a symposium at a local sport conference to reach other sport researchers or create a Facebook page that includes resources for coaches and parents. The list of knowledge translation examples we presented in this chapter is by no means exhaustive. Kinesiology researchers continue to push the boundaries on knowledge translation, with new strategies being tried often, such as quilting, mask making, delivering community forum educational sessions, and developing interactive tools and commercialized products. Equipped with fundamental research tools (many of which were introduced in this book), a strong foundation of ethics, and a guiding research question, the opportunities for synthesizing, disseminating, exchanging, and applying knowledge gained through research are seemingly endless. In the famous words of Dr Seuss, "Oh, the places you'll go!"

Summary

Chapter 12 focused on the various ways that research findings can be disseminated. Traditional approaches to knowledge dissemination, including journal articles and conference presentations, were overviewed. Attention was given to the anatomy of a journal article by linking previous book chapters to the respective components of a standard manuscript. In addition, the chapter featured a range of innovative forms of knowledge translation, such as online videos, fictional narratives, poetic representation, and ethnodrama. In doing so, Chapter 12 emphasized the variety of approaches that are available to kinesiology researchers when communicating their research to others. The importance of presenting research findings in a manner that corresponds to researchers' intended audience was emphasized.

Discussion Questions

1. What is knowledge translation? How might your definition change, or the approach you take to clearly describing it change, if you were describing it to your parents? To your peers? To the local newspaper?

2. In what order would you place the following headings and subheadings to best reflect the order in which they would typically appear in a traditional journal article?
   - Results
   - Method
   - Introduction
   - Literature Review
   - Title
   - Discussion
   - Participants

- Purpose Statement
- Procedures
- Abstract
- Conclusion
- Measures
- Data Analysis
- Measures and Instrumentation
- References

3. What are some challenges researchers might face in choosing not to present their research in a traditional journal article format? What opportunities might this choice present them?

4. Which knowledge translation strategy would work well for a study addressing each of the following purpose statements? Provide justification for your selection.

   - The aim of this study is to evaluate strength, endurance, and hip range of motion in a population of police officers.
   - The purpose of this study is to determine the relationship between infant vitamin D supplementation and bone outcomes at 4 years of age.
   - The goal of this study is to test a new on-ice measurement technique to investigate forward skating in ice hockey.
   - The purpose of this study is to investigate health inequities for women.

5. Although a variety of knowledge translation strategies were presented in this chapter, the approaches that have been discussed do not represent an exhaustive list. In fact, researchers in kinesiology-related fields engage in all sorts of knowledge translation. What are at least two additional specific strategies for each of the innovative knowledge translation subcategories identified in this chapter (i.e., arts-based, text-based, media-based, relationship-oriented)?

Recommended Readings

American Psychological Association. (2010). *Publication manual of the American Psychological Association* (6th ed.). Washington, DC: American Psychological Association.

Canadian Institutes of Health Research. (2015). *Knowledge translation at CIHR*. Retrieved from http://www.cihr-irsc.gc.ca/e/29418.html

Sparkes, A. C., & Smith, B. (2014). *Qualitative research methods in sport, exercise and health: From process to product.* London: Routledge.

Glossary

abstract A typical component of a journal article. A scientific summary of a research study that is concise yet comprehensive and allows readers to survey the contents of an article quickly.

action research An umbrella term or overarching framework for collaborative research approaches that result in direct benefits to participants.

action research spiral A research process for engaging in participatory action research, which involves a spiral of self-reflective cycles that include planning, acting and observing, and reflecting.

alternative hypothesis (H₁) Statements about the strength or direction of a relationship (also called a *research hypothesis*).

Analysis of Covariance (ANCOVA) A statistical analysis used when researchers have control variables that they have identified as important in the analysis.

Analysis of Variance (ANOVA) A statistical analysis that allows researchers to compare two or more groups in one test.

annotated bibliography A summary and critique of the articles, book chapters, and documents that have been identified by the researcher.

applicability An aspect of trustworthiness that refers to the extent to which the findings of a particular qualitative study may be transferable to other contexts or with other participants.

application One of the four fundamental elements of knowledge translation that refers to putting knowledge into practice. The application of knowledge needs to be ethically sound.

armchair walkthrough A process that researchers engage in to obtain methodological coherence in a study, particularly a qualitative study, before conducting the study. Researchers reflect on all aspects of a study (e.g., research questions, data generation options, etc.), and then consider alternative approaches (i.e., different ways to generate data, alternative analysis options, etc.) with the intent of having a well-conceived research plan.

audit trail A strategy to enhance the trustworthiness, rigour, and validation of a qualitative study in which researchers maintain a description of the entire research process for the purpose of having someone external to the study examine the various components of the study.

autoethnography A specific form of ethnography that involves the study of one's own culture.

between-groups Separate (different) groups of participants are examined for each of the different conditions in an experimental study. With between-groups designs, it is important to randomize participants to the conditions.

bimodal A distribution with two peaks or modes.

biohazard Any organism, or its derivative, that could negatively influence another organism.

blinding Hiding or concealing the condition/treatment/manipulation from the participants.

boxplot A standard way of displaying the distribution of data based on the minimum and maximum scores, the first and third quartile, and the median.

bracketing A process whereby researchers work to set aside their own experiences by outwardly acknowledging and recording their own experiences with the phenomenon being studied.

case A system that is bound by time and place.

case study A strategy of inquiry that is focused on studying a case (or cases) within important circumstances.

categorization matrix A process of deductive content analysis in which researchers use existing categories developed from previous theory and research to code text.

central phenomenon The main concept in qualitative research, or a key construct that researchers try to better understand, explore, and describe.

characterizing traits An approach to evaluate qualitative research whereby certain study characteristics *may* suggest high-quality research depending on the context and parameters (e.g., time, purpose) of the study.

chi-square test (χ²) A statistical analysis used to examine the discrepancy in frequencies between groups. Or a comparison between the frequency or ranked data outcome and what would be expected by chance.

closed-ended Interview questions that require participants to choose their answer from a list of defined answers.

coding A systematic organizing of the data into meaningful chunks that, once brought together into something shared, become the significant themes of the research.

collective case study A specific form of case study that includes several cases.

complete observer A specific form of observation whereby researchers have no interactions with the participants and they are typically not seen or noticed by participants.

complete participant A specific form of observation whereby researchers take part in the activity, event, or phenomenon under study.

concurrent mixed methods research design A way to do mixed methods research whereby quantitative and qualitative data are collected at essentially the same time.

concurrent nested designs A concurrent mixed methods research design where the quantitative and qualitative data are given unequal priority or weighting, with one method dominating while the other is nested or embedded within the other method. Typically the nested method is of secondary interest or answers a specific subquestion of interest.

confidentiality The safeguarding of entrusted information.

consistency An aspect of trustworthiness that refers to the dependability of a qualitative study. The focus is on seeking to understand the variability of qualitative study findings or unique experiences.

consolidated criteria for reporting qualitative research (COREQ) An approach to evaluating qualitative research that consists of a 32-item checklist that includes important criteria about the research team, study design, and findings.

construct validity Examines whether the measures used by researchers assess/test what they intended to measure.

constructivism A philosophical worldview that is premised on the notion that multiple realities exist and that meaning is varied and complex.

contingency table A classification system in which two or more groups respond on two or more categories or outcomes.

continuous data Data that can take on any value and range (e.g., the weight of a mouse, a person's maximal energy expenditure, a gymnast's height).

control group Members are not exposed to the manipulation (also called a placebo group).

control variables Variables that could influence the outcome or results of the study. They are measured variables, but are not a main focus of the study.

correlation A statistical technique that allows researchers to determine the relationship between two or more variables.

correlation coefficient These coefficients can range from 0.0 to 1.0 in either a negative or positive direction. The closer the value is to 1.0, the stronger the association between the variables, whereas the closer to 0.0 means there is little to no relationship.

criterion The dependent variable may be called the criterion in correlation study designs.

critical ethnography A specific from of ethnography that includes a political agenda and advocacy.

critical value The point on the scale of the test statistic beyond which the null hypothesis is rejected.

critical value tables A table presenting the critical values based on the p-value or level of confidence.

cross-sectional study Participants are assessed at one point in time.

data saturation A term often used in qualitative data analysis to suggest that no new information will surface from further data generation.

data transformation An option for mixed methods data integration whereby one form of data is converted into the other form of data. Numerical data can be qualitized (i.e., quantitative data is transformed into qualitative data), or non-numerical data can be quantitized (i.e., qualitative data transformed into quantitative data).

deductive data analysis A process by which there is an existing framework or starting list of categories that researchers use to code the data within.

deductive reasoning Opposite approach to inductive reasoning. Researchers start with concrete generalized information often contained within a theory and use this information to explain specific events or circumstances.

degrees of freedom The number of observations that are free to vary.

dependent (or paired) *t*-test When two data points are collected over time (e.g., a pre- and post-test design) or when participants are exposed to the two experimental conditions, a dependent (or paired) t-test would be used. Each participant contributes two data points.

dependent variable The variable that is being affected—it is the outcome being assessed as a result of the independent variable(s) and is the main focus of the study.

descriptive research Problems that are descriptive in nature include the need for describing a phenomena, event, condition, or circumstance whereby no attempt is made to link information or explain outcomes.

discrete data Data that can take on particular values that are either numerical (e.g., number of different exercises in a program) or categorical (e.g., blood pressure in categories of hypertension, hypotension, normal).

discussion A typical component of a journal article that appears after the study results have been presented. Findings are evaluated and interpreted in reference to the research questions, conclusions are stated, and the contribution to the literature is indicated.

dissemination   One of the four fundamental elements of knowledge translation that entails identifying a particular audience and tailoring the message and the medium of knowledge exchange to that audience.

double-blind study   Both the researchers and participants are unaware of who has received the manipulation.

effect sizes   A value calculated to measure the practical significance or meaningfulness of the findings.

empirical phenomenology   A specific form of phenomenology that involves a structural analysis of participant's experiences, which results in a description of the essential structure(s) of the phenomenon.

end-of-project knowledge translation   A way to plan the timing of knowledge translation activities. Sharing knowledge that was gained from a project at the end of a research study, after the project has been completed.

epistemology   A researcher's belief about how we acquire knowledge about truth and reality.

ethical dilemma   An ethical situation in which a researcher is required to perform two or more mutually exclusive actions.

ethical residue   The feeling that a wrong ethical decision might have been made in an ethical dilemma.

ethnodrama   An example of an innovative arts-based knowledge translation strategy. Research data are dramatized through script writing that becomes the basis for a film or theatrical performance.

ethnography   A strategy of inquiry that is focused on understanding cultures or a cultural group.

exchange   One of the four fundamental elements of knowledge translation that includes engagement between researchers and knowledge users that results in mutual learning through planning, producing, disseminating, and applying existing or new research.

experimental group   Members of this group are exposed to some level of manipulation (also called the treatment or intervention group).

expert sampling   Identifying people with known experience and expertise in an area of interest to participate in a study.

explanation problems   These problems exist when researchers can make claims about cause and effect or attempt to answer problems of *why* events and behaviours happen.

explanatory sequential mixed methods design   A sequential mixed methods research design in which the quantitative data are collected in the first phase and the qualitative data are collected in the second phase.

exploratory sequential mixed methods design   A sequential mixed methods research design in which the qualitative data are collected in the first phase and the quantitative data are collected in the second phase.

external validity   The likelihood of seeing similar successes of a treatment or an intervention with other populations, in other contexts, and across time.

extraneous variables   Unmeasured variables that are not controlled for in the study (also called confounding variables). Often identified in the discussion section of the study write-up when researchers attempt to make sense of their findings.

extreme case sampling   A specific form of purposeful sampling whereby researchers sample participants that are deemed outliers to the topic of study.

factorial ANOVA   A statistical analysis that is used when more than one independent variable is manipulated.

fictional narratives   An example of an innovative text-based knowledge translation strategy. Research findings are shared through fiction to engage the reader.

field notes   Written notes recorded by researchers to describe what was observed through their various senses during observations.

five-phase participatory action research approach   A research process for engaging in participatory action research, which involves setting the research question, building trust, data collection, data analysis, and communicating results for action.

frequency distribution   A graph that involves plotting how many times each score occurs (also called a *histogram*).

frequency polygon   The frequency of scores is represented by dots that are connected by a line.

gatherings   An example of a relationship-oriented knowledge translation strategy. A forum of people involved and interested in research that is premised on relationship building and interactions between researchers and various knowledge users.

grounded theory   A strategy of inquiry that is focused on the generation and analysis of data to construct a theory.

group interview   A process of data generation in which researchers engage in a discussion with more than one participant in an effort to better understand their experiences with the topic of study.

guidelines   Suggested practices that allow for flexibility in terms of interpretation and implementation.

histogram   A graph that involves plotting how many times each score occurs (also called a *frequency distribution*).

hypothesis A prediction that is derived from theory, literature, or speculation about the outcome of a study.

independent *t*-test Used when the study has two groups of different participants (each participant contributes one score to the data).

independent variable The variable that is manipulated (also called the treatment variable).

inductive data analysis A process by which researchers identify taxonomies, themes, or theory from the data generated in the research.

inductive reasoning Opposite approach to deductive reasoning. Involves using observations of specific events and circumstances to make predictions about general principles that are tied together and united into theory.

inference If the sample represents a larger group, then the findings can be generalized or *inferred* to the larger group.

instrumental case study A specific form of case study that is focused on studying an issue of interest, which can be understood through a specific case.

integrated knowledge translation A way to plan the timing of knowledge translation activities. Knowledge translation activities are ongoing throughout the entire research process through active engagement between researchers and knowledge users.

interaction The effect of one independent variable on the dependent variable depends on or is explained by a third variable.

internal validity The researchers' ability to claim that any change in an outcome is the result of a treatment or intervention (i.e., manipulation of the independent variable) and not a result of other factors related to the sample, the measures, the techniques, and other possible potential threats.

interpretative phenomenological analysis A specific form of phenomenology that is focused on understanding how experiences of a phenomenon are *perceived* by participants and how people make sense of their social and personal world.

interpretive dance An example of an innovative arts-based knowledge translation strategy. A dance performance is developed to communicate research.

interpretive framework Within the context of qualitative research, theory can be used by researchers to support their interpretation of research findings.

interquartile range Identifies the scores that are the boundaries of the lowest (25th percentile) and highest (75th percentile) of the distribution, or the middle 50% of the scores in a distribution.

interval data Data are ordered, and the intervals between each value are equal (e.g., temperature).

interview guide A defined list of interview questions that is used to ensure that the same (or very similar) questions are asked to all participants.

intrinsic case study A specific form of case study that is focused on studying the complexity of the case.

introduction A typical component of a journal article that eases the reader into the study topic, reviews literature relevant to the topic, and concludes with the research questions and purpose statement.

key terms Typically three to five important words or descriptors that reflect the focus of the study and are used for indexing articles in search engines.

knowledge translation Often referred to as "KT," a dynamic process that includes the synthesis, dissemination, exchange, and ethical application of knowledge.

knowledge user Any individual who is likely to be able to use the knowledge gained through research to make informed decisions about policies, programs, and practices.

kurtosis The degree to which the peak of the data distribution is normal (e.g., mesokurtic), flat (e.g., platykurtic) or pointy (e.g., leptokurtic).

leptokurtic There are few high and low scores with more scores near the centre to create a pointy distribution.

life history A specific form of narrative inquiry that describes the entire life of an individual.

literature map A visual representation or figure that draws together the existing studies and identifies how a particular topic is situated within the broader body of research.

logical validity The quality of researchers' arguments, their application of theory to support the needs for the study, and the appropriate interpretation of results based on the data.

longitudinal study A study in which participants are followed over time.

main effect The effect of an independent variable on a dependent variable while averaging across the levels of any other independent variables or ultimately ignoring the effects of other independent variables.

maximum variation sampling A specific form of purposeful sampling whereby researchers identify individuals that represent a wide range of experiences with respect to the topic of study.

mean The sum of all scores divided by the total number of scores (also called the average).

median   The middle score of a distribution when the scores are ordered by magnitude.

mediator variable   A variable that is proposed to at least partially explain the relationship between an independent and dependent variable.

member check   A strategy to enhance the trustworthiness, rigour, and validation of a qualitative study. Study participants are invited to review the data they generated or emergent study findings, and provided with the opportunity to add, alter, or delete their information and provide feedback on study findings.

mesokurtic   This type of graph represents a normal distribution.

meta-analysis   A technique for research synthesis that involves the identification of a problem to address, a methodology that explains decisions for the literature review and analysis, and an analysis that integrates findings from a number of studies and quantifies the findings in a standard metric called an effect size.

method   A typical component of a journal article that includes details about how the study was conducted, such as participant information, sampling, measures, procedures, and data analysis.

methodological coherence   An approach to evaluate qualitative research in which all components of a research design (e.g., research questions, strategy of inquiry, methods for data generation, data analysis) align with one another.

mixed methods research   An approach to inquiry that systematically and purposefully combines quantitative and qualitative forms of research.

modality   The number of peaks (number of high bars in the histogram) that represent areas of score clusters.

mode   The most frequently occurring or most common score in a data set.

moderator variable   A variable of interest that cannot be manipulated (also called an effect moderator).

musical performances   An example of an innovative arts-based knowledge translation strategy. Music is used to communicate research findings to an audience.

narrative research   A strategy of inquiry that focuses on the stories of individuals.

narratives   An example of an innovative text-based knowledge translation strategy. Often co-constructed between researchers and participants, retelling of experiences and interpretations through a plot that connects events over time (i.e., storytelling).

National 3-Minute Thesis Competition   An example of an innovative media-based knowledge translation strategy. A virtual academic research communication competition for graduate student researchers to present their research ideas and results to the public as efficiently and in as engaging a way as possible.

negative correlation   A relationship that exists when large values for one variable are related to lower values on another variable or vice versa.

negative or discrepant information   A strategy to enhance the trustworthiness, rigour, and validation of a qualitative study whereby results that run counter to main study findings are presented to highlight opposing views or experiences and draw attention to unique perspectives.

negatively skewed   A distribution of scores whereby the lowest frequency of scores clusters closest to the y-axis and the highest frequency of scores are at the far right of the distribution.

neutrality   An aspect of trustworthiness that refers to the degree to which the findings of a qualitative study are based on the participants' meanings and experiences and not a result of researchers' interests and perspectives.

nominal data   Refers to categorically discrete and mutually exclusive data.

nomological network   A web of evidence describing how a measure should be related to measures of other constructs and behaviours.

non-experimental study design   Study design with no randomization to groups, no groups to randomize to, and no manipulation of the independent variable.

non-parametric   The statistical tests used for nominal and ordinal data.

non-probability sampling   Any method that does not use random selection.

normal distribution   A symmetrical data distribution around a centre of scores.

null hypothesis (H$_0$)   States that the independent and dependent variables are not related or that there are no significant differences between groups.

objectivity   Ensures there is reliability or consistency of measurement between different researchers. This is a particularly important concern with observational data collection.

observation   A form of data generation that requires researchers to go into the field, or natural setting, to try to better understand the topic of study by using their various senses. Involves visual and/or audio records and counts of particular behaviours, settings, or interactions and scoring what is seen and heard.

observational protocol   A template that is used to guide researchers' field notes.

observer as participant　A specific form of observation whereby researchers engage in activities with participants, but participation is of secondary importance to actually recording observations.

one-on-one interview　A process of data generation in which researchers engage in a discussion with a single participant in an effort to better understand her or his experiences with the topic of study.

online tools　An example of an innovative media-based knowledge translation strategy. Examples include electronic log books and downloadable apps.

ontology　A researcher's belief in the nature of truth and reality.

open coding　Writing notes and headings in a text as it is being read, with the goal to find a way to describe all aspects of the content.

open-ended　Interview questions that do not have defined answers and require participants to answer the question using their own terms.

oral history　A specific form of narrative inquiry that involves the collection of memories that hold historical significance.

ordinal data　Refers to quantities that have a natural ordering. The ranking of favorite sports or placement of runners finishing a race are both examples of ordinal data.

outliers　A score/value that is extreme or atypical.

parametric tests　A type of statistic based on the assumption that sample data comes from a population that follows a probability distribution based on a fixed set of parameters.

participant as observer　A specific form of observation whereby researchers engage as a participant *and* researcher by taking part in activities and recording observations.

participatory action research (PAR)　An emancipatory research approach that involves the participants in all phases of the research process and results in practical outcomes for the participants.

Pearson product moment correlation (*r*)　A coefficient calculated between one criterion (dependent) and one predictor or correlate (independent) variable and both variables are interval or ratio data types.

peer debrief　A strategy to enhance the trustworthiness, rigour, and validation of a qualitative study. Researchers seek out other professionals (e.g., faculty colleagues, members of a thesis committee) to encourage critical reflection on study findings and push researchers to ensure the results are grounded in the data rather than their own perspectives as researchers.

peer-review process　A manuscript (i.e., research report) that is submitted to a journal for publication gets sent to a few select experts in the research area to be critically reviewed prior to its decision on being accepted for publication. This process plays a significant role in determining which manuscripts get published and therefore disseminated to the academic community.

percentages (%)　Values defined per hundred.

phenomenology　A strategy of inquiry that involves the study of a phenomenon or concept through the exploration of lived experiences.

philosophical worldview　A researcher's set of beliefs about her or his general orientation of the world and the nature of research.

planned comparisons　Tests that are proposed and identified a priori, are based on the alternative hypothesis, and are done to see where the group mean differences are.

platykurtic　Scores are equally distributed across the entire distribution (including more scores in each of the tails) to create a flat distribution.

poetic representation　An example of an innovative text-based knowledge translation strategy. Research data are compressed into a consistent pattern of verse to retell lived experiences through poetry.

population　A well-defined collection of individuals with similar characteristics who are of interest to the researchers. The specific members of a sample are ideally chosen as representation of a population that is of interest for generalizing the findings.

positive correlation　A relationship that exists when large values of one variable are associated with large values of another variable or small values on one variable are associated with small values on another.

positive reporting bias　The selective revealing or suppression of information in research.

positively skewed　A distribution of data in which the highest frequency bar is closest to the *y*-axis and the lowest frequency of scores is at the far right of the graph.

post-hoc tests　Statistical analyses that are done after the main analyses to explore where there are group differences.

post-test only design　The independent variable is introduced to the randomly assigned experimental group participants, and then the effects of the "treatment" versus "no treatment" (or manipulation of the independent variable) are tested by looking at whether the groups are different.

poster presentation　A format for presenting research at a conference. Researchers create posters that depict summaries of their research, which are placed on the walls or on poster stands in a large room during a conference. Researchers stand by their posters and engage with interested individuals who walk around, read the material, and discuss the posters.

postpositivism   A philosophical worldview that is premised on the notion that there is a single reality or objective truth to be discovered through research.

pragmatism   A philosophical worldview that is premised on the idea that researchers need to be concerned with solutions to problems, and as such is not committed to any single notion of reality.

pre-experimental design   A study in which researchers examine *one* group of individuals and provide an intervention during the study.

pre- and post-test design   Design used to examine change in the dependent variable that can be attributed to the independent variable. The aim is to see which group changes more as a result of the manipulation or treatment.

predictive research   Predictive research problems are based on the premise that there is a need to identify relationships among variables.

predictor   The independent variable may be called the predictor in correlation study designs.

principles   Beliefs or moral rules that influence a person's actions.

privacy   A person's right to be free from intrusion by others.

probability sampling   Any method that ensures that the different units in the population have equal probabilities of being chosen.

prolonged engagement   A strategy to enhance the trustworthiness, rigour, and validation of a qualitative study where an extended amount of time is spent with participants "in the field."

purposeful sampling   Sometimes referred to as purposive sampling, this is a process in which researchers recruit a sample of information-rich participants that will intentionally inform an understanding of the topic being studied. It is also a strategy to enhance the trustworthiness, rigour, and validation of a qualitative study.

purposive sampling   Involves identifying units (e.g., people, organizations, teams) that represent a characteristic of interest; as such, the sample is identified with that purpose in mind.

qualitative description   A strategy of inquiry that supports the development of a comprehensive description and summary of a phenomenon or an event.

qualitative research   A research approach in which non-numerical (i.e., qualitative) data are generated and analyzed.

quantitative research   A research approach in which numerical (i.e., quantitative) data are collected and analyzed.

quasi-experimental study design   A study design that shares similarities with the traditional experimental design, but does not include random assignment to treatment or control.

quota sampling   Identifying a certain number or representation needed for the study and then sampling up to that number.

random selection   A process that ensures that every unit (person, team, organization) in the population has an equal probability of being selected for the sample.

randomized control trial (RCT)   Any study that is designed with random assignment of participants, a control group, and manipulation of the independent variable.

range   The distance between the most extreme scores (lowest and highest) in a distribution.

rapport   A close or harmonious relationship between researchers and participants.

ratio data   Interval data with a natural or absolute zero point (i.e., the absence of a trait).

regression analysis   A statistical analysis used to test whether an independent variable (predictor) is able to predict a dependent variable (criterion).

reliability   Indicates that the measure is consistent or repeatable; if any type of assessment is not consistent, then it cannot be trusted. Reliability is an important part of construct validity.

reliable   The degree to which a test is consistent.

repeated measures   Study design in which each subject is involved in all research conditions and usually involves measures taken over time (also called *within-subjects design*).

repeated measures ANOVA   A statistical analysis to use when researchers have two or more time points (e.g., the same people measured a few or more times, such as a baseline assessment, post-intervention, and a follow-up).

research   A structured method used to answer questions and discover new knowledge. Examples of research methods include quantitative, qualitative, and mixed methods research approaches.

research hypothesis   Can be a statement about what treatment group might have higher scores; or statements about the strength or direction of a relationship (also called the *alternative hypothesis*).

research problem   The foundational need for the study that describes the context for the study and the issues that exist in literature, theory, and/or practice.

research question(s)   Broad inquiry statement(s) about the main study variables or central phenomenon.

research synthesis   A detailed literature review that can also stand alone as a research publication if the research question involves an evaluation and integration of published literature on a topic to make empirical and/or theoretical conclusions.

researcher reflexivity   A strategy to enhance the trustworthiness, rigour, and validation of a qualitative study whereby researchers position themselves by reflecting on their background, experiences, and perspectives to consider how their biases may shape or inform their research. Reflexivity consists of two parts: (1) reflecting on one's own experiences with the phenomenon/sample being studied and (2) considering how one's experiences shape the research process.

results   A typical component of a journal article that tells the reader what was found in the study in relation to the study purpose. Results can be presented through printed text, tables, charts, diagrams, maps, and figures.

rich, thick description   A strategy to enhance the trustworthiness, rigour, and validation of a qualitative study. Collecting thorough descriptive data and presenting findings in a rich manner aligns with the meaning-making process of qualitative research and highlights the complexity of experiences.

sample   Represents a group of participants (or organizations, teams, schools, etc.) selected to be in a study.

sample mean   The mean (e.g., average) score of a sample derived from a population. The average of all sample means is the population mean.

sampling frame   The group of accessible people that can be connected with about a study.

science   The discovery of new knowledge.

semi-structured   A term often used in qualitative research to describe interviews that comprise a short set of questions with the flexibility to discuss other topics that are not included in the interview guide.

sequential mixed methods research design   A way to do mixed methods research that involves two distinct phases for the quantitative and qualitative data collection. Data that are collected in the first phase is analyzed and used to inform the second phase.

short film   An example of an innovative arts-based knowledge translation strategy. A brief video that shares research with an audience.

side-by-side comparison   An option for mixed methods data integration whereby quantitative and qualitative data are analyzed separately, and one set of findings is presented followed by the other.

single-subjects design   A single person or a small number of people are studied over a long period of time. The behaviour of an individual is examined over time and established as a "baseline behaviour" that is assessed, a treatment is provided, and then the treatment is withdrawn and the behaviour is assessed again over a period of time.

snowball sampling   A specific form of purposeful sampling whereby individuals or cases involved in a study identify other individuals or cases that they deem appropriate for the study.

social media   An example of an innovative media-based knowledge translation strategy. Social media platforms such as Facebook, Instagram, and Twitter provide ways for researchers to connect, support, and learn from each other by sharing research findings, occurrences, and updates to a readily available audience.

Spearman Rank correlation coefficient (*rho*)   Associations between ordinal or rank-ordered data.

standard deviation (*SD*)   The dispersion or deviation of scores within a distribution.

standard error   A measure of how well the sample represents the population.

standard error of the mean   The standard deviation of the sampling means.

statistics   Objective ways of interpreting observations used to help researchers address questions related to description, prediction and association, and explanation of differences.

stories   An example of an innovative text-based knowledge translation strategy. A medium through which meanings can be communicated in order to make sense of life experiences and convey knowledge.

stratified random sampling   A method of identifying the people in the sample whereby the population (or sampling frame) is divided and grouped on a characteristic before random selection takes place.

structured interview   A data collection tool that is often used to facilitate responses to specific questions that have set answers (i.e., closed-ended).

surveys   A method of data collection that involves the use of paper-and-pencil or online-delivered questions, usually consisting of a mix of rating scales providing ordinal or interval data responses (also called questionnaires).

symposium   A format for presenting research at a conference. Experts in a specific area of research formally gather to present their research on a single topic.

synthesis   One of the four fundamental elements of knowledge translation that contextualizes and integrates findings from individual research studies within the larger body of knowledge on a topic.

systematic sampling   A process whereby researchers use lists or inventories of units in a population (e.g., telephone book, index of registered members) to identify (select) every *N*th entry for the sample, such as every 10th or 100th person.

t-test   Comparisons focused on two groups (regardless of whether they are different groups or the same people measured twice). Tests the difference between group means, while considering the extent to which the means would differ by chance.

taxonomy   A formal qualitative data analysis system for classifying multifaceted and complex phenomenon.

TED talks   An example of an innovative media-based knowledge translation strategy. Short online talks that cover a range of topics with the intent of spreading ideas.

themes   A qualitative data analysis strategy that characterizes the responses of participants and provides insight into the essential components of their experience.

theoretical lens   A perspective in which researchers draw upon theory, or components of a theory, to guide their research.

theory   A set of interlocking causal variables to explain some aspect of our personal, social, or physical realities.

transcribing   The process of taking oral data and reproducing it as faithfully as possible as a written text.

transformative   A philosophical worldview that is premised on the notion that research needs to be closely connected with politics and have an action agenda to advocate for marginalized peoples, such as those who experience inequity based on gender, race, ethnicity, disability, sexual orientation, and socioeconomic status.

triangulation   A strategy to enhance the trustworthiness, rigour, and validation of a qualitative study in which a variety of data sources, perspectives, and methods are used as a way to crosscheck study findings and interpretations.

trimodal   A distribution of data with three peaks/modes.

true experiment   A type of quantitative research design in which participants in the study are randomly assigned to experimental and control groups.

trustworthiness   An approach to evaluate qualitative research. Convincing an audience that study findings are worth paying attention to and worth taking account of.

truth value   An aspect of trustworthiness. The extent to which the results and interpretations in a qualitative study are credible in so much as they reflect participants' meanings and experiences.

two-eyed seeing   A philosophical worldview that bridges Indigenous and Western knowledge. It is rooted in the belief that there are many ways of understanding the world, some represented by various Indigenous knowledge systems and others by European-derived sciences.

Type I error   Researchers make the decision that a manipulation or treatment has been successful when in fact it has not been.

Type II error   Researchers make the decision that the manipulation has failed when in reality it actually did work.

unimodal   A distribution with one mode.

unstructured   A term often used in qualitative research to describe interviews that do not have an interview guide but instead a guiding topic for a conversational discussion.

valid   The degree to which a test measures what is intended to be measured.

validity   A general term used to reflect the degree to which we can have confidence in our conclusions based on the research we conduct.

variability   An index of how the scores vary or disperse (the spread of scores).

variable   An attribute or a characteristic that may vary over time or across cases.

variance   A measure of variability that is calculated as the square of the standard deviation. Variance reflects the dispersion of scores within a distribution and offers insight into the differences among scores within a distribution, as well as the differences or deviation between the scores from the mean of the distribution.

verbal presentation   A format for presenting research at a conference. A researcher speaks in front of an audience at a conference to deliver an overview of her or his research in a short amount of time.

visual art   An example of an innovative arts-based knowledge translation strategy. Engaging the senses to convey information that is difficult to describe in words.

wash-out period   Time between testing sessions in an experiment. There should be sufficient time to wipe out the effects of the previous condition so that participants are essentially starting from their normal baseline at each session.

websites   An example of an innovative media-based knowledge translation strategy. Researchers create a website to share their research and often include updated information about previous and current research projects.

within-subjects design   The same group of participants is examined over time or across conditions (also called *repeated measures*).

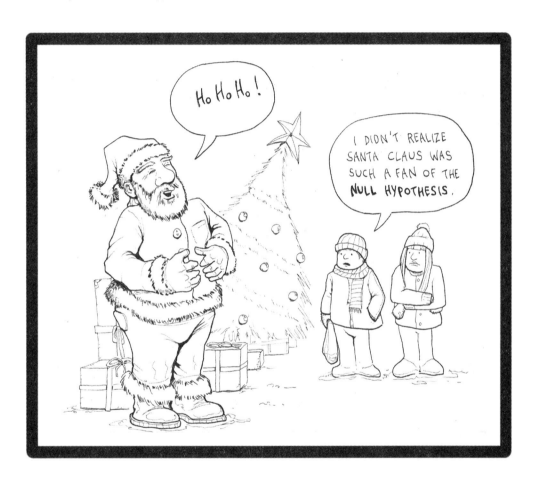

References

CHAPTER 1

Bartlett, C., Marshall, M., & Marshall, A. (2012). Two-eyed seeing and other lessons learned within a co-learning journey of bringing together Indigenous and mainstream knowledges and ways of knowing. *Journal of Environmental Studies and Sciences, 2,* 331–40. doi:10.1007/s13412-012-0086-8

Baumgartner, T. A., & Hensley, L. D. (2012). *Conducting and reading research in kinesiology* (5th ed.). New York: McGraw-Hill.

Baxter-Jones, A. D. G., Kontulainen, S. A., Faulkner, R. A., & Bailey, D. A. (2008). A longitudinal study of the relationship of physical activity to bone mineral accrual from adolescence to young adulthood. *Bone, 43,* 1101–7. doi:10.1016/j.bone.2008.07.245

Bergeron, K., & Lévesque, L. (2014). Designing active communities: A coordinated action framework for planners and public health professionals. *Journal of Physical Activity & Health, 11,* 1041–51. doi:10.1123/jpah.2012-0178

Clark, M. I., Spence, J. C., & Holt, N. L. (2011). In the shoes of young adolescent girls: Understanding physical activity experiences through interpretive description. *Qualitative Research in Sport, Exercise and Health, 3,* 193–210. doi:10.1080/2159676X.2011.572180

Colley, R. C., Garriguet, D., Janssen, I., Craig, C. L., Clarke, J., & Tremblay, M. S. (2011). Physical activity of Canadian adults: Accelerometer results from the 2007 to 2009 Canadian Health Measures Survey. *Health Reports (Statistics Canada, Catalogue 82-003), 22,* 1–9.

Creswell, J. W. (2014). *Research design: Qualitative, quantitative, and mixed methods approaches* (4th ed.). Thousand Oaks, CA: Sage.

Creswell, J. W., & Plano Clark, V. L. (2011). *Designing and conducting mixed methods research* (2nd ed.). Thousand Oaks, CA: Sage.

Deci, E. L., & Ryan, R. M. (2000). The "what" and "why" of goal pursuits: Human needs and the self-determination of behavior. *Psychological Inquiry, 11,* 227–68. doi:10.1207/S15327965PLI1104_01

Easterbrook, G. (2013). *The king of sports: Why football must be reformed*. New York: St. Martin's Press.

Elliott, D. (2007). Forty years of kinesiology: A Canadian perspective. *Quest, 59,* 154–62. doi:10.1080/00336297.2007.10483544

Ferguson, L. J., Kowalski, K. C., Mack, D. E., & Sabiston, C. M. (2014). Exploring self-compassion and eudaimonic well-being in young women athletes. *Journal of Sport and Exercise Psychology, 36,* 203–16. doi:10.1123/jsep.2013-0096

Goodwin, D. L., Krohn, J., & Kuhnle, A. (2004). Beyond the wheelchair: The experience of dance. *Adapted Physical Activity Quarterly, 21,* 229–47.

Holt, N. L, McHugh, T.-L. F., Tink, L. N., Kingsley, B. C., Coppola, A. M., Neely, K. C., & McDonald, R. (2013). Developing sport-based after-school programmes using a participatory action research approach. *Qualitative Research in Sport, Exercise and Health, 5,* 332–55. doi:10.1080/2159676X.2013.809377

Holt, N. L, Spence, J. C., Sehn, Z. L., & Cutumisu, N. (2008). Neighborhood and developmental differences in children's perceptions of opportunities for play and physical activity. *Health & Place, 14,* 2–14. doi:10.1016/j.healthplace.2007.03.002

Magnus, C. R. A., Arnold, C. M., Johnston, G., Dal-Bello Haas, V., Basran, J., Krentz, J. R., & Farthing, J. P. (2013). Cross-education for improving strength and mobility after distal radius fractures: A randomized controlled trial. *Archives of Physical Medicine and Rehabilitation, 94,* 1247–55. doi:10.1016/j.apmr.2013.03.005

Masse, L. C., O'Connor, T. M., Tu, A. W., Watts, A. W., Beauchamp, M. R., Hughes, S. O., & Baranowski, T. (2016). Are the physical activity parenting practices reported by US and Canadian parents captured in currently published instruments? *Journal of Physical Activity & Health, 13,* 1070–8.

Moreside, J. M., & McGill, S. M. (2012). Hip joint range of motion improvements using three different interventions. *Journal of Strength and Conditioning Research, 26,* 1265–73. doi:10.1519/JSC.0b013e31824f2351

Mosewich, A. D., Vangool, A. B., Kowalski, K. C., & McHugh, T.-L. (2009). Exploring women track and field athletes' meanings of muscularity. *Journal of Applied Sport Psychology, 21,* 99–115. doi:10.1080/10413200802575742

Patton, M. Q. (2002). *Qualitative research and evaluation methods* (3rd ed.). Thousand Oaks, CA: Sage.

Riess, K. J., Haykowsky, M., Lawrance, R., Tomczak, C. R., Welsh, R., Lewanczuk, R., . . . Gourishankar, S. (2014). Exercise training improves aerobic capacity, muscle strength, and quality of life in renal transplant recipients. *Applied Physiology, Nutrition, and Metabolism, 39*, 566–71. doi:10.1139/apnm-2013-0449

Sagan, C. (1997). *The Demon-haunted world: Science as a candle in the dark*. London: Headline.

Shields, C. A., Spink, K. S., Chad, K., Muhajarine, N., Humbert, L., & Odnokon, P. (2008). Youth and adolescent physical activity lapsers: Examining self-efficacy as a mediator of the relationship between family social influence and physical activity. *Journal of Health Psychology, 13*, 121–30.

Sparkes, A. C., & Smith, B. (2014). *Qualitative research methods in sport, exercise, and health: From process to product*. London: Routledge.

Strachan, L., Côté, J., & Deakin, J. (2009). An evaluation of personal and contextual factors in competitive youth sport. *Journal of Applied Sport Psychology, 21*, 340–55. doi:10.1080/10413200903018667

Strachan, L., Côté, J., & Deakin, J. (2011). A new view: Exploring positive youth development in elite sport contexts. *Qualitative Research in Sport, Exercise and Health, 3*, 9–32. doi:10.1080/19398441.2010.541483

Strachan, P. H., Kaasalainen, S., Horton, A., Jarman, H., D'Elia, T., Van Der Horst, M. L., . . . Hechman, G. A. (2014). Managing heart failure in the long-term care setting: Nurses' experiences in Ontario, Canada. *Nursing Research, 63*, 357–65. doi:10.1097/NNR.0000000000000049

Sullivan, G. (2005). *Art practice as research: Inquiry in the visual arts*. Thousand Oaks, CA: Sage.

Thomas, J. R., Nelson, J. K., & Silverman, S.J. (2011). *Research methods in physical activity* (6th ed.). Champaign, IL: Human Kinetics.

Tremblay, M. S., & Gorber, S. C. (2007). Canadian Health Measures Survey: Brief overview. *Canadian Journal of Public Health, 98*, 453–56.

Whaley, D. E., & Krane, V. (2011). Now that we all agree, let's talk epistemology: A commentary on the invited articles. *Qualitative Research in Sport, Exercise and Health, 3*, 394–403. doi:10.1080/2159676X.2011.607186

CHAPTER 2

Ajzen, I. (1991). The theory of planned behavior. *Organizational Behavior and Human Decision Processes, 50*, 179–211. doi:10.1016/0749-5978(91)90020-T

Arbour-Nicitopoulos, K. A., Latimer-Cheung, A. E., Buchholz, A. C., Bray, S. R., Craven, B. C., . . . Horrocks, J. (2012). Predictors of leisure time physical activity among people with spinal cord injury. *Annals of Behavioral Medicine, 44*, 104–18. doi:10.1007/s12160-012-9370-9

Balazs, G. C., Pavey, G. J., Brelin, A. M., Pickett, A., Keblish D. J., & Rue, J. P. (2014). Risk of anterior cruciate ligament injury in athletes on synthetic playing surfaces: A systematic review. *American Journal of Sports Medicine*. Epub ahead of print: August 27, 2014, doi:10.1177/0363546514545864

Baumgartner, T. A., & Hensley, L. D. (2012). *Conducting and reading research in kinesiology* (5th ed.). New York: McGraw-Hill.

Baxter-Jones, A. D. G., Eisenmann, J. C., Mirwald, R. L., Faulkner, R. A., & Bailey, D. A. (2008). The influence of physical activity on lean mass accrual during adolescence: A longitudinal analysis. *Journal of Applied Physiology, 105*, 734–41. doi:10.1152/japplphysiol.00869.2007

Blinch, J., Cameron, B. D., Hodges, N. J., & Chua, R. (2012). Do preparation or control processes result in the modulation to Fitts' law for movements to targets with placeholders? *Experimental Brain Research, 223*, 505–15. doi:10.1007/s00221-012-3277-3

Canadian Fitness and Lifestyle Research Institute Bulletin 1: *Physical activity levels of Canadians*. (2014). Available at: http://www.cflri.ca/sites/default/files/node/1374/files/CFLRI_Bulletin%201_PAM%202014-2015.pdf

Charmaz, K. (2006). *Constructing grounded theory*. London: Sage.

Clarke, J., & Janssen, I. (2014). Sporadic and bouted physical activity and the metabolic syndrome in adults. *Medicine and Science in Sports and Exercise, 46*, 76–83. doi:10.1249/MSS.0b013e31829f83a0

Creswell, J. W. (2014). *Research design: Qualitative, quantitative, and mixed methods approaches* (4th ed.). Thousand Oaks, CA: Sage.

Day, R. D., & Gastel, B. (2006). *How to write and publish a scientific paper*. Westport, CT: Greenwood.

Fitts, P. M. (1954). The information capacity of the human motor system in controlling the amplitude of movement. *Journal of Experimental Psychology, 47*, 381–91. doi:10.1037/h0055392

Glazebrook, C. M., Kiernan, D., Welsh, T. N., & Tremblay, L. (2015). How one breaks Fitts' law and gets away with it: Moving further and faster involves more efficient online control. *Human Movement Science, 39*, 163–76. doi:10.1016/j.humov.2014.11.005

Jewett, R., Sabiston, C. M., Brunet, J., O'Loughlin, E. K., Scarapicchia, T., & O'Loughlin, J. (2014). School sport participation during adolescence and mental health in early adulthood. *Journal of Adolescent Health, 55*, 640–4. doi:10.1016/j.jadohealth.2014.04.018

Larsen, K., Cook, B., Stone, M. R., & Faulkner G. E. (2015). Food access and children's BMI in Toronto, Ontario: Assessing how the food environment relates to overweight and obesity. *International Journal of Public Health, 60*, 69–77. doi:10.1007/s00038-014-0620-4

Louveau, A., Smirnov, I., Keyes, T. J., Eccles, J. D., Sherin, J., Rouhani, J., . . . Kipnis, J. (2015). Structural and functional features of central nervous system lymphatic vessels. *Nature.* doi:10.1038/nature14432

Martin Ginis, K. A., Arbour-Nicitopoulos, K. A., Latimer-Cheung, A. E., Buchholz, A. C., Bray, S. R., Craven, B. C., . . . Horrocks, J. (2012). Predictors of leisure time physical activity among people with spinal cord injury. *Annals of Behavioral Medicine, 44*, 104–18. doi:10.1007/s12160-012-9370-9

Martin Ginis, K. A., Latimer-Cheung, A. E., Corkum, S., Ginis, S., Anathasopoulos, P., Arbour- Nicitopoulos, K. P., & Gainforth. H. (2012). A case study of a community-university multidisciplinary partnership approach to increasing physical activity participation among people with spinal cord injury. *Translational Behavioral Medicine, 2*, 516–22. doi:10.1007/s13142-012-0157-0

Martin Ginis, K. A., Phang, S. H., Latimer, A. E., & Arbour-Nicitopoulos, K. P. (2012). Reliability and validity tests of the Leisure Time Physical Activity Questionnaire for People with Spinal Cord Injury. *Archives of Physical Medicine and Rehabilitation, 93*, 677–82. doi: 10.1016/j.apmr.2011.11.005

McGannon, K. R., Gonsalves, C. A., Schinke, R. J., & Busanich, R. (2016). Negotiating motherhood and athletic identity: A qualitative analysis of Olympic athlete mother representations in media narratives. *Psychology of Sport and Exercise, 20*, 51–9. doi:10.1016/j.psychsport.2015.04.010

Mekari, S., Fraser, S., Bosquet, L., Bonnéry, C., Labelle, V., Pouliot, P., . . . Bherer, L. (2015). The relationship between exercise intensity, cerebral oxygenation and cognitive performance in young adults. *European Journal of Applied Physiology, 115*, 189–97.

Mood, D. P., & Morrow, J. R. (2015). *Statistics in human performance.* Scottsdale, AZ: Holcomb Hathaway.

Moola, F., Fusco, C., & Kirsh J. A. (2011). The perceptions of caregivers toward physical activity and health in youth with congenital heart disease. *Qualitative Health Research, 21*, 278–91. doi:10.1177/1049732310384119

Parry, D. C. (2008). The contribution of dragon boat racing to women's health and breast cancer survivorship. *Qualitative Health Research, 18*, 222–33. doi:10.1177/1049732307312304

Passmore, S. R., Burke, J., & Lyons, J. (2007). Older adults demonstrate reduced performance in a Fitts' task involving cervical spine movement. *Adapted Physical Activity Quarterly, 24*, 352–63.

Sabiston, C. M., McDonough, M. H., Sedgwick, W. A., & Crocker, P. R. E. (2009). Muscle gains and emotional strains: Conflicting experiences of change among overweight women participating in an exercise intervention program. *Qualitative Health Research, 19*, 466–80. doi:10.1177/1049732309332782

Simic, L., Sarabon, N., & Markovic, G. (2013). Does pre-exercise static stretching inhibit maximal muscular performance? A meta-analytical review. *Scandinavian Journal of Medicine and Science in Sports, 23*, 131–48. doi:10.1111/j.1600-0838.2012.01444.x

Thomas, J. R., Nelson, J. K., & Silverman, S.J. (2011). *Research methods in physical activity* (6th ed.). Champaign, IL: Human Kinetics.

CHAPTER 3

Annas, G. J., & Grodin, M. A. (Eds.). (1992). *The Nazi doctors and the Nuremberg Code: Human rights in human experimentation.* New York, NY: Oxford University Press.

Arbour, L., & Cook, D. (2006). DNA on loan: Issues to consider when carrying out genetic research with aboriginal families and communities. *Public Health Genomics, 9*, 153–60. doi:10.1159/000092651

Beauchamp, T. L., & Childress, J. F. (2009). *Principles of biomedical ethics* (6th ed.). New York: Oxford University Press.

Canadian Association for Music Therapy. (1999). *Code of ethics.* Waterloo, ON: Wilfrid Laurier University. Retrieved from http://www.musictherapy.ca/about-camt-music-therapy/camt-ethics/

Canadian Council on Animal Care (2015). *CCAC guidelines on: Training of personnel working with animals in science.* Retrieved from http://www.ccac.ca/Documents/Standards/Guidelines/CCAC_Guidelines_on_Training_of_Personnel_Working_With_Animals_in_Science.pdf

Canadian Counselling and Psychotherapy Association (2007). *Code of ethics.* Ottawa, ON: CCA.

Canadian Institutes of Health Research, Natural Sciences and Engineering Research Council of Canada, and Social Sciences and Humanities Research Council of Canada, *Tri-Council Policy Statement: Ethical Conduct for Research Involving Humans,* December 2014. Retrieved from http://www.pre.ethics.gc.ca/pdf/eng/tcps2-2014/TCPS_2_FINAL_Web.pdf

Canadian Medical Association (2004). *CMA code of ethics*. Ottawa, ON: CMA.

Canadian Psychological Association (2000). *Canadian code of ethics for psychologists* (3rd ed.). Ottawa, ON: CPA.

Code of Ethics of the Saskatchewan Kinesiology and Exercises Sciences Association (n.d.). Retrieved March 31, 2014: http://www.skesa.ca/images/pdf/skesa_code_of_ethics.pdf

Cottone, R. R., & Claus, R. E. (2000). Ethical decision-making models: A review of the literature. *Journal of Counseling and Development, 78*, 275–83.

Janes, I. W. C., Snow, B. B. G., Watkins, C. E., Noseworthy, E. A. L., Reid, J. C., & Behm, D. G. (2016). Effect of participants' static stretching knowledge or deception on the responses to prolonged stretching. *Applied Physiology, Nutrition, and Metabolism, 41*(10), 1052–6. doi:10.1139/apnm-2016-0241

Lambert, J. E., Myslicki, J. P., Bomhof, M. R., Belke, D. D., Shearer, J., & Reimer, R. A. (2015). Exercise training modifies gut microbiota in normal and diabetic mice. *Applied Physiology, Nutrition, and Metabolism, 40*(7), 749–52. doi:10.1139/apnm-2014-0452

Lévesque, L., Guilbault, G., Delormier, T., & Potvin, L. (2005). Unpacking the black box: A deconstruction of the programming approach and physical activity interventions implemented in the Kahnawake Schools Diabetes Prevention Project. *Health Promotion Practice, 6*, 64–71. doi:10.1177/1524839903260156

Longtin, R. (2004). Canadian province seeks control of its genes. *Journal of the National Cancer Institute, 96*(21), 1567–9. doi:10.1093/jnci/96.21.1567

Malloy, D. C., Ross, S., & Zakus, D. H. (2003). *Sport ethics: Concepts and cases in sport and recreation* (2nd ed.). Toronto, ON: Thompson Educational Publishing.

McHugh, T.-L. F., Coppola, A. M., & Sinclair, S. (2013). An exploration of the meanings of sport to urban Aboriginal youth: A photovoice approach. *Qualitative Research in Sport, Exercise and Health, 5*, 291–311. do i:10.1080/2159676X.2013.819375

Mosby, I. (2013). Administering colonial science: Nutrition research and human biomedical experimentation in Aboriginal communities and residential schools, 1942–1952. *Histoire sociale/Social history, 46*, 145–72. doi:10.1353/his.2013.0015

Neary, J. P., Malbon, L., & McKenzie, D. C. (2002). Relationship between serum, saliva and urinary cortisol and its implication during recovery from training. *Journal of Science and Medicine in Sport, 5*(2), 108–14. doi:10.1016/S1440-2440(02)80031-7

Paradis, G., Lévesque, L., Macaulay, A. C., Cargo, M., McComber, A., Kirby, R., . . . Potvin, L. (2005). Impact of a diabetes prevention program on body size, physical activity, and diet among Kanien'kehá:ka (Mohawk) children 6 to 11 years old: 8-year results from the Kahnawake Schools Diabetes Prevention Project. *Pediatrics, 115*, 333–9. doi:10.1542/peds.2004-0745

Rothman, D. J. (1982). Were Tuskegee & Willowbrook's studies in nature? *Hastings Centre Report, 12*, 5–7. doi:10.2307/3561798

Smith, L. T. (2012). *Decolonizing methodologies: Research and Indigenous peoples*. New York, NY: Zed books.

Somerville, M. A. (2002). A postmodern moral tale: The ethics of research relationships. *Nature Reviews Drug Discovery, 1*, 316–20. doi:10.1038/nrd773

Thompson, J., Baird, P., & Downie, J. (2001). *The Olivieri Report: The complete text of the report of the independent inquiry commissioned by the Canadian Association of University Teachers*. Toronto, ON: James Lorimer & Company.

Truscott, D., & Crook, K. H. (2013). *Ethics for the practice of psychology in Canada* (revised and expanded edition). Edmonton, AB: The University of Alberta Press.

Welfel, E. R. (2006). *Ethics in counseling and psychotherapy: Standards, research, and emerging issues* (3rd ed.). Belmont, CA: Thomson Brooks/Cole.

Welfel, E. R. (2012). *Ethics in counseling and psychotherapy: Standards, research, and emerging issues* (5th ed.). Belmont, CA: Thomson Brooks/Cole.

Zur, O. (2011). *Gifts in psychotherapy*. Retrieved 05/26/2014 from http://www.zurinstitute.com/giftsintherapy.html.

CHAPTER 4

Campbell, D. T., & Stanley, J. C. (1963). Experimental and quasi-experimental designs for research on teaching. In N. L. Gage (Ed.), *Handbook of research on teaching* (pp. 171–246). Chicago, IL: Rand McNally

Courneya, K. S., Karvinen, K. H., McNeely, M. L., Campbell, K. L., Brar, S., Woolcott, C. G., . . . Friedenreich, C. M. (2012). Predictors of adherence to supervised and unsupervised exercise in the Alberta Physical Activity and Breast Cancer Prevention Trial. *Journal of Physical Activity and Health, 9*, 857–66. doi:10.1186/s12966-014-0085-0

Courneya, K. S., Sellar, C. M., Trinh, L., Forbes, C. C., Stevinson, C., McNeely, M. L., . . . Reiman, T. (2012). A randomized trial of aerobic exercise and sleep quality in lymphoma patients receiving chemotherapy or no treatments. *Cancer Epidemiology, Biomarkers & Prevention, 21*, 887–94. doi:10.1158/1055-9965.EPI-12-0075

Courneya, K. S., Stevinson, C., McNeely, M. L., Sellar, C. M., Friedenreich, C. M., Peddle-McIntyre, C. J., . . . Reiman, T. (2012). Effects of supervised exercise on motivational outcomes and longer term behavior. *Medicine & Science in Sports & Exercise, 44*, 542–9. doi:10.1249/MSS.0b013e3182301e06

Creswell, J. W. (2009). *Research design: Qualitative, quantitative, and mixed methods approaches* (3rd ed.). Los Angeles, CA: Sage.

Creswell, J. W. (2014). *Research design: Qualitative, quantitative, and mixed methods approaches* (4th ed.). Thousand Oaks, CA: Sage.

Field, A., & Hole, G. (2003). *How to design and report experiments.* London, England: Sage.

Guenette, J. A., Martens, A. M., Lee, A. L., Tyler, G. D., Richards, J. C., Foster, G. E., . . . Sheel, A. W. (2006). Variable effects of respiratory muscle training on cycle exercise performance in men and women. *Applied Physiology, Nutrition, and Metabolism, 31*, 159–66. doi:10.1139/H05-016

Herman, K. M., Sabiston, C. M., Mathieu, M. E., Tremblay, A., & Paradis, G. (2015). Correlates of sedentary behaviour in 8- to 10-year-old children at elevated risk for obesity. *Applied Physiology, Nutrition, and Metabolism, 40*, 10–19. doi:10.1139/apnm-2014-0039

Scarapicchia, T., Garcia, E., Andersen, R., & Sabiston, C. M. (2013). The motivational effects of social contagion on exercise participation in young female adults. *Journal of Sport & Exercise Psychology, 35*, 563–75.

Tikuisis, P., Jacobs, I., Moroz, D., Vallerand, A. L., & Martineau, L. (2000). Comparison of thermoregulatory responses between men and women immersed in cold water. *Journal of Applied Physiology, 89*, 1403–11.

Vanderloo, L. M., & Tucker, P. (2015). Weekly trends in preschoolers' physical activity and sedentary time in childcare. *International Journal of Environmental Research and Public Health, 12*, 2454–64. doi:10.3390/ijerph120302454

CHAPTER 5

Cochran, A. J. C., Little, J. P., Tarnopolsky, M. A., & Gibala, M. J. (2010). Carbohydrate feeding during recovery alters the skeletal muscle metabolic response to repeated sessions of high-intensity interval exercise in humans. *Journal of Applied Physiology, 108*, 628–36. doi:10.1152/japplphysiol.00659.2009

Cohen, J. (1988). *Statistical power analysis for the behavioral sciences.* Hillsdale, NJ: Lawrence Erlbaum Associates.

Cooper, H., Hedges, L. V., & Valentine, J. C. (2009). *The handbook of research synthesis and meta-analysis* (2nd ed.). New York, NY: Russell Sage.

Field, A., & Hole, G. (2003). *How to design and report experiments.* London, England: Sage.

Fisher, R. A. (1956). *Statistical methods and scientific inference.* New York: Hafner.

Garriguet, D., Tremblay, S., & Colley, R. (2015). Comparison of Physical Activity Adult Questionnaire results with accelerometer data. *Health Reports, 26*, 11–17.

Gibala, M. J., Little, J. P., MacDonald, M. J., & Hawley, J. A. (2012). Physiological adaptations to low-volume, high-intensity interval training in health and disease. *Journal of Physiology, 590*, 1077–84. doi:10.1113/jphysiol.2011.224725

Ichinose-Kuwahara, T., Inoue, Y., Iseki, Y., Hara, S., Ogura, Y., & Kondo, N. (2010). Sex differences in the effects of physical training on sweat gland responses during a graded exercise. *Experimental Physiology, 95*, 1026–32. doi:10.1113/expphysiol.2010.053710

Moher, D., Liberati, A., Tetzlaff, J., Altman, D. G., & The PRISMA Group (2009). Preferred Reporting Items for Systematic Reviews and Meta-Analyses: The PRISMA Statement. *PLoS Med 6*(7): e1000097. doi:10.1371/journal.pmed1000097

Thomas, J., Nelson, J., & Silverman, S. (2015). *Research methods in physical activity* (7th ed.). Champaign, IL: Human Kinetics.

Tjønna, A. E., Leinan, I. M., Bartnes, A. T., Jenssen, B. M., Gibala, M. J., Winett, R. A., & Wisløff, U. (2013). Low- and high-volume of intensive endurance training significantly improves maximal oxygen uptake after 10-weeks of training in healthy men. *PLoS ONE, 8*, e65382. doi:10.1371/journal.pone.0065382

Vincent, W., & Weir, J. (2012). *Statistics in kinesiology* (4th ed.). Champaign, IL: Human Kinetics.

CHAPTER 6

Colley, R. C., Garriguet, D., Janssen, I., Craig, C. L., Clarke, J., & Tremblay, M. S. (2011). *Physical activity of Canadian adults: Accelerometer results from the 2007 to 2009 Canadian Health Measures Survey.* Health Reports (Statistics Canada, Catalogue 82-003), 22, 1–9.

Henrich, J., Heine, S. J., & Norenzayan, A. (2010). The weirdest people in the world? *Behavioral and Brain Sciences, 33*, 61–83. doi:10.1017/S0140525X0999152X

Hurtubise, J. M., Beech, C., & Macpherson, A. (2015). Comparing severe injuries by sex and sport in collegiate-level athletes: A descriptive epidemiological study. *International Journal of Athletic Therapy and Injury, 20*, 44–50. doi:10.1123/ijatt.2014-0090

Knudson, D., Elliott, B., & Ackland, T. (2012). Citation of evidence for research and application in kinesiology. *Kinesiology Review, 1*, 129–36.

Kowalski, K. C., Crocker, P. R. E., & Faulkner, R. A. (1997). Validation of the Physical Activity Questionnaire for Older Children. *Pediatric Exercise Science, 9*, 174–86.

Messick, S. (1989). Validity. In R. L. Linn (Ed.), *Educational measurement* (3rd ed.; pp. 13-103). New York: Macmillan.

Moher, D., Hopewell, S., Schulz, K. F., Montori, V., Gotzsche, P. C., Devereaux, P. J., . . . Altman, D. G. (2010). CONSORT 2010 explanation and elaboration: Updated guidelines for reporting parallel group randomized trials. *BMJ, 340*, c869. doi:10.1136/bmj.c869

Moore, J. B, Hanes, Jr., J. C., Barbeau, P., Gutin, B., Trevino, R. P., & Yin, Z. (2007). Validation of the Physical Activity Questionnaire for Older Children in children of different races. *Pediatric Exercise Science, 19*, 6–19.

Mullan, E., Markland, D., & Ingledew, D. K. (1997). A graded conceptualization of self-determination in the regulation of exercise behavior: Development of a measure using confirmatory factor analysis procedures. *Personality and Individual Differences, 23*, 745–52. doi:10.1016/S0191-8869(97)00107-4

Plotnikoff, R. C., Courneya, K. S., Sigal, R. J., Johnson, J. A., Birkett, N., Lau, D., . . . Karunamuni, N. (2010). Alberta Diabetes and Physical Activity Trial (ADAPT): A randomized theory-based efficacy trial for adults with type 2 diabetes–rationale, design, recruitment, evaluation, and dissemination. *Trials, 11*, 1–10. doi:10.1186/1745-6215-11-4

Schultz, K. F., Altman, D. G., Moher, D., & CONSORT Group (2010). CONSORT 2010 statement: Updated guidelines for reporting parallel group randomized trials. *Annals of Internal Medicine, 152*, 726–32. doi:10.7326/0003-4819-152-11-201006010-00232

Skelly, L. E., Andrews, P. C., Gillen, J. B., Martin, B. J., Percival, M. E., & Gibala, M. J. (2014). High-intensity interval exercise induces 24-h energy expenditure similar to traditional endurance exercise despite reduced time commitment. *Applied Physiology Nutrition and Metabolism, 39*, 1–4. doi:10.1139/apnm-2013-0562

Troiano, R. P., Berrigan, D., Dodd, K. W., Masse, L. C., Tilert, T., & McDowell, M. (2008). Physical activity in the United States measured by accelerometer. *Medicine and Science in Sports and Exercise, 40*, 181–8. doi:10.1249/mss.0b013e31815a51b3

CHAPTER 7

Atkinson, M. (2008). Triathlon, suffering and exciting significance. *Leisure Studies, 27*, 165–80. doi:10.1080/02614360801902216

Banerjee, A. T., Grace, S. L., Thomas, S. G., & Faulkner, G. (2010). Cultural factors facilitating cardiac rehabilitation participation among Canadian South Asians: A qualitative study. *Heart & Lung: The Journal of Acute and Critical Care, 39*, 494–503. doi:10.1016/j.hrtlng.2009.10.021

Berry, K. A., Kowalski, K. C., Ferguson, L. J., & McHugh, T.-L. F. (2010). An empirical phenomenology of young adult women exercisers' body self-compassion. *Qualitative Research in Sport and Exercise, 2*, 293–312.

Busanich, R., McGannon, K. R., & Schinke, R. J. (2012). Expanding understandings of the body, food and exercise relationship in distance runners: A narrative approach. *Psychology of Sport and Exercise, 13*, 582–90. doi:10.1016/j.psychsport.2012.03.005

Camiré, M., Trudel, P., & Bernard, D. (2013). A case study of a high school sport program designed to teach athletes life skills and values. *The Sport Psychologist, 27*, 188–200.

Caron, J. G., Bloom, G. A., Johnston, K. M., & Sabiston, C. M. (2013). National Hockey League players' experiences with career-ending concussions. *British Journal of Sports Medicine, 47*, e1. doi:10.1136/bjsports-2012-092101.43

Charmaz, K. (2014). *Constructing grounded theory* (2nd ed.). Thousand Oaks, CA: Sage.

Creswell, J. W. (2013). *Qualitative inquiry and research design: Choosing among five approaches* (3rd ed.). Thousand Oaks, CA: Sage.

Cusimano, M. D., Sharma, B., Lawrence, D. W., Ilie, G., Silverberg, S., & Jones, R. (2013). Trends in North American newspaper reporting of brain injury in ice hockey. *PLoS ONE, 8*, e61865. doi:10.1371/journal.pone.0061865

Giacobbi Jr, P., Hausenblas, H., Fallon, E., & Hall, C. (2003). Even more about exercise imagery: A grounded theory of exercise imagery. *Journal of Applied Sport Psychology, 15*, 160–175. doi:10.1080/10413200390213858

Giles, A. R., Castleden, H., & Baker, A. C. (2010). "We listen to our Elders. You live longer that way": Examining aquatic risk communication and water safety practices in Canada's North. *Health and Place, 16*, 1–9. doi:10.1016/j.healthplace.2009.05.007

Giles, A. R., & Darroch, F. E. (2014). The need for culturally safe physical activity promotion programs. *Canadian Journal of Public Health, 105*(4), e317–e319.

Holt, N. L., & Dunn, J. G. (2004). Toward a grounded theory of the psychosocial competencies and environmental conditions associated with soccer success. *Journal of Applied Sport Psychology, 16*, 199–219. doi:10.1080/10413200490437949

Holt, N. L, Spence, J. C., Sehn, Z. L., & Cutumisu, N. (2008). Neighborhood and developmental differences in children's perceptions of opportunities for play and physical activity. *Health & Place, 14*, 2–14. doi:10.1016/j.healthplace.2007.03.002

Humbert, M. L., Chad, K. E., Spink, K. S., Muhajarine, N., Anderson, K. D., Bruner, M. W., . . . Gryba, C. R. (2006). Factors that influence physical activity participation among high-and low-SES youth. *Qualitative Health Research, 16*, 467–83. doi:10.1177/1049732305286051

Huybers-Withers, S. M., & Livingston, L. A. (2010). Mountain biking is for men: Consumption practices and identity portrayed by a niche magazine. *Sport in Society, 13*(7–8), 1204–22. doi:10.1080/17430431003780195

Kentel, J. L., & McHugh, T.-L. F. (2015). "Mean Mugging": An exploration of young Aboriginal women's experiences of bullying in team sports. *Journal of Sport & Exercise Psychology, 37*, 367–78. doi:10.1123/jsep.2014-0291

Knight, C. J., & Holt, N. L. (2014). Parenting in youth tennis: Understanding and enhancing children's experiences. *Psychology of Sport and Exercise, 15*, 155–64. doi:10.1016/j.psychsport.2013.10.010

Kuttai, H. (2010). *Maternity rolls: Pregnancy, childbirth, and disability*. Halifax, NS: Fernwood Publishing.

Leipert, B., Scruby, L., & Meagher-Stewart, D. (2014). Sport, health, and rural community: Curling and rural women: A national photovoice study. *Journal of Rural & Community Development, 9*, 128–43.

LeVasseur, J. J. (2003). The problem of bracketing in phenomenology. *Qualitative Health Research, 13*, 408–20.

MacDonald, D. J., Beck, K., Erickson, K., & Côté, J. (2015). Understanding sources of knowledge for coaches of athletes with intellectual disabilities. *Journal of Applied Research in Intellectual Disabilities, 29*, 242–49. doi:10.111/jar.12174

Mayan, M. J. (2009). *Essentials of qualitative inquiry*. Walnut Creek, CA: Left Coast Press.

McHugh, T.-L. F., Coppola, A. M., Holt, N. L., & Andersen, C. (2015). "Sport is community": An exploration of urban Aboriginal peoples' meanings of community within the context of sport. *Psychology of Sport and Exercise, 18*, 75–84. doi:10.1016/j.psychsport.2015.01.005

Morse, J. M. (2000). Determining sample size. *Qualitative Health Research, 10*, 3–5. doi:10.1080/15459624.2013.843780

Patton, M. Q. (2002). *Qualitative research and evaluation methods* (3rd ed.). Thousand Oakes, CA: Sage.

Rossow-Kimball, B., & Goodwin, D. L. (2014). Inclusive leisure experiences of older adults with intellectual disabilities at a senior centre. *Leisure Studies, 33*, 322–38. doi:10.1080/02614367.2013.768692

Sabiston, C. M., McDonough, M. H., & Crocker, P. R. (2007). Psychosocial experiences of breast cancer survivors involved in a dragon boat program: Exploring links to positive psychological growth. *Journal of Sport and Exercise Psychology, 29*, 419–38.

Sandelowski, M. (1993). Theory unmasked: The uses and guises of theory in qualitative research. *Research in Nursing & Health, 16*, 213–18. doi:10.1002/nur.4770160308

Sandelowski, M. (2000). Focus on research methods—whatever happened to qualitative description? *Research in Nursing and Health, 23*, 334–40.

Stake, R. E. (1995). *The art of case study research*. Thousand Oakes, CA: Sage.

Strachan, L., & Davies, K. (2015). Click! Using photo elicitation to explore youth experiences and positive youth development in sport. *Qualitative Research in Sport, Exercise and Health, 7*, 170–91.

Sutherland, L. M., Kowalski, K. C., Ferguson, L. J., Sabiston, C. M., Sedgwick, W. A., & Crocker, P. R. (2014). Narratives of young women athletes' experiences of emotional pain and self-compassion. *Qualitative Research in Sport, Exercise and Health, 6*, 499–516.

Tamminen, K. A., Faulkner, G., Witcher, C. S., & Spence, J. C. (2014). A qualitative examination of the impact of microgrants to promote physical activity among adolescents. *BMC Public Health, 14*, 1–26. doi:10.1186/1471-2458-14-1206

Tamminen, K. A., & Holt, N. L. (2012). Adolescent athletes' learning about coping and the roles of parents and coaches. *Psychology of Sport and Exercise, 13*, 69–79. doi:10.1016/j.psychsport.2011.07.006

VanWynsberghe, R., & Khan, S. (2007). Redefining case study. International *Journal of Qualitative Methods, 6*, 80–94.

CHAPTER 8

Bradley, E. H., Curry, L. A., & Devers, K. J. (2007). Qualitative data analysis for health services research: Developing taxonomy, themes, and theory. *Health Services Research, 42*, 1758–72. doi:10.1111/j.1475-6773.2006.00684.x

Creswell, J. W. (2013). *Qualitative inquiry and research design: Choosing among five approaches* (3rd ed.). Thousand Oaks, CA: Sage.

Creswell, J. W. (2014). *Research design: Qualitative, quantitative, and mixed methods approaches* (4th ed.). Thousand Oaks, CA: Sage.

Crocker, P. R. E., Mosewich, A. D., Kowalski, K. C., & Besenski, L. J. (2010). Coping: Research design and analysis issues. In A. R. Nicholls (Ed.), *Coping in sport:*

Theory, methods, and related constructs (pp. 53–76). New York: Nova Science Publishers.

Donen, R. M. (2007). *Movement and stillness: Mindfulness and the art of inquiry*. University of Saskatchewan Electronic Theses and Dissertations.

Elo, S., & Kyngäs, H. (2007). The qualitative content analysis process. *Journal of Advanced Nursing, 62*, 107–15. doi: 10.1111/j.1365-2648.2007.04569.x

Ferguson, L., & Philipenko, N. (2016). "I would love to blast some pow music and just dance": First Nations students' experiences of physical activity on a university campus. *Qualitative Research in Sport, Exercise and Health, 8*, 180–93. doi:10.1080/2159676X.2015.1099563

Horton, S., MacDonald, D. J., Erickson, K., & Dionigi, R. A. (2015). A qualitative investigation of exercising with MS and the impact on the spousal relationship. *European Review of Aging and Physical Activity, 12*, 3. doi:10.1186/s11556-015-0148-5

Hseih, H.-F., & Shannon, S. E. (2005). Three approaches to qualitative content analysis. *Qualitative Health Research, 15*, 1277–88. doi:10.1177/1049732305276687

Humble, A. M. (2012). Qualitative data analysis software: A call for understanding, detail, intentionality, and thoughtfulness. *Journal of Family Theory and Review, 4*, 122–37. doi:10.1111/j.1756-2589.2012.00125.x

Kodish, S., & Gittelsohn, J. (2011). Systematic data analysis in qualitative health research: Building credible and clear findings. *Sight and Life, 25*, 52–6.

Kowalski, K. C., Mack, D. E., Crocker, P. R. E., Niefer, C. B., & Fleming, T.-L. (2006). Coping with social physique anxiety in adolescence. *Journal of Adolescent Health, 39*, 275.e9–275.e16. doi:10.1016/j.jadohealth.2005.12.015

Kuttai, H. (2010). *Maternity rolls: Pregnancy, childbirth, and disability*. Halifax, NS: Fernwood Publishing.

Laliberte Rudman, D. (2015). Embodying positive aging and neoliberal rationality: Talking about the aging body within narratives of retirement. *Journal of Aging Studies, 34*, 10–20. doi:10.1016/j.jaging.2015.03.005

Leech, N. L., & Onwuegbuzie, A. J. (2008). Qualitative data analysis: A compendium of techniques and a framework for selection for school psychology research and beyond. *School Psychology Quarterly, 23*, 587–604. doi:10.1037/1045-3830.23.4.587

McArthur, D., Dumas, A., Woodend, K., Beach, S., & Stacey, D. (2014). Factors influencing adherence to regular exercise in middle-aged women: A qualitative study to inform clinical practice. *BMC Women's Health, 14*, 49. doi:10.1186/1472-6874-14-49

McHugh, T.-L., F., & Kowalski, K. C. (2011). "A new view of body image": A school-based participatory action research project with young Aboriginal women. *Action Research, 9*, 220–41. doi:10.1177/1476750310388052

Moola, F. J., & Faulkner, G. E. J. (2014). "A tale of two cases": The health, illness, and physical activity stories of two children living with cystic fibrosis. *Clinical Child Psychology and Psychiatry, 19*, 24–42. doi:10.1177/1359104512465740

Moola, F. J., Faulkner, G., White, L., & Kirsh, J. (2015). Kids with special hearts: The experience of children with congenital heart disease at Camp Woodland. *Qualitative Research in Sport, Exercise, and Health, 7*, 271–93. doi:10.1080/2159676X.2014.926968

O'Reilly, E., Tompkins, J., & Gallant, M. (2001). "They ought to enjoy physical activity, you know?": Struggling with fun in physical education. *Sport, Education, and Society, 6*, 211–21.

Patton, M. Q. (2002). *Qualitative research and evaluation methods* (3rd ed.). Thousand Oaks, CA: Sage.

Poland, B. D. (1995). Transcription quality as an aspect of rigor in qualitative research. *Qualitative Inquiry, 1*, 290–310.

Sabiston, C. M., Sedgwick, W. A., Crocker, P. R. E., Kowalski, K. C., & Mack, D. E. (2007). Social physique anxiety in adolescence: An exploration of influences, coping strategies, and health behaviors. *Journal of Adolescent Research, 22*, 78–101. doi:10.1177/0743558406294628

Sparkes, A. C., & Smith, B. (2014). *Qualitative research methods in sport, exercise and health: From process to product*. London: Routledge.

Stake, R. E. (1995). *The art of case study research*. Thousand Oakes, CA: Sage.

Taylor, S. L., Werthner, P., & Culver, D. (2014). A case study of a parasport coach and a life of learning. *International Sport Coaching Journal, 1*, 127–38. doi:10.1123/iscj.2013-0005

Tjong, V. K., Murnaghan, M. L., Nyhof-Young, J. M., & Ogilvie-Harris, D. J. (2013). A qualitative investigation of the decision to return to sport after anterior cruciate ligament reconstruction: To play or not to play. *American Journal of Sports Medicine, 42*, 336–42. doi:10.1177/0363546513508762

Webster, F., Perruccio, A. V., Jenkinson, R., Jaglal, S., Schemitsch, E., Waddell, J. P., . . . Davis, A. M. (2015). Understanding why people do or do not engage in activities following total joint replacement: A longitudinal qualitative study. *Osteoarthritis and Cartilage, 23*, 860–7. doi:10.1016/j.joca.2015.02.013

Witcher, C. S. G. (2010). Negotiating transcription as a relative insider: Implications for rigor. *International Journal of Qualitative Methods, 9*, 122–32.

Woods, M., Paulus, T., Atkins, D. P., & Macklin, R. (2016). Advancing qualitative research using qualitative data analysis software (QDAS)? Reviewing potential versus practice in published studies using ATLAS.ti and NVivo, 1994–2013. *Social Science Computer Review, 34*, 597–617. doi:10.1177/0894439315596311

CHAPTER 9

Agha, A., Liu-Ambrose, T. Y. L., Backman, C. L., Leese, J., & Li, L. C. (2015). Understanding the experiences of rural community-dwelling older adults in using a new DVD-delivered Otago Exercise Program: A qualitative study. *Interactive Journal of Medical Research, 4*, e17. doi:10.2196/ijmr.4257

Bailey, K. A., Cline, L. E., & Gammage, K. L. (2016). Exploring the complexities of body image experiences in middle age and older adult women within an exercise context: The simultaneous existence of negative and positive body images. *Body Image, 17*, 88–99. doi:10.1016/j.bodyim.2016.02.007

Balish, S., & Côté, J. (2014). The influence of community on athletic development: An integrated case study. *Qualitative Research in Sport, Exercise and Health, 6*, 98–120. doi:10.1080/2159676X.2013.766815

Côté, J. (1999). The influence of the family in the development of talent in sport. *The Sport Psychologist, 13*, 395–417.

Creswell, J. W. (2014). *Research design: Qualitative, quantitative, and mixed methods approaches* (4th ed.). Thousand Oaks, CA: Sage.

Davies, D., & Dodd, J. (2002). Qualitative research and the question of rigor. *Qualitative Health Research, 12*, 279–89. doi:10.1177/104973230201200211

Ferguson, L. J., Kowalski, K. C., Mack, D. E., & Sabiston, C. M. (2014). Exploring self-compassion and eudaimonic well-being in young women athletes. *Journal of Sport and Exercise Psychology, 36*, 203–16. doi:10.1123/jsep.2013-0096

Guba, E. G. (1981). Criteria for assessing trustworthiness of naturalistic inquiries. *Educational Communication and Technology, 29*, 75–91.

Haverkamp, B. E. (2005). Ethical perspectives on qualitative research in applied psychology. *Journal of Counseling Psychology, 52*, 146–55. doi:10.1037/0022-0167.52.2.146

Kirby, A. M., Lévesque, L., & Wabano, V. (2007). A qualitative investigation of physical activity challenges and opportunities in a northern-rural, Aboriginal community: Voices from within. *Pimatisiwin: A Journal of Aboriginal and Indigenous Community Health, 5*, 5–24.

Morse, J. M. (1999). The armchair walkthrough. *Qualitative Health Research, 9*, 435–6. doi:10.1177/104973299129121956

Morse, J. M., Barrett, M., Mayan, M., Olson, K., & Spiers, J. (2002). Verification strategies for establishing reliability and validity in qualitative research. *International Journal of Qualitative Methods, 1*, 13–22. doi:10.1177/160940690200100202

Patton, M. Q. (2002). *Qualitative research and evaluation methods* (3rd ed.). Thousand Oaks, CA: Sage.

Protudjer, J. L. P., Dumontet, J., & McGavock, J. M. (2014). My voice: A grounded theory analysis of the lived experience of type 2 diabetes in adolescence. *Canadian Journal of Diabetes, 38*, 229–36. doi:10.1016/j.jcjd.2014.05.008

Schinke, R. J., Smith, B., & McGannon, K. R. (2013). Pathways for community research in sport and physical activity: Criteria for consideration. *Qualitative Research in Sport, Exercise and Health, 5*, 460–8.

Seale, C. (1999). *The quality of qualitative research*. London: Sage.

Shannon, C. S. (2016). Exploring factors influencing girls' continued participation in competitive dance. *Journal of Leisure Research, 48*(4), 284–306.

Sparkes, A. C., & Smith, B. (2009). Judging the quality of qualitative inquiry: Criteriology and relativism in action. *Psychology of Sport and Exercise, 10*, 491–7. doi:10.1016/j.psychsport.2009.02.006

Sparkes, A. C., & Smith, B. (2014). *Qualitative research methods in sport, exercise and health: From process to product*. London: Routledge.

Thomas-MacLean, R., Spriggs, P., Quinlan, E., Towers, A., Hack, T., Tatemichi, S., . . . Tilley, A. (2010). Arm morbidity and disability: Reporting the current status from Canada. *Journal of Lymphoedema, 5*, 33–8.

Thomas-MacLean, R., Towers, A., Quinlan, E., Hack, T., Kwan, W., Miedema, B., . . . Graham, P. (2009). "This is a kind of betrayal": A qualitative study of disability after breast cancer. *Current Oncology, 16*, 26–32. doi:10.3747/co.v16i3.389

Tong, A., Sainsbury, P., & Craig, J. (2007). Consolidated criteria for reporting qualitative research (COREQ): A 32-item checklist for interviews and focus groups. *International Journal for Quality in Health Care, 19*, 349–57. doi:10.1093/intqhc/mzm042

Wozniak, L., Soprovich, A., Mundt, C., Johnson, J. A., & Johnson, S. T. (2015). Contextualizing the proven effectiveness of a lifestyle intervention for type 2 diabetes in primary care: A qualitative assessment based on the RE-AIM framework. *Canadian Journal of Diabetes, 39*, S92–S99. doi:10.1016/j.jcjd.2015.05.003

Yi, K. J., Landais, E., Kolahdooz, F., & Sharma, S. (2015). Factors influencing the health and wellness of urban Aboriginal youths in Canada: Insights of in-service professionals, care providers, and stakeholders. *Framing Health Matters, 105*, 881–90.

CHAPTER 10

Andrew, S., & Halcomb, E. J. (Eds.). (2009). *Mixed methods research for nursing and the health sciences.* Chichester: Wiley-Blackwell.

Bélanger, M., Caissie, I., Beauchamp, J., O'Loughlin, J., Sabiston, C., & Mancuso, M. (2013). Monitoring activities of teenagers to comprehend their habits: Study protocol for a mixed-methods cohort study. *BMC Public Health, 13*, 649. doi:10.1186/1471-2458-13-649

Bills, K. J. (2012). Just a walk in the park, or is it? A case study analysis of a Seniors Community Park in Oak Bay, British Columbia. (Master's thesis). Available from ProQuest Dissertations and Theses Global. (MR94765)

Brunet, J., & Sabiston, C. M. (2011). Self-presentation and physical activity in breast cancer survivors: The moderating effect of social cognitive constructs. *Journal of Sport & Exercise Psychology, 3*, 759–78.

Brunet, J., Taran, S., Burke, S., & Sabiston, C. M. (2013). A qualitative exploration of barriers and motivators to physical activity participation in women treated for breast cancer. *Disability and Rehabilitation, 35*, 2038–45. doi:10.3109/09638288.2013.802378

Castonguay, A. L., Sabiston, C. M., Crocker, P. R. E., & Mack, D. E. (2014). Development and validation of the Body and Appearance Self-Conscious Emotions Scale (BASES). *Body Image, 11*, 126–36. doi:10.1016/j.bodyim.2013.12.006

Castonguay, A. L., Sabiston, C. M., Kowalski, K. C., & Wilson, P. M. (2016). Introducing an instrument to measure body and fitness-related self-conscious emotions: The BSE-FIT. *Psychology of Sport and Exercise, 23*, 1–12. doi:10.1016/j.psychsport.2015.10.003

Creswell, J. W. (2014). *Research design: Qualitative, quantitative, and mixed methods approaches* (4th ed.). Thousand Oaks, CA: Sage.

Creswell, J. W., & Plano Clark, V. L. (2011). *Designing and conducting mixed methods research* (2nd ed.). Thousand Oaks, CA: Sage.

Ferguson, L. J., Kowalski, K. C., Mack, D. E., Wilson, P. M., & Crocker, P. R. E. (2012). Women's health-enhancing physical activity and eudaimonic well-being. *Research Quarterly for Exercise and Sport, 83*, 451–63. doi:10.1080/02701367.2012.10599880

Harvey, W. J., Reid, G., Bloom, G. A., Staples, K., Grizenko, N., Mbekou, V., . . . Joober, R. (2009). Physical activity experiences of boys with and without ADHD. *Adapted Physical Activity Quarterly, 26*, 131–50.

Henrich, J., Heine, S. J., & Norenzayan, A. (2010). The weirdest people in the world? *Behavioral and Brain Sciences, 33*, 61–83. doi:10.1017/S0140525X0999152X

Huynh, E., Rand, D., McNeill, C., Brown, S., Senechal, M., Wicklow, B., . . . McGavock, J. (2015). Beating diabetes together: A mixed-methods analysis of a feasibility study of intensive lifestyle intervention for youth with type 2 diabetes. Canadian *Journal of Diabetes, 39*, 484–90. doi:10.1016/j.jcjd.2015.09.093

Knudson, D., Elliott, B., & Ackland, T. (2012). Citation of evidence for research and application in kinesiology. *Kinesiology Review, 1*, 129–36.

Mason, J. (2006a). Six strategies for mixing methods and linking data in social science research. In *Real Life Methods, Sociology.* University of Manchester.

Mason, J. (2006b). Mixing methods in a qualitatively driven way. *Qualitative Research, 6*, 9–25. doi:10.1177/1468794106058866

McTaggart-Cowan, H. M., O'Cathain, A., Tsuchiya, A., & Brazier, J. E. (2012). Using mixed methods research to explore the effect of an adaptation exercise on general population valuations of health states. *Quality Life Research, 21*, 465–73. doi:10.1007/s11136-011-9994-4

Mercer, K., Giangregorio, L., Schneider, E., Chilana, P., Li, M., & Grindrod, K. (2016). Acceptance of commercially available wearable activity trackers among adults aged over 50 and with chronic illness: A mixed-methods evaluation. *JMIR mHealth and uHealth, 4*, e7. doi:10.2196/mhealth.4225

Mistry, C. D., Sweet, S. N., Rhodes, R. E., & Latimer-Cheung, A. E. (2015). Text2Plan: Exploring changes in the quantity and quality of action plans and physical activity in a text messaging intervention. *Psychology & Health, 30*, 839–56. doi:10.1080/08870446.2014.997731

Naylor, P.-J., McConnell, J., Rhodes, R. E., Barr, S. I., Ghement, I., & Scott, J. (2014). Efficacy of a minimal dose school fruit and vegetable snack intervention. *Journal of Food & Nutritional Disorders, 3*, 4. doi:10.4172/2324-9323.1000147

Naylor, P.-J., Tomlin, D., Rhodes, R., & McConnell, J. (2014). Screen Smart: Evaluation of a brief school facilitated and family focused intervention to encourage children to manage their screen-time. *Child & Adolescent Behavior, 2*, 1. doi:10.4172/jcalb.1000124

Rhodes, R. E., Murray, H., Temple, V. A., Tuokko, H., & Higgins, J. W. (2012). Pilot study of a dog walking randomized intervention: Effects of a focus on canine exercise. *Preventive Medicine, 54*, 309–12. doi:10.1016/j.ypmed.2012.02.014

Robinson, D. B., & Randall, L. (2016). Smooth sailing or stormy seas? Atlantic Canadian physical educators on the state and future of physical education. *Canadian Journal of Education, 39*, 1–31.

Sparkes, A. C. (2015). Developing mixed methods research in sport and exercise psychology: Critical reflections on five points of controversy. *Psychology of Sport and Exercise, 16*, 49–59. doi:10.1016/j.psychsport.2014.08.014

Tremblay, M. S., LeBlanc, A. G., Carson, V., Choquette, L., Connor Gorber, S., Dillman, C., . . . Spence, J. C. (2012). Canadian sedentary behaviour guidelines for the early years (aged 0-4 years). *Applied Physiology, Nutrition, and Metabolism, 37*, 370–80. doi:10.1139/H2012-019

Wilson, P. M., Rodgers, W. M., Loitz, C. C., & Scime, G. (2006). "It's who I am . . . really!" The importance of integrated regulation in exercise contexts. *Journal of Applied Biobehavioral Research, 11*, 79–104. doi:10.1111/j.1751-9861.2006.tb00021.x

Wilson, P. M., Sabiston, C. M., Mack, D. E., & Blanchard, C. M. (2012). On the nature and function of scoring protocols used in exercise motivation research: An empirical study of the behavioral regulation in exercise questionnaire. *Psychology of Sport and Exercise, 13*, 614–22. doi:10.1016/j.psychsport.2012.03.009

Woodgate, R. L., & Sigurdson, C. M. (2015). Building school-based cardiovascular health promotion capacity in youth: A mixed methods study. *BMC Public Health, 15*, 421–31. doi:10.1186/s12889-015-1759-5

Yeung, E., Woods, N., Dubrowski, A., Hodges, B., & Carnahan, H. (2015). Sensibility of a new instrument to assess clinical reasoning in post-graduate orthopaedic manual physical therapy education. *Manual Therapy, 20*, 303–12. doi:10.1016/j.math.2014.10.001

CHAPTER 11

Boog, B. W. M. (2003). The emancipatory character of action research, its history and the present state of the art. *Journal of Community & Applied Social Psychology, 13*, 426–38. doi:10.1002/casp.748

Brydon-Miller, M., Kral, M., Maguire, P., Noffke, S., & Sabhlok, A. (2011). Jazz and the banyan tree: Roots and riffs on participatory action research. In N.K. Denzin & Y.S. Lincoln (Eds.), *The SAGE handbook of qualitative research* (4th ed., pp. 387–400). Thousand Oaks, Sage Publications.

Canadian Parks and Recreation Association (2009). *Everybody gets to play™ First Nations, Inuit & Métis Supplement.* Ottawa, ON, Canada.

Carpenter, A., Rothney, A., Mousseau, J., Halas, J., & Forsyth, J. (2008). Seeds of encouragement: Initiating an Aboriginal youth mentorship program. *Canadian Journal of Native Education, 31*, 51–69.

Castleden, H., Morgan, V. S., & Lamb, C. (2012). "I spent the first year drinking tea": Exploring Canadian university researchers' perspectives on community-based participatory research involving Indigenous peoples. *The Canadian Geographer/Le Géographe Canadien, 56*, 160–79. doi:10.1111/j.1541-0064.2012.00432.x

Etowa, J. B., Bernard, W. T., Oyinsan, B., & Clow, B. (2007). Participatory action research (PAR): An approach for improving Black women's health in rural and remote communities. *Journal of Transcultural Nursing, 18*(4), 349–57. doi:10.1177/1043659607305195

Frisby, W. (2011). Promising physical activity inclusion practices for Chinese immigrant women in Vancouver, Canada. *Quest, 63*, 135–47. doi:10.1080/00336297.2011.10483671

Frisby, W., Maguire, P., & Reid, C. (2009). The 'f' word has everything to do with it: How feminist theories inform action research. *Action Research, 7*, 13–29. doi:10.1177/1476750308099595

Frisby, W., Reid, C. J., Millar, S., & Hoeber, L. (2005). Putting "participatory" into participatory forms of action research. *Journal of Sport Management, 19*, 367–86.

Giesbrecht, E. M., Miller, W. C., Mitchell, I. M., & Woodgate, R. L. (2014). Development of a wheelchair skills home program for older adults using a participatory action design approach. *BioMed Research International*, 1–13. doi:10.1155/2014/172434

Henrich, J., Heine, S. J., & Norenzayan, A. (2010). The weirdest people in the world? *Behavioral and Brain Sciences, 33*, 61–83. doi:10.1017/S0140525X0999152X

Kemmis, S., & McTaggart, R. (2008). Participatory action research: Communicative action and the public sphere. In N.K. Denzin & Y.S. Lincoln (Eds.), *Strategies of qualitative inquiry* (3rd ed., pp. 271–330). Thousand Oaks, CA: Sage Publications.

Lavallée, L., & Lévesque, L. (2013). Two-eyed seeing: Physical activity, sport, and recreation promotion in Indigenous communities. In J. Forsyth, & A. R. Giles (Eds.), *Aboriginal peoples & sport in Canada: Historical foundations and contemporary issues* (pp. 206-228). Vancouver: UBC Press.

Lewin, K. (1946). Action research and minority problems. *Journal of Social Issues, 2*, 34–46. doi:10.1111/j.1540-4560.1946.tb02295.x

McGannon, K. R., Busanich, R., Witcher, C. S. G., & Schinke, R. J. (2014). A social ecological exploration of physical activity influences among rural men and women across life stages. *Qualitative Research in Sport, Exercise and Health, 6*, 517–36. doi:10.1080/2159676X.2013.819374

McGannon, K. R., & Smith, B. (2015). Centralizing culture in cultural sport psychology research: The potential of narrative inquiry and discursive psychology. *Psychology of Sport and Exercise, 17*, 79–87. doi:10.1016/j.psychsport.2014.07.010

McHugh, T.-L. F., Kingsley, B. C., & Coppola, A. M. (2013). Enhancing the relevance of physical activity research by engaging Aboriginal peoples in the research process. *Pimatisiwin: A Journal of Aboriginal and Indigenous Community Health, 11*, 293–305.

Messner, M. A., & Musto, M. (2014). Where are the kids? *Sociology of Sport Journal, 3*, 102–22. doi:10.1123/ssj.2013-0111

Oosman, S., Smylie, J., Humbert, L., Henry, C., & Chad, K. (2016). Métis community perspectives inform a school-based health promotion intervention using participatory action research. *Engaged Scholar Journal: Community-Engaged Research, Teaching, and Learning, 1*, 58–76. doi:10.15402/esj.v1i2.112

Reid, C., Tom, A., & Frisby, W. (2006). Finding the 'action' in feminist participatory action research. *Action Research, 4*, 315–32. doi:10.1177/1476750306066804

Schinke, R. J., McGannon, K. R., Watson, J., & Busanich, R. (2013). Moving toward trust and partnership: An example of sport-related community-based participatory action research with Aboriginal people and mainstream academics. *Journal of Aggression, Conflict and Peace Research, 5*, 201–10. doi:10.1108/jacpr-11-2012-0012

Schinke, R. J., Smith, B., & McGannon, K. R. (2013). Pathways for community research in sport and physical activity: Criteria for consideration. *Qualitative Research in Sport, Exercise and Health, 5*, 460–8.

Stringer, E. T., & Genat, W. J. (2004). *Action research in health.* New Jersey: Pearson Education Inc.

CHAPTER 12

American Psychological Association. (2010). *Publication manual of the American Psychological Association* (6th ed.). Washington, DC: American Psychological Association.

Baskin, C. (2005). Storytelling circles: Reflections of Aboriginal protocols in research. *Canadian Social Work Review, 22*(2), 171–87.

Bérubé, M., Choinière, M., Laflamme, Y. G., & Gélinas, C. (2016). Acute to chronic pain transition in extremity trauma: A narrative review for future preventive interventions (part 2). *International Journal of Orthopaedic and Trauma Nursing.* Advance online publication. doi:10.1016/j.ijotn.2016.04.001

Block, B. A., & Weatherford, G. M. (2013). Narrative research methodologies: Learning lessons from disabilities research. *Quest, 65*(4), 498–514. doi:10.1080/00336297.2013.814576

Canadian Institutes of Health Research. (2015). *Knowledge translation at CIHR.* Retrieved from http://www.cihr-irsc.gc.ca/e/29418.html

Clandinin, D. J., & Connelly, F. M. (2000). *Narrative inquiry: Experience and story in qualitative research.* San Francisco, CA: Jossey-Bass.

De Almeida Vicente, A., Shadvar, S., Lepage, S., & Rennick, J. E. (2016). Experienced pediatric nurses' perceptions of work-related stressors on general medical and surgical units: A qualitative study. *International Journal of Nursing Studies, 60*, 216–24. doi:10.1016/j.ijnurstu.2016.05.005

Dell, C. A. (2011). Voices of healing: Using music to communicate research findings. In *Innovations in knowledge translation: The SPHERU KT casebook,* 10–14.

Fitts, P. M. (1954). The information capacity of the human motor system in controlling the amplitude of movement. *Journal of Experimental Psychology, 47*, 381–91. doi:10.1037/h0055392

Glesne, C. (1997). That rare feeling: Re-presenting research through poetic transcription. *Qualitative Inquiry, 3*(2), 202–21.

Gregg, M. J., O., J., & Hall, C. R. (2016). Examining the relationship between athletes' achievement goal orientation and ability to employ imagery. *Psychology of Sport and Exercise, 24*, 140–46. doi:10.1016/j.psychsport.2016.01.006

Haines-Saah, R. J., Oliffe, J. L., White, C. F., & Bottorff, J. L. (2013). "It is just not part of the culture here": Young adults' photo-narratives about smoking, quitting, and healthy lifestyles in Vancouver, Canada. *Health & Place, 22*, 19–28. doi:10.1016/j.healthplace.2013.02.004

Ho, K., & Peter Wall Workshop Participants. (2014). Harnessing the social web for health and wellness: Issues for research and knowledge translation. *Journal of Medical Internet Research, 16*(2), e34. doi:10.2196/jmir.2969

Killham, M. E., Kowalski, K. C., & Duckham, R. L. (2015). Self-compassion and women athletes' body appreciation and intuitive eating experiences. *Journal of Exercise, Movement, and Sport, 47*(1).

Moola, F., Johnson, J., Lay, J., Krygsman, S., & Faulkner, G. (2015). "The heartbeat of Hamilton": Researcher's reflections on Hamilton children's engagement with visual research methodologies to study the environment. *International Journal of Qualitative Methods, 14*, 1–14. doi:10.1177/1609406915611560

ParticipACTION. (2016). *Are Canadian kids too tired to move? The 2016 ParticipACTION Report Card on Physical Activity for Children and Youth.* Retrieved from www.participACTION.com/reportcard

Rice, C., Chandler, E., Harrison, E., Liddiard, K., & Ferrari, M. (2015). Project Re-Vision: Disability at the edges of representation. *Disability & Society, 30*, 513–27. doi:10.1080/09687599.2015.1037950

Robinovitch, S. N., Feldman, F., Yang, Y., Schonnop, R., Leung, P. M., Sarraf, T., . . . Loughin, M. (2013). Video capture of the circumstances of falls in elderly people residing in long-term care: An observational study. *The Lancet, 381*(9860), 47–54. doi:10.1016/S0140-6736(12)61263-X

Salsberg, J., Parry, D., Pluye, P., Macridis, S., Herbert, C. P., & Macaulay, A. C. (2015). Successful strategies to engage research partners for translating evidence into action in community health: A critical review. *Journal of Environmental and Public Health*, 1–15. doi:10.1155/2015/191856

Sanchez-Ramirez, D. C., Malfait, B., Baert, I., van der Leeden, M., van Dieën, J., Lems, W. F., . . . Verschueren, S. (2016). Biomechanical and neuromuscular adaptations during the landing phase of a stepping-down task in patients with early or established knee osteoarthritis. *The Knee, 23*, 367–75. doi:10.1016/j.knee.2016.02.002

Saunders, D., Richer, N., Jehu, D., Paquet, N., & Lajoie, Y. (2015). The influence of an anterior load on attention demand and obstacle clearance before, during, and after an obstacle crossing. *Journal of Sport & Exercise Psychology, 37*(Supplement), S59.

Sparkes, A. C., & Smith, B. (2014). *Qualitative research methods in sport, exercise, and health: From process to product.* London: Routledge.

Speechley, M., DeForge, R. T., Ward-Griffin, C., Marlatt, N. M., & Gutmanis, I. (2015). Creating an ethnodrama to catalyze dialogue in home-based dementia care. *Qualitative Health Research, 25*(11), 1551–9. doi:10.1177/1049732315609572

Spier, R. (2002). The history of the peer-review process. *Trends in Biotechnology, 20*(8), 357–8. doi:10.1016/S0167-7799(02)01985-6

Stamatakis, K. A., McBride, T. D., & Brownson, R. C. (2010). Communicating prevention messages to policy makers: The role of stories in promoting physical activity. *Journal of Physical Activity and Health, 7*(Supplement 1), S99–107.

West, K., & Bloomquist, C. (2015). Poetic re-presentations on trust in higher education. *The Canadian Journal for the Scholarship of Teaching and Learning, 6*(2), 1–22. doi:10.5206/cjsotl-rcacea.2015.2.5

Woollings, K., McKay, C., Kang, J., Meeuwisse, W., & Emery, C.A. (2014). Injury rates, mechanisms, and risk factors for injury in youth rock climbers. *British Journal of Sports Medicine, 48*, 672. doi:10.1136/bjsports-2014-093494.303

Index